Introduction to
Information Systems for Health Information Technology

THIRD EDITION

Nanette B. Sayles, EdD, RHIA, CCS, CDIP, CHDA, CHPS, CPHI, CPHIMS, FAHIMA
and Lauralyn Kavanaugh-Burke, DrPH, RHIA, CHES, CHTS-IM

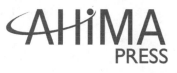
AHIMA
PRESS

ISBN: 978-1-58426-626-6

AHIMA Product No.: AB103417

AHIMA Staff:
Jessica Block, MA, Production Development Editor
Chelsea Brotherton, MA, Assistant Editor
Megan Grennan, Managing Editor
Caitlin Wilson, Project Editor

Cover image: ©Click Bestsellers, Shutterstock

For more information, including updates, about AHIMA Press publications, visit **http://www.ahima.org/education/press**.

American Health Information Management Association
233 North Michigan Avenue, 21st Floor
Chicago, Illinois 60601-5809
ahima.org

Contents

Detailed Contents

Chapter 3   Databases   27

Chapter 4   System Selection   43

Chapter 5   System Implementation   69

Chapter 6   Computers in HIM   85

Chapter 9   Electronic Health Record

Chapter 13   Security
217

Nanette B. Sayles, EdD, RHIA, CCS, CDIP, CHDA, CHPS, CPHI, CPHIMS, FAHIMA

Dr. Sayles has a bachelor of science degree in medical record administration, a master of science in health information management, a master's degree in public administration, and a doctorate in adult education. Dr. Sayles has more than 10 years of experience as a health information management practitioner with roles in hospitals, a consulting firm, and a computer vendor. She has 20 years of health information management education experience. She was the 2005 American Health Information Management Association (AHIMA) Triumph Educator award winner. She has held numerous offices and other volunteer roles for AHIMA, the Georgia Health Information Management Association (GHIMA), the Alabama Association of Health Information Management (AAHIM), the Middle Georgia Health Information Management Association (MGHIMA), and the Birmingham Regional Health Information Management Association (BRHIMA). These positions include: AHIMA Educational Strategies Committee, AHIMA Co-Chair RHIA Workgroup, GHIMA Director, and President of MGHIMA. Dr. Sayles has published a number of health information management textbooks and is currently the associate professor of health information management at East Central College in Union, Missouri.

Lauralyn Kavanaugh-Burke, DrPH, RHIA, CHES, CHTS-IM

Dr. Burke earned her bachelor of science degree in health record administration with a minor in biology from York College of Pennsylvania, a master of science degree in Community Health Education from West Virginia University, and received her doctor of public health (DrPH) with a concentration in epidemiology from Florida A&M University. She has more than 35 years of management experience in hospital health information departments, coding consulting and DRG analysis, health education programs, and teaching in both health information technology and management programs. Through her extensive experience, Dr. Burke's main areas of interest are hospital disaster preparedness, bioterrorism and infectious diseases, and the implementation of technology in health information management. In addition to her degrees, she also a certified health education specialist (CHES) and certified in implementation management for health information technology (CHTS-IM). She has published in the Journal of the American Health Information Management Association, Perspectives in Health Information Management and Educational Perspectives in Health Information Management and is the author of the medical science chapter of Cengage Learning's Professional Review Guide for the RHIA and RHIT Examinations. Dr. Burke has also held positions and participated in committees within the Northwest Florida Health Information Management Association (NWFHIMA) and the Florida Health Information Management Association (FHIMA). She currently is an assistant professor in the Division of Health Informatics and Information Management at Florida A&M University.

Acknowledgments

From Nanette Sayles:

This book is dedicated to my husband, Mark, and my daughter, Rachel, who are my biggest supporters. I love you both. Thanks to AHIMA Press for your vote of confidence in publishing this book. Thanks, Lauralyn, for your partnership on this book. You have made it better. To the students and faculty who use this book, I hope you find it a valuable resource.

From Lauralyn Kavanaugh-Burke:

This book is dedicated to my husband, John K. Burke, Jr. and my late parents, Lieutenant Colonel (Ret.) Richard D. and Cathryn C. Kavanaugh for their unconditional love, unwavering support, and encouragement in my educational journey and achieving this personal goal. A special thank you to Dr. Nanette Sayles for inviting me to coauthor the third edition of this great textbook. It has been a challenging and worthwhile experience. To all who use this book, may it provide the stepping stone in a long and productive career.

AHIMA Press and the authors would like to thank Judy Ferraro, RHIA, and Linda Galocy, MS, RHIA, FAHIMA, for their review and feedback on this book.

Introduction to Computers in Health Information Management

Learning Objectives

- Identify and discuss the impact of computers on healthcare.
- Discuss the history of computers in healthcare.
- Compare and contrast the similarities and differences among the Internet, intranet, and extranet as used in healthcare.
- Explain data analytics and health informatics and how information systems (ISs) apply.

Key Terms

Certified health data analyst (CHDA)
Computer on wheels (COW)
Clinical pathways
Clinical practice guidelines
Cloud computing
Dashboards
Data
Data analytics

Data mining
Descriptive statistics
Dumb terminals
Electronic health record (EHR)
Evidence-based medicine
Extranet
Financial applications
Health informatics
Health information exchange (HIE)

Inferential statistics
Information
Information system (IS)
Intranet
Mainframe computers
Patient safety
Personal computer (PC)
Point of care (POC)
Predictive modeling

Computer use in healthcare and health information management (HIM) is not a new concept. Computers have been used in patient care, public health, and research since the 1960s. Even though the HIM profession has relied on data since the time of the first paper health record, the way that the data—raw facts and figures—are collected, stored, and shared has changed dramatically with the implementation of information systems. An information system (IS) is an automated system that uses computer hardware and software to record, manipulate, store, recover, and disseminate data (that is, a system that receives and processes input and provides output). These changes range from data interaction among individuals and departments to system-wide networks and hospital information systems that span several states. It is the role of the HIM professional to enter, analyze, use, and maintain data at all levels of ISs and networks in hospitals and other healthcare facilities. This responsibility can be a challenge as technology changes, quickly requiring constant updating of skills and knowledge. Adoption and implementation of the technology in a healthcare facility generally move at a much slower rate. For example, electronic health records, defined in the next section, have been around for decades but have only recently been implemented in many healthcare facilities. ISs now play a major role in healthcare. This chapter covers the history of computers in healthcare, the impact of computers on healthcare, an introduction to health informatics, and an introduction to data analytics.

History of Computers in Healthcare

The first computers in healthcare used punch-card systems prior to the 1960s. Punch cards were cards with holes punched in them to represent data to be read by the computer. At that time, computers were large machines that filled entire rooms and needed extreme cooling controls; these machines used vacuum tubes rather than microchips for memory. Much of the healthcare-related computers used in those days involved data entry.

Early Information Systems

The first ISs installed in the 1960s were mostly financial applications, which were among the few software systems available and were some of the simplest software packages. Financial applications are software applications that handle patient accounts, budgets, and other financial activities. With the use of mainframe computers throughout hospitals, the healthcare industry was beginning to experience the benefits computers could provide. Mainframe computers are large computers that are used by the government and other organizations that require speed and the ability to process large amounts of data. Although the trend has been to use smaller computers, some mainframe computers are still in use.

In the 1970s, technology evolved and the memory capability of computers increased. In the late 1970s, the healthcare industry began to use departmental ISs, such as those used in the laboratory, radiology, and HIM departments. See chapters 6 and 7 for details on ISs.

In HIM departments, computers were used to help the personnel with master patient index (MPI) functions and abstracting, which are further discussed in chapter 7. Most of the computers used were dumb terminals. In dumb terminals, all of the processing is performed at the server or mainframe, whereas with personal computers (PCs) some or all of the processing is performed on the PC. Some advanced HIM departments in the 1970s began having employees input patient data into the dumb terminals, capturing various patient or clinical data for reporting purposes. Previously, all abstracting of data from the health record was done by the HIM technicians on paper abstracts. These abstracts were then mailed to the various reporting agencies for data entry and report creation. The ability to abstract patient data once into a computer system, which then could be used to send the abstracts to several agencies or used to generate several reports, was innovative for the time. Using the old paper abstracts for reporting purposes was a time-consuming process for the personnel, and having the computer system available to print much of the data regarding patient demographics, which was already contained within the IS, saved abstractors a great deal of time. The new ISs also decreased the possibility of errors made when transcribing by hand any notes from the primary record to a secondary source. The computerized abstract printed the reports directly from the system in available ad hoc formats as directed so that reports could be customized.

The 1980s and 1990s saw even more advancement in computers' memory capacity and speed. The physical size of the computers and their costs decreased while memory and the amount of storage increased at tremendous rates. Use of computers in business continued to increase, and purchases of home computers multiplied during this period. The PCs for consumers became more affordable, making the computer a machine that home users could enjoy and not just a tool for business and industry. The PC is a computer that has a central processing unit (CPU), computer memory, and storage devices for data. The CPU is also known as a microprocessor, which is a microchip that processes the information and the code (instructions) used by a computer; it is the "brains of a computer." Information is data that have been manipulated into something meaningful.

During the 1990s, wired networking among hospital departments became more common, and computers and other digital devices helped facilities share data more quickly and with greater ease. The 1990s also saw data entry being performed using technologies such as barcoding of data, speech recognition, touch screens, light pens, and microphones. Hospital departments—such as admissions, business offices, quality improvement offices, and utilization management—that worked closely with the HIM departments were networked so that data were shared and less time was spent rekeying data. This network made these departments more efficient, and data sharing within hospitals became popularized.

Modern Information Systems

Today wireless devices, such as tablets and cellular phones, are used throughout the healthcare facility. Many of these wireless devices are small and are easily carried to nursing units for patient care at the bedside by healthcare practitioners. Wireless computers are often seen at the **point of care (POC)**, the place or location where the physician administers services to the patient, such as the patient's bedside. One type of device used at the POC is the **computer on wheels (COW)**—also referred to as wireless on wheels (WOW)—which involves a wireless computer mounted on a mobile cart that can be moved from patient to patient. Using the COW at the POC improves documentation because it is done as soon as the care occurs. It also gives current information to other healthcare professionals involved in the patient's care. One of the downsides to wireless computers is that they are easy targets for both physical and virtual theft.

Healthcare facilities have been working toward the **electronic health record (EHR)** for decades as they have implemented other ISs that feed data into the EHR. The EHR is an electronic record of health-related information on an individual that conforms to nationally recognized interoperability standards and that can be created, managed, and consulted by authorized clinicians and staff across more than one healthcare organization. Many healthcare facilities, however, began the transition to the EHR after the American Recovery and Reinvestment Act of 2009. This law enacted an incentive program known as Meaningful Use, which gave healthcare providers who met the requirements financial incentives for implementing the EHR and using it in a meaningful way.

Within the HIM industry, computers helped increase employee productivity. Since the end of the 1990s, most HIM department employees have used PCs at their workstations to better perform their HIM roles within the facility. Some HIM departmental employees may use laptops, tablets, or other portable devices to perform their work. There are risks in using the portable devices, as they can be easily stolen. See chapter 13 for additional information about these risks.

Today, cloud computing is a way to store data and run applications for many healthcare facilities. **Cloud computing** is a system that operates on a computer that is owned and maintained by a vendor. Storing data in the cloud facilitates sharing of information, which is important to healthcare. The data storage is at a remote location, and information is moved via the Internet. The Internet enables physicians, HIM professionals, and others to access patient and other information for patient care, billing, and other purposes. The Internet comprises thousands of networks with millions of computers linked together to share data and information. It allows patient information as well as administrative information to be shared outside the facility with insurers, healthcare providers, and others.

Many facilities have a private network, known as an intranet, that is used by their own employees and other authorized individuals. The **intranet** is a private information network that is similar to the Internet in that it uses Internet technologies; however, its servers are located inside a firewall or security barrier so that the general public cannot gain access to information housed within the network, distinguishing it from the Internet. The firewall built around the intranet will prevent unauthorized access to it or restricted parts of the website. (See chapter 13 for a description of a firewall.) A facility's intranet might give updates on upcoming events, house the bylaws and rules and regulations as well as the policies and procedures of the facility, provide a repository for forms, and contain an employee directory, map of the facility, or other items helpful for employees. It can also provide users with a site search engine for items not found in the contents page.

Healthcare facilities may also have an extranet. An **extranet** uses a system of connections of private Internet networks outside an organization's firewall and uses Internet technology to enable collaborative applications to allow external users to access the IS. This system can be used by healthcare organizations to allow patients to access health information and schedule appointments and by vendors to allow healthcare facilities to monitor the status of orders.

CHECK YOUR UNDERSTANDING 1.1

1. A patient can access his test results by using the _____.
   a. Intranet
   b. Extranet
   c. COW
   d. Meaningful Use

(Continued)

CHECK YOUR UNDERSTANDING 1.1 (Continued)

2. Cloud computing refers to _____.

    a. Data that is inaccurate or incomplete
    b. Using a computer that is owned and managed by a vendor
    c. Flexibility that is built into the IS
    d. Outdated information that is purged from an IS

3. The American Recovery and Reinvestment Act of 2009 encouraged _____.

    a. Implementation of wireless devices
    b. Implementation of the EHR
    c. Transition away from mainframes
    d. Creation of an intranet

4. The use of computers in healthcare began in the _____.

    a. 1950s
    b. 1960s
    c. 1970s
    d. 1980s

5. Where would an employee access the form to request reimbursement recent travel?

    a. Internet
    b. Intranet
    c. Extranet
    d. WOW

Impact of Computers on Healthcare

The healthcare industry continues to grow in size and in complexity. Without computers to aid in the management of patient data, the healthcare industry would not be able to obtain the information needed to function in this complex environment. Technology allows the healthcare industry to use data in ways that enhance patient care, research, business practices, education, and public health. These ways include identifying effective medications or treatments, monitoring for epidemics, improved decision making, and sharing information between healthcare providers at other healthcare facilities. Technology has also enabled significant changes in such areas as patient safety, quality of patient care, and access to information.

Impact of Technology on Patient Care

The impact that ISs have on patient care is seen in multiple ways including

- Actual care provided to the patient
- Patient engagement in healthcare
- Creation of evidence-based medicine
- Creation of practice guidelines
- Patient safety

The care provided to the patient has been improved in multiple ways through the use of technology. The EHR provides immediate access to the patient's past medical history, current test results, allergies, and so forth. It also reminds physicians of tests that should be considered and helps with the quality of documentation. Chapter 9 provides more information about the benefits of EHRs.

Health information exchange (HIE) is the exchange of health information electronically between providers and others with the same level of interoperability. It allows healthcare providers access to patient information even if the previous health records are located with healthcare providers with other facilities whether local or in other states. Figure 1.1 shows an example of how an HIE links various healthcare providers in the local area. See chapter 11 for more information on HIE.

Figure 1.1. Health information exchange

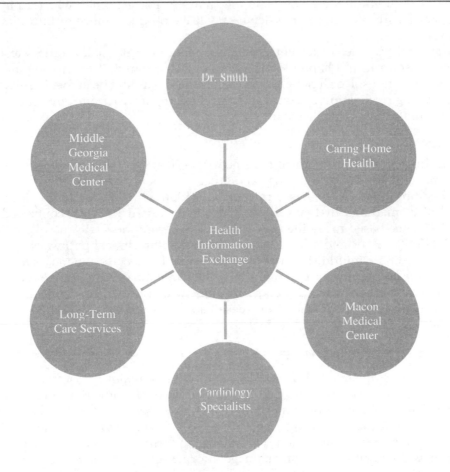

Today patients are more engaged in their own healthcare than ever before. Patients use the Internet to research their symptoms, diseases, treatments, and medications. They also use the Internet to communicate with their healthcare provider, schedule appointments, check test results, access a summary of their care, and more. These practices will be discussed in chapter 10. One of the most important impacts that technology can have on patient care is supporting patient safety efforts.

Patient Safety

Patient safety is a hot topic in healthcare and has been since the publication of *To Err Is Human: Building a Safer Health System* by the Institute of Medicine (now known as National Academies of Medicine). This report was published in 1999 and related that up to 98,000 people died each year in hospitals as a result of preventable medical errors (IOM 1999). This report prompted the healthcare industry to take steps to improve patient safety.

Patient safety has been enhanced through the use of technology. Examples of these efforts include:

- Use of barcodes to verify patient identification for medication administration (see chapter 8)
- Checking medications ordered against allergies and other medications (see chapter 8)
- Improved data quality through edits and standardization (see chapter 2)
- Clinical provider order entry (see chapter 8)

With the paper health record, the capturing of data on the patient's care and then analyzing the data was very difficult, time-consuming, and costly. Now with the EHR and other technologies research and data analysis can be performed using the databases. The EHR along with data mining (discussed later in this chapter) offers healthcare providers valuable knowledge, such as drugs with serious complications, best treatment for a condition or disease, and so forth.

Technologies such as the EHR eliminated illegibility issues that were found in the handwritten patient health record and that can lead to errors in medication dosage and other patient safety issues. Technology can also help reduce or even eliminate incomplete information. For example, when a physician orders a medication in the paper health record, the physician may leave off a key piece of information such as the route of administration.

With the use of clinical provider order entry, which is where the physician orders tests, medications, and other procedures (discussed in chapter 8), the physician is prompted to provide all of the required information. Technology cannot solve all patient care issues; there may still be errors in software, issues with usability of a system, wrong medication ordered, and more. It can, however, improve patient outcomes and give patient confidence in the healthcare system.

Evidence-Based Medicine

Research concerning drugs and other medical treatments is critical to patient care. Physicians and other healthcare providers need to know that the drugs and other treatments used are effective. One of the ways this is accomplished is through evidence-based medicine. Evidence-based medicine describes healthcare services based on clinical methods that have been thoroughly tested through controlled, peer-reviewed biomedical studies. Evidence-based medicine uses data analysis from the EHR and other ISs. The findings from the review of data in the EHR and other ISs are used to develop clinical pathways. Clinical pathways are a tool designed to coordinate multidisciplinary care planning for specific diagnoses and treatments. For example, if a patient has an acute myocardial infarction, the clinical pathways define the best practices for treatment. Another tool is the clinical practice guidelines, which provide a detailed, step-by-step guide used by healthcare practitioners to make knowledge-based decisions related to patient care and issued by an authoritative organization such as a medical society.

Impact on the HIM Profession

Technological advancements implemented in healthcare have had a major impact on the HIM profession. For decades, the health record had not changed significantly. With the advent of department ISs such as the laboratory IS (see chapter 8) laboratory reports were computer generated, printed out, and then filed in the health record. This began the slow transition to the EHR. Today many facilities utilize the EHR to capture, store, and manage patient information. This change in format has enabled the HIM department to use technology to process the health record and manage information to perform many tasks including

- Assigning diagnosis and procedures codes
- Managing the MPI
- Managing registries
- Transcribing documents such as the discharge summary
- Analyzing the health record
- Documentation of release of information activities
- Computer-assisted coding

Before the EHR, these functions were slow, methodical, tedious, and labor-intensive. Using ISs to perform management of information tasks saves time and money and reduces the number of employees needed (thereby saving employers salary costs).

Some healthcare facilities use a virtual HIM department, in which (when the EHR is available) coders, transcriptionists, and other HIM professionals can work from home. A virtual HIM department lowers the employer's costs associated with occupying office space and benefits both employers and employees in other ways. Working virtually allows employees to save on transportation costs, allows them more flexibility in their job, can lessen distractions, and may lead to improved job satisfaction. Studies have shown that the productivity of remote employees is higher than that of employees who worked on-site (Tiny Pulse 2016; Bloom 2015).

Another option is providing HIM services at a centralized location rather than having staff at each individual healthcare facility. For example, ABC Hospital System has hospitals in Macon, Atlanta, and Columbus, Georgia. All three of these hospitals utilized the EHR. ABC Hospital System could centralize their HIM services in Atlanta. As a result, most of the HIM services for all three hospitals can be performed in Atlanta, eliminating the need for three HIM directors, coding staff and space in all locations, and so forth.

There are downsides to both the virtual and centralized departments. In both models, there are limited HIM professionals and staff that can support the physicians, committees, and other staff onsite and there can be increased security when employees access data remotely. In the case of the centralized department, scanning of paper documents may be performed at the remote location, increasing privacy and security concerns with the transportation. The virtual department model relies on employees to be self-motivated, as a supervisor is not overseeing them in person. Another concern is the difficulty in collaboration among staff members across various locations. While existing communication tools can help facilitate remote communication, they do not always achieve the same effect as face-to-face collaboration (Forbes Technology Council 2017).

The skills required by the HIM professional have changed significantly in light of technological advancements. The HIM skills of today include system implementation, databases, data governance, legal health record, data analysis, data mining, healthcare informatics, and much more. The HIM profession has changed from one that is focused on processing health records to one that is focused on data and information that can be used to monitor quality of patient care, patient outcomes, and more. With the paper health record, aggregating health data and turning it into information was difficult because the HIM professional had to review each health record and collect data before it can be turned into information. With the EHR, data can easily be manipulated and turned into information. Many new roles, such as data integrity analyst, data analyst, and mapping specialist, have been created as a result. See chapter 15 for more on HIM roles.

Introduction to Health Informatics

Health informatics is "a scientific discipline that is concerned with the cognitive, information-processing, and communication tasks of healthcare practice, education, and research, including the information science and technology to support these tasks" (Greenes and Shortliffe 1990). It is an interdisciplinary field whose goal is to improve healthcare. This field of study uses ISs to manipulate and use information to improve healthcare. This is only possible because the data are stored in the ISs. This improvement takes the form of development of standards as well as clinical pathways and clinical practice guidelines discussed earlier in this chapter. Standards are a scientifically based statement of expected behavior against which structures, processes, and outcomes can be measured. Standards are covered in more detail in chapter 12. In order to get quality information, quality data are needed. See chapter 2 for more about data collection and data quality.

Introduction to Data Analytics

With the data collected through the EHR and other ISs, HIM professionals and others are able to turn data into information through the use of data analytics. Data and information, as defined earlier, are not interchangeable. An example of data is "33% of the patients have commercial insurance." This is a fact about numbers, but it does not provide context or meaning. The statement "33% of the patients have commercial insurance, which is a 2% increase over this point last year" identifies not only the specific number of patients but also how the number has changed and in what period. Data analytics is the science of examining raw data with the purpose of drawing conclusions about that information. This information can then be used to make business decisions concerning which services to provide and how to improve patient care.

Data analytics is becoming more important to healthcare and HIM. The American Health Information Management Association (AHIMA) sponsors the certified health data analyst (CHDA) certification. This advanced certification covers data management, data analytics, and data reporting (CCHIIM 2017).

Data analytics can be divided into three categories: descriptive, predictive, and prescriptive. Descriptive analytics addresses the past to determine what has already occurred. Predictive analytics addresses the future to predict what will likely occur. Prescriptive analytics concerns what to do with what you have learned (Crocket and Eliason 2016).

A number of tools are used in data analytics, including data mining, statistics, dashboards, predictive modeling, descriptive statistics, and inferential statistics. These tools utilize ISs to manipulate and analyze the data contained in the database. The data are used for research, monitoring the quality of patient care, and much more.

Data mining is the process of extracting and analyzing large volumes of data from a database for the purpose of identifying hidden and sometimes subtle relationships or patterns and using those relationships to predict behaviors. It uses data to determine differences in the way physicians practice medicine, determine changes in the patients being seen, and more. Refer to chapter 3 for additional information.

Dashboards are reports of process measures to help leaders follow progress to assist with strategic planning. The dashboard provides the status on key measures. For example, a hospital chief financial officer might want to know the total charges of unbilled claims, accounts receivable, accounts payment, percentage of patients with various insurers, and so forth. These figures would change automatically as payments are received, bills are submitted, and so forth. This allows the user to have the most current information in one location. This information may be displayed in line graphs, pie charts, and other displays. The dashboard would allow the user to monitor these key measures closely. An example of a dashboard is found in figure 1.2.

Figure 1.2. Sample dashboard

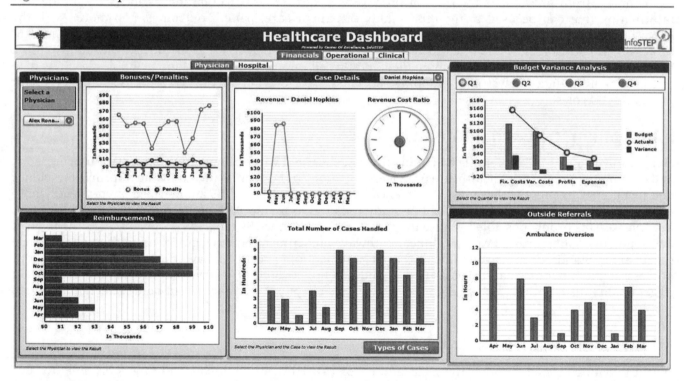

Source: InfoStep 2010.

Descriptive statistics is a set of statistical techniques used to describe data, such as means, frequency distributions, and standard deviations; statistical information describes the characteristics of a specific group or a population, such as the mean costs for patients who have had an appendectomy.

Inferential statistics is a set of statistical techniques that allows researchers to make generalizations about a population's characteristics on the basis of a sample's characteristics, such as HIM professionals' continuing education efforts.

Predictive modeling is a process used to identify patterns that can be used to predict the odds of a particular outcome based on the observed data. Predictive models use historical data in order to predict what is likely to happen in the future. For example, it might be used to predict the number of inpatient beds needed.

A healthcare facility can use one or more of these tools to perform data analytics. The choice(s) would be based on the objectives. For example, a hospital can have a dashboard showing key indicators like hospital census. This census data would be displayed as descriptive statistics.

CHECK YOUR UNDERSTANDING 1.2

1. AHIMA's certification related to data analytics is _____.

   a. CHDA
   b. RHIA
   c. RHIT
   d. CCS

2. _____ is used to assess the status of key indicators.

   a. Predictive modeling
   b. The annual report
   c. Data mining
   d. The dashboard

3. Applied informatics will assist in improving _____.

   a. Population health
   b. Data collection
   c. Processes
   d. Patient care

4. A trend seen in HIM is _____.

   a. The elimination of HIM functions
   b. The ability for staff to be able to work from home
   c. Bringing staff back into the department to work
   d. To return to the basics of HIM

5. Determine the true statement about health informatics.

   a. Health informatics is solely the responsibility of HIM.
   b. The goal of health informatics is to improve processes.
   c. Health informatics is a multidisciplinary field.
   d. Health informatics is being replaced by data analytics.

Real-World Case

Sophie is the HIM director at Pine Ridge Medical Center. Pine Ridge is part of a five-hospital chain and two health clinics known as Hometown Health. She earned her RHIA certification 20 years ago, prior to any computerization. In fact, the hospital implemented the EHR only 6 months ago. Sophie is feeling overwhelmed with all of the changes that the EHR has caused and is struggling to adapt. Now the hospital wants to expand the emergency room, which is next door to the HIM department. In order to make space for this expansion, the decision has been made to send the transcriptionists and coders home to work. New employees will have to work at the site for a minimum of 6 months to ensure the quality of their work before being able to work at home. Another reason behind this decision is that Hometown Health plans to centralize the HIM departments of their five healthcare facilities over the next 2 or 3 years. This stage would begin the transition to the virtual department.

REVIEW QUESTIONS

1. To make conclusions about a population, use _____.

   a. Descriptive statistics
   b. Inferential statistics
   c. Predictive modeling
   d. Data modeling

2. The field that uses technology to manipulate and use information to improve healthcare is known as _____.

   a. Data analytics
   b. Data modeling
   c. Population health
   d. Health informatics

3. The first ISs used in healthcare were _____.

   a. Financial applications
   b. EHR
   c. Dashboard
   d. Mainframes

4. Identify the true statement about the intranet.

   a. It is a synonym for Internet.
   b. It is used to communicate with vendors.
   c. It is used to access employee resources.
   d. It is used by patients.

5. The impact of ISs specifically on HIM professionals includes _____.

   a. Improving patient safety
   b. Improving access to health information
   c. The need to assign diagnosis and procedure codes
   d. Skills required

6. Identify the true statement about the EHR.

   a. The EHR allows flexibility by not requiring recognized standards.
   b. The EHR stores information about the population, not individuals.
   c. The EHR implementation was encouraged through the Meaningful Use program.
   d. The EHR is available only to HIM professionals.

7. The point of care documentation is improved because _____.

   a. It uses evidence-based medicine.
   b. It is created as soon as the care is provided.
   c. It uses clinical practice guidelines.
   d. It uses wireless technology.

8. Wired networking became popular in the _____.

   a. 1960s
   b. 1970s
   c. 1980s
   d. 1990s

9. The facility wants to use historical data to determine what will happen in the future. This is known as
   _____.

   a. Descriptive statistics
   b. Inferential statistics
   c. Predictive modeling
   d. Data modeling

10. Data analytics tools include

    a. Clinical pathway
    b. Dashboard
    c. Barcodes
    d. EHR

References

Bloom, N. A., J. Liang, J. Roberts, and Z. J. Ying. 2015. Does working from home work? Evidence from a Chinese experiment. *The Quarterly Journal of Economics* 130(1). https://doi.org/10.1093/qje/qju032.

Commission on Certification for Health Informatics and Information Management (CCHIIM). 2017. Candidate Guide. https://www.ahima.org/~/media/AHIMA/Files/.../Recertification_Guide.ashx.

Crocket, D. and B. Eliason. 2016. What is data mining in healthcare? https://www.healthcatalyst.com/wp-content/uploads/2014/05/Healthcare-Data-Mining.pdf.

Dooling, J. A., K. Osborne, and L. A. Wiedemann. 2014. Defining the basics of health informatics for HIM professionals. *Journal of AHIMA* (85)9:66.

Forbes Technology Council. 2017. 13 Pros and Cons of Having a Distributed Workforce. Forbes. https://www.forbes.com/sites/forbestechcouncil/2017/08/03/13-pros-and-cons-of-having-a-distributed-workforce/#15e8601313d9

Greenes R. A. and E. H. Shortliffe. 1990. Medical informatics: an emerging academic discipline and institutional priority. *JAMA* (263)8: 1114–20.

InfoStep. 2010 (July). "Healthcare_Infostep.jpg." Digital Image. Wikimedia Commons. https://commons.wikimedia.org/wiki/File:Healthcare_Infostep.JPG.

Institute of Medicine. 1999. To Err Is Human: Building a Safer Health System. http://www.nationalacademies.org/hmd/~/media/Files/Report%20Files/1999/To-Err-is-Human/To%20Err%20is%20Human%201999%20%20report%20brief.pdf.

TinyPulse. 2016. What Leaders Need to Know About Remote Workers: Surprising Differences in Workplace Happiness and Relationships. https://cdn2.hubspot.net/hubfs/443262/TINYpulse_What_Leaders_Need_to_Know_About_Remote_Workers.pdf?t=1462203875281.

Information Integrity and Data Quality

Learning Objectives

- Identify the various data sources that populate the electronic health record.
- List and give an example of each of the American Health Information Management Association data quality management model characteristics.
- Choose the appropriate field type for a data element.
- Make recommendations to address data quality and data integrity issues.

Key Terms

AHIMA data quality management model
Authorship
Back-end speech recognition (BESR)
Data accessibility
Data accuracy
Data capture
Data cleansing
Data comprehensiveness
Data consistency
Data currency
Data definition

Data granularity
Data integrity
Data mapping
Data precision
Data quality
Data quality management
Data quality measure
Data relevancy
Data timeliness
Direct data entry
Edit check
Front-end speech recognition (FESR)

Hot spot
Natural language processing
Peer review
Physician advisor (PA)
Primary data source
Qualitative analysis
Quantitative analysis
Secondary data source
Speech recognition
Structured data fields
Template-based data entry
Unstructured data fields
Version control

Patient history has been recorded on paper for centuries; written records of treating the sick date back to the Middle Ages. Although these documents are not what are currently thought of as quality health records, they show that patient care was recorded. The history of healthcare and the importance of recording written data are a part of the foundation that has been expanded into the complex healthcare delivery systems currently in place. The importance of data quality in healthcare cannot be overstressed or overstated. Every piece of information from the health record is vital to patient care. The healthcare provider must read, review, analyze, and compare the patient's health record to similar cases to make a plan for the patient's care and administer treatment accordingly. Therefore, it is critical that all information is timely, accurate, and complete.

The data contained within the health record by itself would be raw data or figures; however, when these data are organized and presented to produce meaning, this results in information. Healthcare providers must rely on information so that patient care can be provided at the highest level. A health record containing only raw data is a record full of numbers and other documentation that has little meaning to anyone. These data must have meaning attached to them; once this occurs, these data become useful information that can be used by the practitioners to treat the patient.

For example, a routine laboratory report contains a list of test results for a patient. The normal range scale for each test is listed next to the results, thus giving it meaning and translating it into information. For example, a complete blood count would have a hematocrit, hemoglobin, white blood cell count, and other blood cell measurements. The hematocrit will have a range such as 34–46. If the normal range scale is not listed and there is no knowledge of where the normal ranges fall, it remains raw data because the numbers have no meaning.

Most health records are documented with the best information available at the time by healthcare providers and personnel who are trained on how to appropriately document within health records and to use electronic health records (EHRs) and databases accordingly. However, errors can still be made when documenting, computer problems can transpire, or other data mishaps can occur. Because of the possibility of errors related to data, the quality of information must be a priority in healthcare. Content in this chapter includes data sources, screen design, data integrity, data quality management, and data integrity issues.

Data Sources

Data that populate the EHR come from many sources. Data sources can be categorized into primary and secondary data sources.

Primary Data Sources

Primary data sources come directly from the original source, such as the patient when talking about symptoms or the reason for coming to the healthcare facility. The health record is also considered to be a primary source of data as the physicians and other healthcare providers document the treatments, observations, and care provided. The highest quality of data will always come from the primary source, which is the original source of the information.

Secondary Data Sources

Secondary data sources are derived from the primary data sources, such as the health record. Secondary data sources include indices, registries, and other databases. A registry is a collection of care information related to a specific disease, condition, or procedure that makes health record information available for analysis and comparison. Secondary data are typically used to conduct research, address population health issues, and for administrative purposes such as monitoring for possible fraud (Sharp 2016, 173).

Screen Design

Screen design is an important part of data quality as it influences data capture, which is discussed in the next section. Poor screen design can confuse users if instructions are not provided, if the data fields are not in a logical order, and if users are entering data in different ways. An example of an illogical order of the data fields is the placement of the first name at the top of the page and the last name at the bottom. In another example, users might enter data in different ways in response to the data element "state": they could enter the full state name (Georgia) or the abbreviation (GA). This variance would make data retrieval and analysis difficult. For more on screen design, refer to chapter 5.

Data Capture

Data capture is the process of recording healthcare-related data in a health record system or clinical database. The healthcare practitioners who input data into the health record are responsible for the quality of data they enter into the EHR or other information system (IS). Poor data capture result in not only poor quality of care but also poor business decisions. For example, if the patient's weight is entered incorrectly, the wrong dosage of a medication may be administered. The adage garbage in, garbage out (GIGO) is applicable to the documentation of healthcare data. There are a number of ways that data are captured to help prevent the "garbage." These methods include direct data entry, template-based data entry, speech recognition, and natural language processing.

Direct Data Entry

Direct data entry includes a number of manual data entry methods such as keyboard, mouse, or other devices for entering data into the computer. A number of data field types are available for use in an IS. Some of these field types can contribute to data quality by limiting the number of choices, by limiting the appropriate entries, and further specifying the data required.

Many vendors use hot spots throughout their software applications to make the data fields as user-friendly as possible. A hot spot is a type of help message that is triggered when the cursor is placed on top of a data field. For example, the cursor changes to another symbol, such as a hand, which indicates another level of choices from which the user can select. The help message displayed by the hot spot is specific for the data field. It provides an explanation for that data field and what data are needed. The valid entries, number of characters, and other attributes are controlled by the data dictionary, which is discussed further in chapter 3. The field types are selected based on the type of data collected and the flexibility of data entry required. The field type also depends on whether or not structured or unstructured data are needed.

Unstructured Data Fields

Unstructured data fields use data elements that allow for free text entry, which means that the user can type in any data that he or she chooses. Examples of unstructured data include a description of the procedure performed or a patient's explanation of his medical history. Unstructured data complicates data retrieval and analysis, so structured data are preferred. For example, different terms could be used by different users.

Text box fields allow the user to type free text into the field, so they are not limited to allowed choices. The data dictionary can limit the types of characters allowed, such as A through Z or 0 through 9, as well as the number of characters. The type of data collected in the text box will dictate the number of characters allowed. For example, the last name field might be limited to 40 alphabetic characters. The address field would accept both numbers and letters. A text field in which the physician enters his or her findings might allow 500 or even 1,000 characters. The text box is unstructured data.

Structured Data Fields

Structured data fields guide the user during the data entry process, limiting what a user can enter into the field. A number of different types of structured data fields can be used, including radio buttons, drop-down boxes, check boxes, and more. Some of these fields, such as drop-down boxes and radio buttons, have proved to be an effective and efficient method for capturing data, thus improving productivity. Other types of user-friendly aids within the health record are examples located near a data field to show the user a suggested response format for a data field. For example, there may be a question mark by the field that when clicked tells the user more about what data should be entered and in what format.

Drop-Down Menus

One type of structured data field is the drop-down menu, which is frequently used in EHRs. The user simply clicks on the arrow to the right (or left) of a data field and a drop-down menu appears with several choices. The choices can be controlled by the healthcare facility based on its needs. For example, a community hospital may populate the drop-down menu choices in the service field as medical, surgical, and obstetrical, while a large teaching facility may list medical, surgical, transplant, cardiology, nephrology, and many more. Another use for a drop-down menu is patient type such as inpatient, outpatient, and emergency.

Once selected, the data field is automatically populated with the user's selection. A drop-down menu can be used for countless numbers of data fields within the health record. It is used in many documents, such as the admission record or the face sheet, the financial record, or the history and physical examination. Drop-down menus save time because the entire data field item does not have to be typed in the data field. They improve consistency because everyone enters data the same way. For example, the state of Georgia is selected from the drop down box consistently as "Georgia" rather than being entered by some users as GA and others as Georgia.

Check Box

The check box is a type of data field that displays a comprehensive list of approved answers for the data element. The user can choose zero, one, or many of the options. For example, if the check box field is part of the cardiac section of the history, the options may be murmurs, gallops, and rubs. The user can then choose all the options that apply to the patient. As with the drop-down field, the choice of options must be comprehensive.

Radio Buttons

Radio buttons are a type of data field that also identifies a comprehensive list of choices, much like the check box. The difference is that the user can choose only one of the options. This type of field is for data for which only one option should be chosen, such as gender. In this case, the choices are generally: male, female, and unknown.

Numeric Field

A numeric field allows for the entry of numbers. The number of characters and range can be controlled through the data dictionary. It could control the format, such as decimal points and currency. The values in the numeric fields must be able to be added and subtracted, as with age, weight, and so forth. Dates, even though they are entered as numbers, would not be considered numeric because they are not added, subtracted, or otherwise mathematically manipulated.

Date Field

A date field allows for the entry of valid dates. "Valid" does not mean that the date is correct but rather means that an invalid date (for example, February 30) cannot be entered.

Time Field

A time field allows for the entry of valid times. It would prevent 26 hours in a day or 70 minutes in an hour. This does not mean that the time is correct but rather means an invalid time cannot be entered.

Autonumbering

Autonumbering means that the IS assigns a number in numeric order. This type of field is used for the health record number and the patient account number. For example, the health record numbers would be assigned in numeric order, such as 12-34-56, 12-34-57, and 12-34-58.

Template-Based Data Entry

Template-based data entry is a cross between free text and structured data entry. The user can pick and choose data that are entered frequently, thus requiring the entry of data that change from patient to patient. It assists the healthcare provider by providing direction in what is to be documented. For example, if a physician is documenting a history and physical examination, the template will instruct the physician to document a review of system, history of present illness, physical examination, impression, plan, and other required components. The template helps ensure that all required categories of data are collected.

Speech Recognition

Speech recognition, which also may be known as voice recognition, is technology that translates speech to text. The text must be edited, as speech recognition software may misunderstand words and therefore translate speech into text incorrectly. There are two strategies to editing documents created by speech recognition: front-end speech recognition and back-end speech recognition. Dictation with front-end speech recognition (FESR) occurs when the physician or the dictator is the editor of the document that is dictated. The advantage to FESR is that the authenticated document is available in the health record quickly. The downside is that the physicians and other healthcare providers must be trained in how to edit documents. This takes away from the time available to see patients or read radiology reports.

The strategy known as back-end speech recognition (BESR) is the specific use of speech recognition technology in which the physician dictates in the traditional manner and an editor listens to the audio and reviews the document created. Because the dictated documents do not have to be transcribed, the role of transcriptionist is evolving to the role of an editor, who will edit the document to correct any errors created by speech recognition. The document is sent to the dictating physician for approval following the editing process. The advantage of BESR is that the physician is not required to take the time to perform the editing.

Natural Language Processing

Natural language processing is the technology that converts human language (structured or unstructured) into data that can be translated then manipulated by computer systems. It is sophisticated enough to be able to identify key words needed to perform specific tasks such as computer-assisted coding (see chapter 7). This technology basically teaches the meaning of a word or phrase to a software application after several uses. For example, the system would learn how to assign the appropriate procedure code for new procedure. This is done by a statistical algorithm, as the applications can then compare and code these similar expressions accurately and quickly.

Data Integrity

Data integrity is the extent to which healthcare data are complete, accurate, consistent, and timely.

Data quality is the reliability and effectiveness of data for its intended uses in operations, decision making, and planning. Thus, data quality focuses on using the data, whereas data integrity is about the data itself. When designing an IS, steps should be taken to build in data quality. There are a number of tools that can help accomplish this, including required fields, edit checks, user-friendly data field, and field type. To ensure data integrity within the patient's health record, there are many methods that users can build into their paper-based or electronic systems. Because most health records are electronic, they will be the focus of discussion in the sections that follow.

Required Fields

The data fields within an IS for capturing data are individual blank fields required to be populated with patient data. A required field is a preset field in which data must be entered before the IS will allow the user to proceed. If these data fields were on paper, the user would interview the patient for data and type the data into the blanks on the paper to complete the data fields. There would be no alerts to let the user know that a data field was skipped or omitted, or if wrong data were entered into a field during entry. With an electronic IS, the user may not be able to skip ahead on the screen, although some systems may allow the user to override the required field to enter other data, and then come back to enter data in this field later. The existence of required fields is one of many reasons why the EHR is the preferred method for capturing data.

The healthcare facility, working with the IS vendor, determines which data fields should be set as required, if any. It is good practice to set fields as required for information that is essential for patient care, a facility's needs, or other reporting purposes. The healthcare facility must weigh the benefits and disadvantages of required fields to determine what essential information is needed because the user can get frustrated by an excessive number of required fields.

Edit Check

Many ISs have functionality within the software to minimize errors and aid in data accuracy. An **edit check** is a standard feature in many applications' data entry and data collection software packages. Edit checks are preprogrammed definitions of each data field set up within the application. So, as data are entered, if any data are different from what has been preprogrammed, an edit message appears on the screen. For example, edit message would prevent a user from entering a body temperature of 254 degrees. This edit message is sometimes called a flag because it signals that the user needs to verify the data being entered to ensure that the criteria of the field are met. This serves as a quality verification of data being entered into the system as part of the data collection process.

Edit checks can check for illogical data, such as when a patient's gender does not match patient gender-specific procedure documented. For example, a message flag would appear on the screen indicating that a hysterectomy cannot be performed on a male patient. The user would then check the health record for a correct diagnosis and procedure as well as check the patient's gender and determine which information is correct and which needs to be edited. Another example of an illogical data edit is a blood pressure of 543/87.

Edits also can make sure that the type of data entered and its format is valid for that data element. For example, the discharge date should be a valid date. The discharge data would also be entered in MMDDYYYY format such as 10101963. Even though the system stores it in MMDDYYYY format, the system may display it in a more user-friendly view, such as 10/10/1963.

CHECK YOUR UNDERSTANDING 2.1

1. Which of the following is a data integrity tool?
   a. Cloning copy/paste
   b. Natural language processing
   c. Speech recognition
   d. Required field

(Continued)

2. Within an IS, which tool can be accessed by the user to get more information about the data field?

   a. Help screen
   b. Edit check
   c. Hot spot
   d. Automatic save

3. Identify the field type that is BEST for entering gender.

   a. Drop-down box
   b. Check box
   c. Radio buttons
   d. Text box

4. Identify the primary data source.

   a. Data set
   b. Health record
   c. Registry
   d. Index

5. Identify the BEST field type for service.

   a. Drop-down box
   b. Check box
   c. Radio button
   d. Text box

Data Quality Management

Data quality management is defined as "the business processes that ensure the integrity of an organization's data during collection, application (including aggregation), warehousing, and analysis" (Davoudi et al. 2015). Collection in data quality management refers to the way that data elements are gathered. Application is the reason for collecting the data. Warehousing involves the methods used to store the data. Analysis entails converting data into information (Davoudi et al. 2015). The American Health Information Management Association (AHIMA) data quality management model (figure 2.1) displays the components of data quality management and the characteristics of data quality.

Data Accessibility

Data accessibility means that data items are easily obtainable by authorized users. Data can be accurate and relevant, but if it is not accessible to the healthcare providers when needed, then it is of no use. With the paper health record, the accessibility is limited because the health record may be in use by another provider, or may be in transit between patient care areas. In the EHR, the health records are immediately accessible to multiple users at the same time unless the system is down. In case of system downtime, data must still be accessible; a business continuity plan must be in place to address what happens during downtime. For more information on the business continuity plan, see chapter 12.

Data Accuracy

The patient's health record must be accurate and complete. Data accuracy means that data are free of identifiable errors. A multitude of problem areas can prevent a health record from being an accurate record; however, quantitative and qualitative analyses are two methods used to help prevent inaccurate data from occurring frequently within a health record.

   Quantitative analysis is a review of the health record to determine its completeness and accuracy. It is used by health information management (HIM) professionals as a method to detect whether elements of the

Figure 2.1.   AHIMA data quality management model functions and characteristics

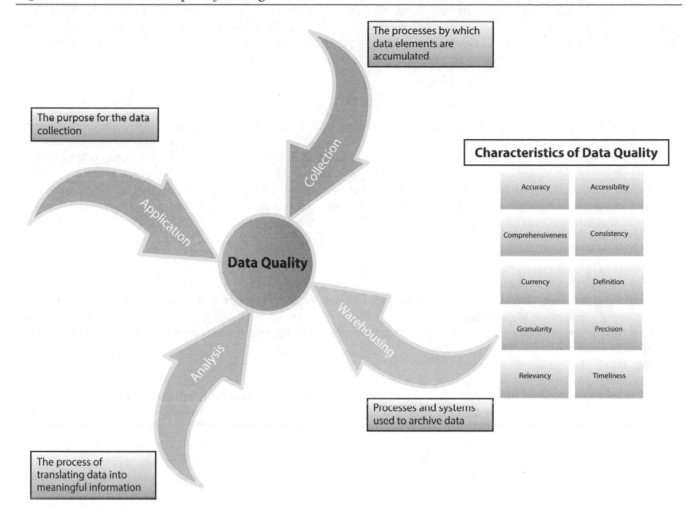

The processes by which data elements are accumulated

The purpose for the data collection

Characteristics of Data Quality

Accuracy	Accessibility
Comprehensiveness	Consistency
Currency	Definition
Granularity	Precision
Relevancy	Timeliness

Data Quality

Collection

Application

Warehousing

Analysis

Processes and systems used to archive data

The process of translating data into meaningful information

Source: Davoudi et al. 2015.

patient's health record are missing. This may mean that a report could be missing entirely or a section of a report is missing, such as a few hours of progress notes. In quantitative analysis, the reviewer determines whether or not the reports are present or absent from the health record.

A qualitative analysis is a review of the health record to ensure that standards are met and to determine the adequacy of entries documenting the quality of care. While reviewing a health record, the reviewer considers whether the health record appropriately documents the care provided. The reviewer would also look at issues such as legibility, whether only approved abbreviations are used, and if all required components are in the discharge summary or other document. HIM professionals look at legibility, use of abbreviations, patient identification, and so forth. Physicians, nurses, and others review the actual quality of the documentation.

When qualitative and quantitative reviews are performed retrospectively, it is difficult to make changes when problems are found. Concurrent reviews allow deficiencies to be identified during the course of the patient's care and therefore the documentation can be addressed in the health record. When documentation issues are found, the problem documentation can be used as teaching points to show the medical staff and other practitioners who document within health records what should be written, so that future documentation can improve.

Inaccurate data are useless, are expensive, and can be harmful to patients. Data form much of the body of knowledge used by medical professionals, epidemiologists, policymakers, and public health officials in decision making. These decisions affect patient lives, policies on healthcare reform, and other major issues regarding health. Resources are allocated at local, state, and national levels based on data collected and entrusted to be accurate. Accurate data are needed to evaluate patient outcomes and quality of life, and to determine satisfaction issues and implement procedures for improvement.

Some errors in the accuracy of the health record are obvious. Spelling errors are the most common obvious errors and often occur in paper-based health records. As more facilities, including hospitals, clinics, and physician offices, become computerized, fewer spelling errors are seen thanks to spell check. Data errors are often made by carelessness, such as transposition of digits when typing a string of numbers. For example:

Physician order: Penicillin 250 mg

Transposed physician order: 520 mg

If the nurse was hurriedly typing in the order for the patient, it is easy to see how the numbers could be transposed. It is also easy to see how this type of error can be missed when proofing the data entry because the same numbers are there but out of order. Depending on the transposition, there could be serious consequences.

Another data accuracy issue arises when many patients have the same last name or the same first name, raising the possibility that duplicate health record numbers could be assigned to more than one patient. During the admission process, the patient must be questioned to make sure that two different patients with the same or similar name have a different health record number.

Data Comprehensiveness

Data comprehensiveness means that the patient's health record must be complete, meaning that all required data are included. Many governmental and accreditation organizations and medical staffs have standards that mandate complete health records. Incomplete health records (missing documents or missing data, or even missing entries or signatures) would not serve any purpose. Any item or element that is not in the patient's health record that should be there is considered missing and qualifies as incomplete data, making the record incomplete.

The HIM profession has been monitoring incomplete patient records since the beginning of record keeping because it is a sound practice of good documentation. Not only is this legally advisable but the primary reason is for the quality of the continuity of patient care. Without accurate and complete data in the health record, practitioners cannot accurately treat the patient. It is in the best interest of the patient and the healthcare facility as well as all practitioners to ensure that all clinical data on the patient's care are contained in the health record. This is again why HIM professionals perform a detailed review of health records, with a quantitative and qualitative review to ensure that records are comprehensive. Reviews help ensure that the healthcare facility meets legal and regulatory requirements and that the documentation within the health records will reinforce this if ever questioned. Complete documentation also is needed for billing and reimbursement. If there are data missing, there is good reason for the claim to be rejected or denied by a third-party payer.

HIM professionals are trained to conduct quantitative analysis and qualitative analysis within a health record. If during a qualitative review of a record there appears to be documentation that does not reflect best practice, if the notes appear to have a lapse in time covered, or if something does not look right, the HIM technician will submit the health record for review by a physician advisor (PA). The PA is hired by the healthcare facility to act as a liaison between the HIM or others and the patient's physician. The PA reviews health records for various reasons, including qualitative reviews, utilization reviews, quality reviews, surgical case and tissue reviews, other pathological reviews, and a host of blood and laboratory reviews for various medical staff and hospital committees. Typically, several physicians serve as PAs on an annual basis and are usually from diverse backgrounds, such as pathology, surgery, medicine, and other disciplines so that reviews can be a true peer review.

Peer review is a review by like professionals, or peers, established according to an organization's medical staff bylaws, organizational policy and procedure, or the requirements of state law. The peer review system allows medical professionals to candidly critique and criticize the work of their colleagues without fear of reprisal, as the feedback comes from the committee, not a specific individual. An example of a true peer review would be a cardiologist reviewing a health record that was documented by another cardiologist and not a physician from any other discipline. Peer review is at its best whenever physicians of the same discipline review each other. However, this is not always possible, especially in small healthcare facilities. These qualitative, quantitative, and peer reviews are more easily performed with the EHR as data are more readily accessible to authorized reviewers. Additionally, the data in EHRs are complete since the EHR can prevent the user from moving forward if required information is missing. In the paper environment, data elements on forms are frequently left blank, so the review process has greatly benefited from the conversion from a paper-based record to the EHR.

Whether data are entered into fields located as entries on a page in a paper-based record or as entries in an EHR, all data must be entered to be considered comprehensive. If data do not apply, a field usually has several options for the user to choose (such as Not Applicable, Not Given, or Not Known) so there are no blank fields in the health record. Using one of the aforementioned options signals that the user has read the option, but there is not a designation that applies from the choices given, and the field was not skipped or left blank unintentionally.

Data Consistency

Data consistency ensures that like data are the same on each document or computer screen. For example, in the paper health record, the patient's date of birth is listed on many different documents. It is easy for someone to write the wrong age on a document, which would create different ages on different documents. With the EHR, the date of birth is entered once and is displayed on multiple screens.

Data Currency

Data currency ensures that data are up to date. A data value is up to date if it is current for a specific point in time, and it is outdated if it was current at a preceding time but incorrect at a later time. Patient care must be provided based on current information. For example, a patient's chest x-ray study from six weeks ago has little to no value when a physician is treating the patient's pneumonia. The physician needs a current chest x-ray study to evaluate the patient's condition.

Data Definition

The data definition is the specific meaning of a healthcare-related data element. Defining each data element provides the foundation that allows everyone to interpret and collect the data in the same way.

Data Granularity

Data granularity describes the level of detail at which the attributes and values of healthcare data are defined. The required level of detail depends on the circumstances of the patient's care. For example, the documentation in the health record for a patient who is being treated for cardiac disease will describe the patient's cardiac condition much more detail than if the patient had a disease in another body system.

Data Precision

Data precision ensures that there is justification for the need to collect the data, such as for patient care, data analysis, billing, and other operational tasks. In order to be useful, the data must be defined for precise understanding. Meanings can vary by department, facility, or another factor, supporting the need for a standard definition to avoid confusion. For example, "admission time" can be the time the patient arrived at the hospital, the time the patient's information was entered into the IS, or the time the patient arrived in their room. In addition, if the patient is first seen in the emergency room or when the IS is down, the time of admission would be impacted. Therefore, "admission time" should be defined, and the definition should be made available to all users.

Data Relevancy

Data relevancy is the extent to which healthcare-related data are useful for the purposes for which they were collected. Thus, only data that are needed or are expected to be needed in the future are collected. The type of data is determined by the needs of the healthcare facility. In the case of the health record, relevant data should include demographic data, administrative data, and clinical data. Demographic data are basic information about the patient, such as name, address, and date of birth. Administrative data include consent forms, insurance information, and authorizations to release health information. Clinical data includes information about the patient's care, such as symptoms, test results, physician observations, and treatment performed. The data needed in the health record vary by setting (hospital, emergency department) and service (surgical, medical, obstetrical). The data collected should support the patient's care; for example, one would generally not collect data such as patient's eye color or shoe size.

Data Timeliness

Data timeliness means that data should be recorded in an appropriate period of time after the event and should be available to the user when needed. The healthcare facility determines the appropriate period of time for each data element based on accreditation, state licensure, and other requirements. The timeliness of data entry is of utmost importance and represents one aspect of data quality. Healthcare providers should document the care of the patient at or near the time that the care is provided; however, there is no established standard timeframe for documentation. Timeliness ensures that the information is available to the other care providers and improves the accuracy of the information in the health record as well. The care provider will better remember the details of the care provided when it is documented immediately. This way, the information will not be forgotten or confused with that of another patient. Best practice is to complete documentation of the care provided to one patient before moving on to the next. The documentation must reflect the exact time and date when care was performed. Inaccurate accounting of the treatment may reflect poor quality of care as well as poor documentation of care. Users of the patient's health record depend on accurate and timely data, so it is important that the actual time of care is recorded. It also helps to meet accreditation standards that list requirements on the timeliness of documents such as the history and physical examination.

The signatures or initials of the healthcare practitioners who oversee each event during a patient's stay, such as verbal and written orders, should be recorded. This verifies that the practitioner has overseen the treatment or plans for treatment and that these plans have been carried out. The timeliness of authentication (a provider's signature or initials) is just as important as the patient's treatment because it represents proof of care, not to mention satisfying medicolegal requirements and billing and claims reimbursement after the patient's discharge.

Data Integrity Issues

Efforts should be made to prevent data integrity issues in order to have the best data available for decision making. Failure to do so can result in poor quality patient care and bad business decisions. These efforts include data cleansing, data mapping, and a number of documentation integrity issues.

Data Cleansing

Data cleansing is the process of checking internal consistency and duplication as well as identifying outliers and missing data. In other words, data cleansing means looking for errors or problems with the data, such as duplicate patients. There may be outliers, which is an extreme statistical value that falls outside the normal range. For example, if a research study has captured the number of continuing education hours that registered health information technicians report and most reported somewhere in the range of 20 and 250 hours but one reported 1,500 hours, then the 1,500 hours would be an outlier. An outlier is not necessarily an error, but it should be evaluated for accuracy because of the impact that it has on the mean and other statistical analysis of the data. Another consideration when performing data cleansing is missing data, such as when the number of continuing education hours is not reported. Efforts should be taken to complete any missing data that is identified. Failure to perform cleansing may lead to poor data integrity.

Data Mapping

Data mapping allows for connections between two systems. For example, the *International Classification of Diseases, Ninth Revision, Clinical Modification* and *International Classification of Diseases, Tenth Revision, Clinical Modification* have similar concepts but are not identical. If the concepts in the two systems are not linked appropriately, there will be problems with data integrity. For example, a link has been established when the codes for an open appendectomy in each coding system are identified as equivalent codes for each other. For additional information on data mapping, refer to chapter 14.

Documentation Integrity Errors

Data integrity of documentation can be compromised in many ways in ISs like the EHR, such as when a revision is made to an operative report and it is unclear which is the most current report. These integrity errors affect patient identification, authorship, dictation, amendments, cloning, and copying and pasting. These errors not only harm the integrity of the data but can lead to poor quality of care and allegations of fraud and abuse.

Patient Identification

Patient identification errors occur when patient A's health information is documented in patient B's health record. This mistake can lead to serious patient care errors for both patients. Healthcare facilities should use methods that help ensure the identity of patients, such as algorithms, biometrics, and photography (AHIMA Work Group 2013).

Authorship

Authorship is the origination or creation of recorded information attributed to a specific individual or entity acting at a particular time. In other words, documentation in the EHR or other health record must be credited to the individual who created it. This is typically done through the use of a unique user identifier and a password. When the digital signature is created, it indicates that the data have been reviewed and approved by the physician or other care provider. A digital signature is an electronic signature that binds a message to a particular individual and can be used by the receiver to authenticate the identity of the sender. Failure to link the documentation to the proper author makes it difficult to determine who actually recorded it when multiple healthcare providers are involved in the patient's care (AHIMA Work Group 2013). It is important to identify the author because the documentation is used for legal reasons to prove what the healthcare professional did or did not do. Authorship is important in other areas, too, including coding, because generally only the patient's physician documentation is used in coding.

Dictation Errors Without Editing

If speech recognition is utilized, and the documents are not edited after their creation to ensure accuracy, then there may be problems with data integrity. The speech recognition software may misinterpret and the health record could include incorrect medications and other incorrect words (AHIMA Work Group 2013).

Copying and Pasting

One of the ways to speed data entry is through the copy and paste functions. Data from one patient's health record can be copied and pasted into another patient's health record or data from the same patient's previous hospitalization may be moved to their current hospitalization. Copying and pasting are commonly done for routine procedures, radiology results, and other common entries for which the same information is used over and over again. Benefits include legibility, being consistent in what is documented, and ensuring that the documentation is complete (AHIMA 2014, 3). However, there are risks associated with this, so this practice is not always recommended. For example, the physician may copy and paste a preoperative order from one patient's record to another's. In the order copied from the first patient's record, there may be a medication inappropriate for the second patient. If not caught, the patient may be given this medication in error. Copying can also be used in moving data, such as diagnoses and medication, between different visits of the same patient. For example, data can be moved from a patient's October 1 visit to their December 30 visit. Although this function speeds data entry, there is a data quality risk if the information copied may not completely apply to the patient's care. When this happens, the patient's health record contains erroneous information that can impact the quality of care.

Amendments to the Health Record

The data contained in the health record must be amended when changes are necessary, such as correcting mistakes, attaching addendums, making late entries, and replacing a draft (unsigned) copy of a document with a final (signed) copy. For example, if the patient's blood type is entered in the EHR as A+ but it is actually B–, then the blood type must be corrected.

Once a health record entry is signed, the document should be locked to prevent further alterations. The system should also lock the entire record from edits at a predetermined point, such as 30 days after discharge. To amend the health record, it would have to be unlocked by an authorized user so that the necessary changes can be made. There should also be policies in place regarding who has the ability to amend. For example, the HIM professional may be able to correct the spelling of the patient's name or a transposition in the social security number, but only the physician would be able to correct his clinical documentation. The deleted information should not be permanently deleted so that it can be retrieved if needed. Late entries and addendums should be clearly labeled so that it is clear when the documentation was created (Davoudi et al. 2015).

The erroneous information should not be completely deleted; rather, there should be a way to identify that the health record was altered. The best practice is to create a second version of the document. Version control is necessary to manage the various documents. Version control in healthcare is the process whereby a healthcare facility ensures that only the most current version of a patient's health record is available for viewing, updating, and so forth. However, there must be a way for authorized users to be able to view the previous version to see what was changed. This would be necessary in court cases and other legal circumstances.

Data Quality Measure

Data quality measure is a "mechanism to assign a quantitative figure to quality of care by comparison to a criterion. Quality measurements typically focus on structures or processes of care that have a demonstrated relationship to positive health outcomes" (Davoudi et al. 2015). For example, when steps are taken to reduce postoperative infections, the data quality measure would address issues, such as use of antibiotics and wound care. These are used to compare actual patient information to a standard created by an accreditation organization, government agency, or other group to determine the quality of care provided. The data can be aggregated (compiled) and be used to compare healthcare facilities against state or national scores.

CHECK YOUR UNDERSTANDING 2.2

1. The identification of the individual who recorded a progress note in the health record is known as _____.

   a. Edit check
   b. Data integrity
   c. Version control
   d. Authorship

2. Checking for missing information and outliers is known as _____.

   a. Edit check
   b. Qualitative analysis
   c. Data cleansing
   d. Quantitative analysis

3. Documentation integrity issues includes _____.

   a. Amendments
   b. Data precision
   c. Edit check
   d. Data capture

4. Which characteristic of data quality addresses the level of detail of the data collected?

   a. Data relevancy
   b. Data precision
   c. Data accuracy
   d. Data granularity

5. Which attribute of data quality addresses availability of the data collected?

   a. Data relevancy
   b. Data consistency
   c. Data accessibility
   d. Data granularity

Real-World Case

In order to improve patient safety and efficiency, XYZ Hospital recently implemented a clinical provider order entry (CPOE) system. One of the functions of the CPOE system is to notify physicians of any problems at the time that an order is entered. Days after the CPOE system was implemented, Dr. Smith ordered medication X for a patient named Mary Johnson. Immediately, the CPOE came back with a message stating that medication X was contraindicated (not recommended) for patients on medication Y and that Mary was taking medication Y. Dr. Smith realized that he had almost ordered a medication that could have significantly harmed Mary. He was able to delete the order of medication X and order medication Z instead. Mary received her medication in a timely manner and was discharged from the hospital in two days.

REVIEW QUESTIONS

1. Identify the type of data field that is most appropriate for the health record number.

   a. Numeric field
   b. Autonumbering field
   c. Text box field
   d. Radio button field

2. What is the benefit of front-end speech recognition?

   a. It does not impact the physician.
   b. The document is available immediately upon completion of the dictation.
   c. It speeds availability of the document.
   d. It eliminates data quality issues.

3. A missing document would fall under what type of data quality characteristic?

   a. Comprehensiveness
   b. Accuracy
   c. Consistency
   d. Definition

4. What data quality characteristic ensures that data support the reason for the collection of the data?

   a. Precision
   b. Currency
   c. Constancy
   d. Definition

5. The fact that there is missing data would be identified in _____.

   a. Authorship
   b. Data analysis
   c. Data mapping
   d. Data cleansing

6. The identification of who documented a note in the health record is known as _____.

   a. Patient identification
   b. Authorship
   c. Authentication
   d. Validation

7. Identify the statement that is true about amending a health record.

   a. Anyone should be able to alter the health record at any time.
   b. The author of an entry should be able to alter the health record at any time.
   c. Any documentation deleted should be retrievable if needed.
   d. Health records cannot be amended.

8. Ensuring that only the most recent report is available for viewing is known as _____.

   a. Documentation integrity
   b. Authorship
   c. Validation
   d. Version control

(Continued)

REVIEW QUESTIONS (*Continued*)

9. Edit checks ensure that _____.

   a. The format is appropriate for the data element
   b. The data entered is accurate for that patient
   c. The health record is complete
   d. The data entered is at the level appropriate for the situation

10. Qualitative analysis reviews the quality of _____.

   a. Forms in the health record
   b. Screen design
   c. Documentation in the health record
   d. The data dictionary

References

American Health Information Management Association (AHIMA). 2014. Appropriate Use of the Copy and Paste Functionality in Electronic Health Records. http://library.ahima.org/PdfView?oid=300306.

AHIMA Work Group. 2013. Integrity of the Healthcare Record: Best Practices for EHR Documentation (2013 update). http://bok.ahima.org/doc?oid=300257#.WjxsKeRy5jo.

Davoudi, S., J. A. Dooling, B. Glondys, T. D. Jones, L. Kadlec, S. M. Overgaard, K. Ruben, and A. Wendicke. 2015. Data Quality Management Model (2015 update). http://bok.ahima.org/doc?oid=107773#.WjxlEORy5jo.

Sharp, M. 2016. Secondary Data Sources. Chapter 7 in *Health Information Management Technology: An Applied Approach*, 5th ed. Edited by N. B. Sayles and L. L. Gordon. Chicago: AHIMA.

Learning Objectives

- Assist in the development of a database.
- Develop and manage the data dictionary.
- Develop queries to retrieve data contained in the database.
- Read and understand an entity-relationship diagram.
- Identify the primary key contained in an entity.
- Differentiate between a data repository and a data warehouse.
- Expound on the ways that data mining can be useful.
- Complete simple normalization of data.
- Differentiate between the various types of data.

Key Terms

Boolean search
Clinical data repository (CDR)
Computer-aided software engineering (CASE)
Conceptual data model
Data control language (DCL)
Data definition language (DDL)
Data dictionary
Data field
Data flow diagram (DFD)
Data manipulation
Data manipulation language (DML)
Data mart
Data mining
Data modeling
Data repository

Data set
Data standards
Data warehouse
Database
Database administrator (DBA)
Database management system (DBMS)
Database table
Entity-relationship diagram
File
Foreign key
Hierarchical database model
Java
Key field
Logical data model
Mask
Metadata

Multidimensional database model
Natural language queries
Network database model
Normalization
Object-oriented database model
Online analytical processing (OLAP)
Physical data model
Primary key
Query
Query by example (QBE)
Record
Standards development organization (SDO)
Structured query language (SQL)
Use case
Wildcard search

A database is defined as an organized collection of data, text, references, or pictures in a standardized format, typically stored in a computer system for multiple applications. Healthcare facilities collect and store a tremendous amount of administrative, financial, and clinical data. A database can assist the healthcare facility in many ways, including the following:

- Facilitate data sharing
- Streamline workflow
- Assist in clinical decision making
- Provide information for managerial decision making
- Provide data for data analysis

Databases allow data to be stored in one place and accessed by many different systems and end-users. This consolidation reduces the redundancy of data and improves data consistency because data are entered into the database once, and any screen, report, or system can access that data element. One-time data entry improves the consistency of data, which improves data quality and, ultimately, patient care. Additionally, the use of a database allows for the standardization of data forms, names of data elements, and documentation, which makes moving from transitioning between various screens and various information systems (ISs) easier for the users.

A database requires a database administrator (DBA) to manage it. The DBA is the individual responsible for the technical aspects of designing and managing databases. The DBA is responsible for designing the database as well as managing the database after implementation (Amatayakul 2016, 393).

Requirements for Establishing a Database

The healthcare facility must develop a database that meets its needs. These needs are identified by researching the needs of the users and the external stakeholders, such as the Joint Commission, state licensing agencies, and the Centers for Medicare and Medicaid Services. The data elements stored in the database must meet the requirements of data sets. A data set is a list of recommended data elements with uniform definitions that are relevant for a particular use. For example, the Uniform Hospital Discharge Data Set (UHDDS) is used by acute-care hospitals to capture and report the minimal data required for all inpatient discharges. The UHDDS includes patient name, discharge disposition, date of admission, diagnosis and procedure codes, and much more. As this is only the minimum amount of data to be collected, the healthcare facility can add other data elements to meet the needs of the organization, such as accreditation, research, state licensure, and other needs. The data elements may be administrative, such as patient name and health record number; financial, such as the charge for the hospital room or the laboratory test performed; or clinical, such as history of present illness or follow-up plan.

Once all of the necessary individual data elements are determined, a common data definition should be developed for each data element. As discussed in chapter 2, this definition would be utilized to collect data consistently throughout the healthcare facility. For example, time of discharge could be the time that the discharge order is written, the time the discharge is entered into the IS, or the time the patient walks out of the hospital.

Database Management System

A database cannot function without a database management system (DBMS) to manipulate and control the data stored within the database to meet the needs of the user. It controls the ability to create, read, write, and delete data stored in the database. There are six DBMS functions, listed as follows:

- Moving where data is stored in database
- Managing concurrent data access by multiple users, including provisions to prevent simultaneous updates from conflicting with one another
- Managing transactions so that each transaction's database changes are an all-or-nothing unit of work. In other words, if the transaction succeeds, all database changes made by it are recorded in the database
- Support for a query language, which is a system of commands that a database user employs to retrieve data from the database

- Provisions for backing up the database and recovering from failures
- Security mechanisms to prevent unauthorized data access and modification (Oppel 2004)

The parts of the DBMS include data definition language, data manipulation language, data control language, and data dictionary.

The **data definition language (DDL)** is a special type of software used to create the tables within a relational database (defined later in this chapter). It translates how data are stored in the computer from the physical view (physical structure of the database) to the logical view (one that is understandable by the user). It is "used to define data structures and modify data. For example, DDL commands can be used to add, remove, or modify tables within a database" (HIMSS 2017, 64).

The **data manipulation language (DML)** is a special type of software used to retrieve, update, and edit data in a relational database. The DML accesses, makes changes to, and retrieves data from the database. These capabilities can easily be performed in a database without the user being an experienced computer programmer. It is a "family of computer languages, including commands permitting users to manipulate data in a database" (HIMSS 2017, 70). To retrieve data, a query is generated. As discussed earlier, the term query is used to describe selecting records that meet specific criteria. Queries may also perform calculations on the data, such as calculating the average length of stay. Queries can also screen data for inclusion or exclusion. Four user methods to access data contained in the database are natural language queries, query by example, structured query language, and data dictionary. The **data control language (DCL)** controls access to data within a database.

Natural Language Queries

Natural language queries use common words to tell the database which data are needed. For example, the user may enter a query by typing "list all of the patients whose principal procedure is 0F140D3." This command would generate a list of patients who had the principal procedure. Another example may be, "how many patients were discharged on October 1, 20XX?" To process the query, the system searches key words in the question in order to fulfill the request. Some ISs may allow the use of voice recognition, thus eliminating the need to type in the request.

Query by Example

Query by example (QBE) is a query method whereby the user only has to point and click to choose tables and fields contained in the database. The IS then allows the user to choose whether the entries that meet those criteria should be included or excluded from the query. For example, the user may choose the patient table and discharge date as the field. The user can then tell the IS to include patients discharged January 1, 20XX through January 31, 20XX. Only the patients with a discharge date within that range would be included in the results of the query. **Boolean search** capabilities such as "and," "or," and "not" may be used in the QBE database to narrow down the data to specifically what the user needs. For example, the query could retrieve patients who had a principal diagnosis of cholecystitis "and" a principal procedure of laparoscopic cholecystectomy. Truncation, such as the **wildcard search**, may be used to look for variations in the word (Oracle n.d.). For example, the user could search for patients whose admission date is greater than, or before, a specific date. The wildcard would be used to indicate that the query should identify data that meet the partial information provided. For example, a query of 0F140D% would retrieve all codes that start with the specified characters such as 0F140D3, 0F140D4, 0F140D5, 0F140D6, and so on. Other query tools include the greater than and less than options to retrieve data that meets the criteria 0F140D. Different characters may be used as wildcards in different databases.

Structured Query Language

A common data retrieval tool is **structured query language (SQL)**, the standard language for the relational database. SQL defines data elements and manipulates and controls data. The data definition components of SQL allow the user to create tables, delete tables, and show how something is viewed. **Data manipulation** allows the user to add and delete rows in a table and to sort, find, and compare. Another function of the data manipulation component is to update data. SQL is the programming language that manages a user's access and what the user can do. Examples of SQL commands typed by the programmer are CREATE TABLE, SELECT, WHERE, COUNT, and UPDATE PATIENT (Oppel 2004).

An SQL query that assumes a table with the name Patients and the columns ID, FirstName, LastName, and DateAdded can be used as follows:

- To retrieve all the records and all the columns
  Select * from Patients

- To retrieve all the records and only the FirstName column
  Select FirstName From Patients

- To retrieve all the records and all the columns ordered by LastName Descending
  Select * From Patients Order By LastName desc

- To retrieve all the records and all the columns that were added before 1/1/2014
  Select * From Patients Where DateAdded < '1/1/2014'

- To select only the records where the FirstName is equal to Mark
  Select * from Patients Where FirstName = 'Mark'

Data Dictionary

The **data dictionary** is a descriptive list of the names, definitions, and attributes of data elements to be collected in an IS or database whose purpose is to standardize definitions and ensure consistent use. It also helps to control the quality of data. The data dictionary improves data consistency because it ensures that fields have the same meaning and format throughout the organization. It helps create consistent data field names, data field definitions, field length, and element values (AHIMA 2017, 7). Examples of how the data dictionary supports data consistency are provided in table 3.1.

Table 3.1.   Examples of how data dictionary assists in data consistency

Data Element	Example
Field name	The unique identifier given to a specific patient encounter is called encounter number in all ISs, not account number and not billing number.
Field definition	Discharge time is the time the order was written, not the time the discharge is entered into the system or the time that the patient leaves the nursing unit.
Field length	The field length of the account number is 10 digits in all ISs, not 8 in some and 12 in others.
Element values	The insurance type for Medicare is M in all ISs, not MCR.

The data dictionary assists in improving

- Data quality
- Data integrity
- Documentation
- Data analysis
- Data reuse (AHIMA 2016)

The data contained in the data dictionary is known as metadata. **Metadata** is descriptive data that characterize other data to create a clearer understanding of their meaning and to achieve greater reliability and quality of information. Some of the metadata contained in the data dictionary includes, but is not limited to, the following:

- Names of data elements
- Definition
- Source of data

- Length of field
- Allowable range as appropriate
- Valid values
- Access restrictions
- Length of field (Amatayakul 2017, 315)

The data dictionary may also control if a mask is used and, if so, what form it takes. Table 3.2 shows an abbreviated sample of a data dictionary. The data dictionary defines any masks to be used. A mask is a format in which data are displayed. This display is different from how the data are stored in the database. For example, if a patient's home telephone number is entered as 5555555555, numbers could appear as (555) 555-5555. Another example of where a mask could be used is social security number. The social security number of 123456789 could be entered and it appears in the system as 123-45-6789.

Table 3.2.   Abbreviated data dictionary

Field Name	Last Name	First Name	Health Record Number	Date of Birth	Gender
Data type	Text	Text	Text	Alphanumeric	Alphanumeric
Format	A–Z	A–Z	0–9	MM-DD-YYYY	M, F, U
Field size	25	25	10	8	1
Range			0000000001–0009999999		
Required	Yes	Yes	Yes	Yes	Yes

Data Standards

Data standards allow us to share data in a uniform way. Data standards include data content standards and data exchange standards. These standards are created by a standards development organization (SDO). An SDO is a private or government agency involved in the development of healthcare informatics standards at a national or international level. Data content standards are clear guidelines for the acceptable values for specified data fields. These standards make it possible to exchange health information using electronic networks. Without standards, sharing data between healthcare facilities is difficult because facilities could name and define the same data element differently. Data content standards make it possible to share information by ensuring that users interpret data in the same way.

Data exchange standards are protocols that help ensure that data transmitted from one system to another remain comparable. Data exchange standards are critical as the nationwide health information network is created so that information can be shared across providers and other users of health information to facilitate quality patient care. See chapter 12 for more information on standards for ISs.

CHECK YOUR UNDERSTANDING 3.1

1. The best choice for field type to assign the health record number is _____.
   a. Alphanumeric
   b. Numeric
   c. Autonumbering
   d. Alphabetic

(Continued)

CHECK YOUR UNDERSTANDING 3.1 (*Continued*)

2. The term used to describe breaking data elements into the level of detail needed to retrieve the data is

   a. Normalization
   b. Data definitions
   c. Primary key
   d. Database management system

3. Information collected on a single patient is found in a _____.

   a. File
   b. Record
   c. Row
   d. Field

4. What is the term used when queries are limited by words such as "and"?

   a. Boolean search
   b. Natural language queries
   c. SQL
   d. Data dictionary

5. Which component defines the length of a field?

   a. Data manipulation language
   b. Data definition language
   c. Data dictionary
   d. Data control language

6. The user entered the social security number as 123456789 and it was displayed as 123-45-6789. This is an example of a _____.

   a. Query
   b. DBMS
   c. Mask
   d. Wildcard

Data Modeling

Data modeling is the process of determining the users' information needs and identifying relationships among the data. The model should be based on the organization's strategic plan and should identify the data elements to be collected and the relationship between them. It contains all of the entities appropriate for the healthcare facility and shows the technical database structure to be used in the database. There are three levels of data models—conceptual data model, physical data model, and logical data model.

The conceptual data model is not tied to a particular database model, but rather defines the requirements for the database to be developed. This conceptual data model is the basis for the logical and physical data models.

The physical data model shows how the data are physically stored within the database. The users are not involved with this level of the database because of its technical complexity.

The logical data model is a "complete representation of data requirements and the structural business rules that govern data quality in support of project's requirements" (HHS n.d., 1). In other words, it ensures that the data are available and in a useful format for the intended purpose. For example, the nursing department would look at the data differently than the HIM department and the HIM department would look at it differently than the marketing department.

The data-modeling tools used in the logical data model vary by the type of database involved, but may include the entity-relationship diagram. Data modeling generally includes the entity-relationship diagram or the semantic object model. The **entity-relationship diagram** is a common type of data modeling that focuses on relationships between entities. An entity is a person, location, thing, or concept that is to be tracked in the database. In healthcare, entities would include such items as patient, physician, and laboratory test. Each entity has attributes, which are facts or data about the entity. Some examples of attributes of the entity patient include:

- Health record number (primary key)
- Last name
- First name
- Middle initial
- Street address
- City
- State
- Zip code
- Home phone
- Cell phone
- Work phone
- Date of birth
- Social security number

Each entity would have a unique identifier. A patient's unique identifier could be the health record number. In an entity-relationship diagram, entities are linked together to show relationships between the two. There are several types of relationships, such as one-to-one, one-to-many, and many-to-many. An example of a one-to-one relationship is a lab test and its result. The following are examples of the one-to-many relationships:

- A patient may have many physicians.
- A patient may have many laboratory tests.
- A physician may have many patients.

In a many-to-many relationship a patient can have many lab tests and a lab test can be performed on many patients. Additional examples of these relationships are shown in figures 3.1 and 3.2.

Figure 3.1.   One-to-one relationship: Patient has one attending physician

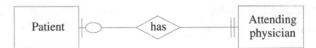

Figure 3.2.   One-to-many relationship: Patient can have many consulting physicians

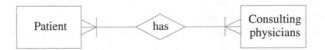

Data-Modeling Tools

A number of tools can be used to create the data model. **Computer-aided software engineering (CASE)** is designed to create many of the diagrams and other tools used in the data model. CASE can develop tools such as the entity-relationship diagrams described as well as **data flow diagrams (DFDs)**. A DFD is a diagram that shows how data moves (input, storage, output) within the database. The DFD is a way to show management and other nontechnical users the system design. It is also a way to introduce the overall design of the system without getting bogged down in the details. These details can be shown on other diagrams. Unfortunately, developing and updating a DFD are time-consuming, and the DFD may be difficult to design if the user does not have the necessary level of detail or if the data flow is constantly changing.

Another tool for data modeling is the use case. The use case is a technique that is used to develop scenarios based on how users will use the data and functionality to assist in developing ISs that support the information requirements. These ISs include the databases that support them. For example, a use case might be created to show how the user would retrieve information or generate a report. Specifically, it might show how to create a list of healthcare claims requiring coding. This use case identifies the data elements needed, the flow of information, and more.

Common Database Models

The database model is a description of the structure used to organize data in a healthcare-related database such as an electronic health record. This is different from data modeling, which is the process of determining what data is needed. There are a number of database models available, including relational, hierarchical, network, object-oriented, and multidimensional (Morley and Parker 2017, 505–506).

Relational Database Model

The most common database model used is the relational database model. In the relational database, data are stored in tables. It is named for the relationships that are created when there are data elements, such as health record number, in common between the tables. The database table contains all data related to a particular subject or concept, such as a patient, and is made up of the records and fields. In the table, the data are stored in rows and columns much like a spreadsheet. The data in a database is stored in a file. A file is a collection of digital data stored in the database. In healthcare, a file contains information on patient care, patient accounts, employee files, or another subject. Within the file are multiple records.

Within the relational database model, each row in the database table is called a record. A record is all the data that has been collected on an individual patient, employee, patient account, or a specific transaction. This data is stored in a data field. A data field is a predefined area within a healthcare database in which the same type of information is usually recorded. Examples of data fields collected in healthcare include patient last name, health record number, gender, diagnosis, procedure, and date of birth. The computer screen should provide a definition of the field, instructions on how to enter data into the field such as format, and valid characters.

The data collected in each field can take a number of formats based on the type of data. Types of fields include the following:

- Alphabetic fields accept only alphabetic characters. Data elements of this field type include patient name and city.
- Numeric fields accept only numbers that can be calculated. This would include charges, but would not include zip codes and the health record number, as these numbers cannot be calculated (added, subtracted, and so on).
- Alphanumeric fields accept alphabetic characters, numbers, or a combination of the two. Examples of alphanumeric fields include street address, zip codes, and phone numbers.
- Time and date fields contain only a date or time.
- Autonumbering fields create a unique number that will never be assigned again. This could be the health record number or a unique number assigned to a patient visit.

Before the data elements go into a database, the fields should be normalized. Normalization is breaking the data elements into the level of detail desired by the healthcare facility. For example, last name and first name should be in separate fields, as should city, state, and zip code. This allows the user to search or otherwise manipulate any of the data elements. Conversely, if the city and state were stored in the same field, the user would not be able to run reports or query the database based on state; because the name of the city varies widely in length, the computer does not know where the city ends and where the state begins. For example, the name of the city of Opp, Alabama is much shorter than San Luis Obispo, California. The latter also has three words in the name, so the computer cannot be made to look for a space or a number of characters. By breaking the city and state into different fields, searches by city or state can be done with ease. See table 3.3 for examples of normalized and unnormalized data.

Database administrators and others are able to display information about the data onscreen when a user has a request for particular data. The information is requested through a query, which is a search for data that meet specific criteria the user requests within subsets of the database. The queries sort and filter the data to display all records that meet the criteria for user review. For example, the user could query all patients discharged by Dr. Smith in 20XX. The patients could then be sorted by diagnosis, procedure,

Table 3.3.   Examples of normalized and unnormalized data

Normalized Data	Unnormalized Data
Last name First name Middle initial Address City State Zip	Last name, first name Middle initial Address City, state, zip

date of discharge, or other data element that exists in the database. If the results of the query are too voluminous, the criteria for the search can be narrowed to provide further filtering for a more desirable result. For example, the patients who received an appendectomy could be limited to Medicare patients or Dr. Smith's patients.

Key Field

A key field is a field in a table that holds a unique identifier to ensure that each data entry in the database table is different. This unique identifier is generally called the primary key. In the electronic health record (EHR) and other clinical ISs, this unique identifier is typically the health record number. Within the database, the tables organize the information from all records into rows and columns or cubes and use the primary key to locate the information. With the use of the primary key such as the health record number, then all of the patient's health information can be linked together.

When a primary key from one table is found in another table, the second primary key is called a foreign key. For example, the patient table would have a primary key of health record number but the physician table primary key may also be in the table so that the patient's attending physician can be identified. Once the attending physician is identified, then all of the physician's information, such as specialty, address, and phone number, can also be retrieved. Other examples of primary keys found in healthcare are a billing number or a physician identification number.

When a certain data field is designated as a primary key, this means that a search for certain criteria values of this field will speed up the process. Furthermore, in a relational model two tables can be matched by using the search criteria, so searching can be done across tables. The relational database has a number of advantages. First, it is flexible because the file is not tied to a specific application. The relational database allows the database administrator to control access to certain tables in order to provide security for the data contained in that database. Also, because data are entered only once, data consistency and quality are improved. This one-time data entry improves not only the quality of the data but also the efficiency of the healthcare organization. Finally, because data are stored in a single location, the user will have the most current data available. See table 3.4 for an example of the table in the relational database.

Table 3.4.   Example of table in a relational database

Medical Record Number	Last Name	First Name	DOB	Admitting Date	Discharge Date
123456	Smith	Harry	10/10/1963	04/17/2018	04/21/2018
234567	Jones	Patricia	11/08/1956	05/14/2018	05/27/2018
345678	Adams	Georgia	01/31/1930	04/23/2018	04/25/2018
134534	Warren	Mallory	03/12/2008	05/01/2018	05/04/2018

Hierarchical Database Model

The **hierarchical database model**, like the name implies, structures the data in a hierarchy very similar to that used for an organizational chart. To use the analogy of a tree, the trunk of the tree would be the starting point or the initial query by the user, and as the search narrows or goes forward, each branch of the tree becomes smaller, progressing outward toward the leaves of the tree, which represent the end point of the search. Each piece of data in the database is called a node. Pointers indicate where in this tree structure the data are stored. A parent-child relationship is created by the relationships developed by the pointer. The relationship can be described as one-to-many. This means that a parent can have many nodes but a child can have only one parent (Harrington 2016, 604).

As mentioned before, in the hierarchical data model, access to data starts at the top of the hierarchy and moves downward. For example, in figure 3.3, the hierarchy moves from patient, to laboratory test, and then to name of test. In that example, the node patient is parent to three child nodes. These three nodes are laboratory test, attending physician, and radiology examination. The node laboratory test has four child nodes. Then at the next level, laboratory test becomes a parent to four children: name of test, date of test, time of test, and test results.

The hierarchical database model is not always user-friendly because it may require developers of the IS to predetermine the queries that will be needed rather than write a query ad hoc (as needed). Another disadvantage of this model is that the user must understand both the physical and logical data models (Abdelhak and Hanken 2016, 299).

Figure 3.3. Example of a hierarchical data model

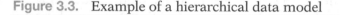
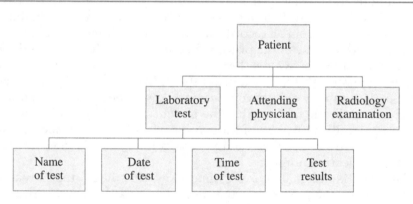

Network Database Model

The **network database model**, illustrated in figure 3.4, uses pointers to connect data. The nodes are called owners and members rather than parent and child nodes, as in the hierarchical database model. A member node in the network database model can have more than one owner, unlike in the hierarchical database model (Abdelhak and Hanken 2016, 299).

Figure 3.4. Example of a network database model

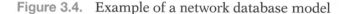
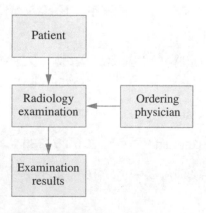

Object-Oriented Database Model

The object-oriented database model handles text, images, audio, video, and other objects. These images and other nontext items are stored as objects. An object is the basic component in an object-oriented database that includes both data and their relationships within a single structure. Each data element is called a variable. The object-oriented database uses programming tools such as Java, a programming language that was designed to be used on the Internet and that runs some of the functions of Internet applications. When the users access the webpage, a window appears asking the user to install the Java applet, which are programs that reside on HTML web pages.

Two concepts related to the object-oriented model are encapsulation and inheritance. Encapsulation is defining the characteristics of an object. For example, a laboratory test would have a name, test result, time, and date. In the object-orientated database, an object can inherit properties from another object when the characteristics are similar. This characteristic is called inheritance. An example of this is physician and resident physician. Both have the data elements of name, address, specialty, phone number, and others in common as they are both physicians (Abdelhak and Hanken 2016, 300).

Multidimensional Database Model

A multidimensional database model is used in data warehouses. The data are collected from multiple sources, such as other databases, and then summarized. This enables data analysis using a wide range of data. The multidimensional database is designed to quickly access this summarized data (Morley and Parker 2017, 506).

Data Repository and Data Warehouse

Data in healthcare facilities are collected in many different systems, both clinical and administrative. The data from these ISs are frequently centralized into a single database. Two options for this single database are the data repository and data warehouse.

Data Repository

A data repository is an open-structure database (not dedicated to the software of any particular vendor or data supplier) in which data from multiple ISs are stored so that an integrated, multidisciplinary (includes a variety of healthcare providers) view of the data can be achieved in a single source. The data repository is updated by the various ISs in real time, thus providing users with access to the most current information available. This real-time access to data is called online or real-time transaction processing.

The data repository may store clinical, administrative, and financial information data. Other data repositories store one specific type of data. For example, a data repository for a laboratory or pharmacy IS stores only clinical information. This centralized data repository is called a clinical data repository (CDR). For example, a query could identify all of the patients who took a specific medication and had to be admitted to the hospital as a result of an adverse effect. CDRs that use object-oriented databases may include video, audio, images, and other types of data. The primary key is used to link the data between the various data repositories.

Data Warehouse

A data warehouse is a database that makes it possible to access data from multiple databases and combine the results into a single query and reporting interface. Like the data repository, it stores data from many different systems, and it includes historical and current information. Data warehouses hold an abundance of data from many different source systems and are designed for specific types of analyses, such as patient care or business. The source systems will vary depending on how the data warehouse will be used. For example, a data warehouse may be designed to look for trends in patient care. This type of data warehouse will require information from all of the clinical ISs, the financial IS, the clinical provider order entry, and other ISs. These systems would be chosen for inclusion in the data warehouse because they provide data on the care provided to the patient, the costs of that care, the tests ordered, and the alerts identified. It does not include systems like the chart locator and chart deficiency systems used in the HIM department because these systems have no bearing on identifying trends in patient care.

Additional uses of a data warehouse in healthcare include identifying best practices in patient care, such as which medication is the most effective; identifying data that can provide the competitive advantage, such as which services or physicians generate the most revenue; and improving efficiency. A data warehouse can also be used in quality management to look for trends in problem areas, such as nosocomial infections; identifying patterns in coding practices, such as comparing hospital medical necessity denials to national rates; looking for particular diagnoses, procedures, services, or physicians that may have a compliance problem; and investigating other HIM-related issues.

The data warehouse is updated periodically rather than in real time like the EHR or the data repository. There should be a predetermined policy about the frequency of the updates and how long data should be retained.

Data Mart

A **data mart** is a subset of the data warehouse designed for a single purpose or specialized use. The data mart performs the same type of analysis as a data warehouse; however, the scope of the data is narrower. The healthcare facility may choose to develop the data warehouse before the data mart, or the data mart can be developed first, or both can be developed at the same time. This order of development depends on the needs of the organization. Examples of how a data mart may be used include patient satisfaction and medical research. Patient satisfaction would not require the patient-specific information that would be stored in the data warehouse, but it would include the types of services, the nursing unit, and other basic information in addition to the patient survey or other patient satisfaction information collected. The data mart can be used in research because it can be used to provide deidentified information and the limited information required to conduct the research and thus can protect the confidentiality of the patient by providing only the minimum information necessary.

Data Mining

Data mining is the process of extracting and analyzing large volumes of data from a database for the purpose of identifying hidden and sometimes subtle relationships that would be unnoticed without the analysis. Data mining may also be called database exploration or information discovery. Data mining is important because it turns data into meaningful information. Data mining requires sophisticated software, tools, and techniques, such as anomaly detection, association rule learning, cluster analysis, classification analysis, and regression analysis:

- Anomaly detection: In anomaly detection, the goal is to identify data that does not follow expectations. This can be used to identify fraud and or other issues that need investigation.

- Association rule learning: This type of data mining identifies interesting relationships between two concepts in the database. For example, it may identify that patients who are treated with drug A have a better outcome than patients who are treated with drug B.

- Cluster analysis: Cluster analysis is identifying concepts that have traits in common. For example, monitoring the treatment practices of physicians for a specific diagnosis or procedure.

- Classification analysis: Classification analysis is a method of identifying important information about the data in the database by grouping data much like grouping diagnoses and procedures. This grouped data can then be used in the cluster analysis described earlier.

- Regression analysis: This method identifies the dependency between variables such as patients, diagnoses, patient type, and more (van Rijmenam 2014).

Once the data pattern, dependency, or trait has been identified, the facility must decide how to use the information.

Online Analytical Processing

Online analytical processing (OLAP) is a data access architecture that allows the user to retrieve specific information from a large volume of data. The use of OLAP turns the data warehouse into a decision support tool because it can analyze large amounts of data quickly. It does this in one of three ways: drilling down into the data, consolidation, or "slicing and dicing." Drilling down is going deeper and deeper into the data. For example, drilling down could entail looking at the cancer rate from across the country, then at the cancer rate Georgia, then in Macon, and then within the zip code 31052. Consolidation refers to the aggregation of data, which is just the opposite of drilling down. "Slicing and dicing" is looking at the data from multiple viewpoints. For example, a healthcare facility could look at their reimbursement by payer type (Medicare, Medicaid) and then look at it by service (medical, surgical, obstetric) (Hall 2015, 477). OLAP enables the healthcare facility to use operational data that it already has in order to make strategic decisions.

Common Uses and Examples in Healthcare and Health Information Management

Healthcare facilities collect an abundance of data and retain these data for years. Unless the data are turned into information, they have no real value to the healthcare facility. HIM professionals work together with database administrators, other information technology staff, and the end users to ensure that the data stored within the data warehouse will meet the needs of the users. The HIM professional is often a liaison between the information technology staff and the end user. The HIM professional can be involved in data mining by defining the data to be collected and stored in the data warehouse. The HIM professional can build data quality into the databases contained in the data warehouse. This can be done by building a data dictionary, populating drop-down boxes, building edits, and by building other data quality measures into the system. Examples of how data mining can be used in healthcare, including HIM, include identifying

- Best practices in patient care
- Medication adverse effects
- Potential fraud and abuse violations
- Patterns of mortality and morbidity
- Patterns of denials

Having this type of information enables the healthcare facility to use new information to improve services, patient care, and other functions. As more data are entered, the healthcare facility can continue to run analyses to determine if other patterns appear.

CHECK YOUR UNDERSTANDING 3.2

1. In a database model the concept of patient is an example of a(n) _____.

   a. Entity
   b. Relationship
   c. Data flow diagram
   d. CASE software

2. What tool would one use to illustrate how data moves through the IS?

   a. Data dictionary
   b. Entity-relationship diagram
   c. Data flow diagram
   d. Data standard

3. An attribute is _____.

   a. An assumption about an entity
   b. A fact about an entity
   c. Defined by the data dictionary
   d. A type of data model

4. The database model that uses a table as the basis for the design is _____.

   a. Relational
   b. Network
   c. Hierarchical
   d. Object-oriented

5. What should be created in order to show how users will use the IS?

   a. Data flow diagram
   b. Use case
   c. Data model
   d. OLAP

Real-World Case

Janice has been given the responsibility of creating and managing the data dictionary for the laboratory IS that is being implemented. There are a number of existing ISs that have their own data dictionaries. The data from the laboratory IS will be part of a clinical data repository. She decided that she needs to start from scratch to make the data dictionary the best it can be. She is reviewing the data dictionaries from the other ISs used at the healthcare facility but she does not always use the same terminology and format that are used in the other ISs.

CHAPTER REVIEW

1. The role of the database management system is to _____.

   a. Control and manipulate the database
   b. Collect data
   c. Report data
   d. Delete data when the need for it is over

2. An advantage to a database is that it _____.

   a. Controls the data stored in it
   b. Reduces redundancy
   c. Stores data using flat files
   d. Establishes data sets

3. The date of birth is an example of a _____.

   a. File
   b. Record
   c. Data field
   d. Key field

4. Select the key field for the physician entity.

   a. Last name
   b. Address
   c. Unique identifier
   d. Date of birth

5. What is used to retrieve a list of all of Dr. Smith's patients?

   a. Data definition
   b. Data dictionary
   c. Metadata
   d. Query

6. Data about data is known as _____.

   a. Metadata
   b. Data definition
   c. Query
   d. Mask

7. The data model that addresses the data requirements is the _____.

   a. Logical data model
   b. Conceptual data model
   c. Relational database
   d. Physical data model

8. The hierarchical database relationships are called _____.

   a. Structured
   b. Parent and child
   c. Table
   d. Owners and members

9. Java is used in what type of database?

   a. Relational
   b. Object-oriented
   c. Multidimensional
   d. Hierarchical

10. Data repositories are _____.

   a. A proprietary database
   b. Used solely for clinical data
   c. A database used solely for video and audio
   d. An open-structure database

References

Abdelhak, M., and M. A. Hanken. 2016. *Health Information: Management of a Strategic Resource*. St. Louis, MO: Saunders Elsevier.

Amatayakul, M. K. 2017. *Health IT and EHRs: Principles and Practice*, 6th ed. Chicago: AHIMA.

Amatayakul, M. K. 2016. Health Information Systems Strategic Planning. Chapter 13 in *Health Information Management: Concepts, Principles, and Practice*, 5th ed. Edited by P. Oachs and A. Watters. Chicago: AHIMA.

American Health Information Management Association. 2017. Health Data Analysis Toolkit. http://bok.ahima.org/PdfView?oid=107504.

American Health Information Management Association. 2016. Managing a Data Dictionary (2016 update). http://library.ahima.org/doc?oid=302014.

Department of Health and Human Services (HHS). n.d. Practices Guide: Logical Data Modeling. Accessed February 5, 2018. https://www2.cdc.gov/cdcup/library/hhs_cplc/26%20-%20Logical%20Data%20Model/EPLC_Logical_Data_Model_Practices_Guide.pdf.

Hall, J. A. 2015. *Accounting Information Systems*. 9th ed. Boston, MA: Cengage Learning.

Harrington, J. 2016. *Relational Database Design and Implementation*. 4th ed. Cambridge, MA: Elsevier.

Health Information Management Systems Society. 2017. *HIMSS Dictionary of Health Information Technology Terms, Acronyms, and Organizations*, 4th ed. Boca Raton, FL: CRC Press.

Morley, D., and C. S. Parker. 2017. *Understanding Computers: Today and Tomorrow, Comprehensive*, 16th ed. Boston, MA: Cengage Learning.

Oppel, A. 2004. *Databases DeMYSTiFieD: A Self-Teaching Guide*. Emeryville, CA: McGraw-Hill Osborne.

Oracle. n.d. Performing Query-by-Example and Query Count. Accessed February 5, 2018. https://docs.oracle.com/cd/A60725_05/html/comnls/us/fnd/10gch314.htm.

van Rijmenam, M. 2014. "Five Data Mining Techniques That Help Create Business Value." *Datafloq* (blog). February 1, 2014. https://datafloq.com/read/data-mining-techniques-create-business-value/121.

Chapter 4

System Selection

Learning Objectives

- Identify the steps in the system selection process.
- Develop the request for proposal.
- Explain how the decision matrix will assist in the most appropriate selection for the healthcare entity.
- Collect data to be used in the systems analysis process.

Key Terms

Acceptance testing
Alpha site
Best of breed
Best of fit
Beta site
Bidders' conference
Change management
Chief information officer (CIO)
Cloud computing
Critical path
Escrow
External scanning
Feasibility study
Force majeure
Functional requirements
Gantt chart

Go-live
Information systems project
   steering committee
Information system strategic
   planning
Intangible benefits
Integrated information systems
Interface
Internal scanning
Payment milestones
Project
Project definition
PERT chart
Project management
Project manager
Project team

Request for information (RFI)
Request for proposal (RFP)
Scope creep
Site visits
SMART methodology
Software license
Source code
Status reports
Systems analysis
System development life cycle
   (SDLC)
System selection
Tangible benefits
Testing
User task force
Weighted decision matrix

System selection is determining which information system (IS) will be purchased. The system selection process begins with the idea that the healthcare facility should consider obtaining a particular IS, such as the master patient index. The process continues until the contract has been signed. The complexity of the system selection process varies widely, from selecting a standard off-the-shelf software product like a word processor to the very complex implementation of an electronic health record (EHR) system. The length of time required thus varies from a few minutes to a year or more. The number of people involved will also vary based on who is impacted by the IS and the complexity of the IS to be selected.

System selection is part of the system development life cycle (SDLC), a model used to represent the ongoing process of developing (or purchasing) ISs. The SDLC is a structured process that can be useful by identifying users' needs and alternatives, selecting the IS, system implementation, and other steps in managing IS. SDLC requires the involvement of people throughout the healthcare facility, including those who use the system. The use of people throughout the healthcare facility who are impacted by the healthcare facility ensures that the needs of all the users and the healthcare facility are met. There are a number of different models for the SDLC. The one used in this chapter (shown in figure 4.1) has four steps: planning and analysis, design, implementation, and support and evaluation (Wager et al. 2013). The focus of this chapter will be the first two stages: planning and analysis, and design.

Figure 4.1. System development life cycle (SDLC) diagram

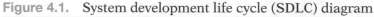

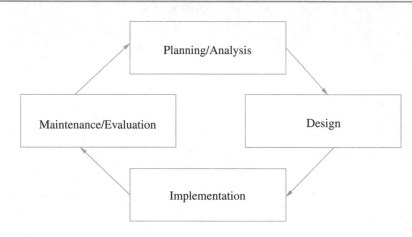

Planning and Analysis Phase

During the planning and analysis phase of the SDLC the project is defined, a formal structure for project management is created, and the needs of the healthcare facility are identified. The phase begins with initiation, which is when the decision is made to obtain the IS. This decision may come about because of an IS strategic plan, the obsolescence of an existing IS, or some other reason.

One thing to keep in mind during the planning process is that any IS selected should support the healthcare facility's business objectives. An example of a business objective might be to provide high-quality care. The specific IS to be implemented should be identified and prioritized during the IS planning process, as more ISs are usually identified than the healthcare facility's resources can handle. Information system strategic planning means identifying ISs needed to meet the healthcare facility's business objectives. IS strategic planning is defined as "the process of identifying and assigning priorities to the application of information technology that will assist an organization in executing its business plans and achieving its strategic goals and objectives" (Austin and Boxerman 2003, 259). For example, if a healthcare facility business objective is to meet a goal of improved quality of care, then the healthcare facility should look for an IS that would support this goal, such as the EHR or clinical provider order entry (CPOE). The EHR would improve the quality of care because of the immediate access to patient information, as well as the use of alerts and other features. The CPOE would improve care because the orders would be immediately available to the ancillary department, and the healthcare provider would be able to take advantage of reminders and alerts regarding contraindications, the need for laboratory tests to monitor blood levels, and so on. Part of the IS strategic planning process is performing a needs assessment. The needs assessment evaluates the need for the various ISs under consideration. The needs assessment should include a comparison of costs to benefits received.

Steps included in the planning and analysis phase are as follows:

1. Planning
2. Organizing the project
3. Defining scope of project
4. Systems analysis

Planning

Planning is the most critical step in the system selection process. A major IS selection requires a lot of collaborative work by many people across a healthcare facility. A lack of planning can cause problems with the system, which can ultimately cause the system to fail or delay the implementation date, thus costing the healthcare facility money and wasting resources. An example of poor planning is ordering hardware without evaluating the space. Insufficient space can prohibit hardware installation when there is not enough electrical wiring, inadequate space, or some other problem with the physical plant. The most common reasons for failure are:

- Poor planning and direction
- Insufficient communication
- Ineffective management
- Failure to meet the needs of stakeholders
- Lack of involvement from executive leadership
- Lack of skills by staff
- Weak methodology and tools (Gulla 2012)

Another reason for failure is the lack of end-user involvement. Employees who are involved in the system selection and implementation are more likely to embrace the IS than those who are not.

If a healthcare facility spends more time and energy from the beginning of the IS selection project, it will be better positioned to succeed. Adequate planning is demonstrated, in part, when the healthcare facility has the necessary staff, money, and other resources, as well as an understanding of what is needed and identification of desired outcomes from the outset of the project. Planning for an IS is a complex process and involves the following:

- Conducting a feasibility study
- Setting the budget
- Setting the goals and objectives
- Identifying the project manager and team
- Obtaining buy-in from management and users

Conducting a Feasibility Study

A feasibility study is conducted by the healthcare facility to determine if a proposed IS is an appropriate option to meet the objectives of the healthcare facility. For example, the healthcare facility could investigate the feasibility of implementing an EHR to support an objective to improve the quality of care. The study examines the costs, the benefits, and any expected problems and then determines whether or not to proceed with the proposed IS. The benefits should be both tangible and intangible. Tangible benefits are easy to quantify in dollars and include eliminating duplicate tests, no longer having to purchase health record file folders, and not microfilming paper records. Intangible benefits cannot be quantified monetarily. An example of an intangible benefit would be improved quality of care. If the benefits do outweigh the costs, then the project should be considered.

Setting the Budget

Developing the budget for a system selection project is important as cost is a key determining factor in deciding whether or not to implement an IS. The budget should be comprehensive and as accurate as possible because it is used in the decision-making process. The budget should include system selection and implementation expenses as well as the cost of maintaining the IS for a specified period of time, such as two to five years. Additionally, the budget should include items such as cost of software, upgrading infrastructure, hardware, training, renovations to the physical plant, maintenance of the IS, project management, consultant expenses, and travel expenses for site visits.

Goals and Objectives

Goals and objectives for the IS must be established as part of the planning process. The goals and objectives identify what the healthcare facility wants to accomplish with the implementation of the proposed system and how these goals will be achieved. These IS goals should be based on the healthcare facility's business goals. As with any goals, they should be realistic and attainable.

One strategy for writing goals is the **SMART methodology**, which stands for

- **S**pecific,
- **M**easurable,
- **A**ttainable,
- **R**elevant, and
- **T**ime-based

A specific goal tells you the what, who, where, when, which, and why. A measurable goal provides something that you can use to compare the actual outcome to the goal to determine if it has been met. An attainable goal is one that you have the skills and resources to accomplish. A relevant goal is one that, while challenging, can be accomplished given the time and other factors. A timely goal is one that provides a deadline to meet (Swenson 2016, 677).

Examples of SMART goals include the following:

- To provide new employee orientation to 100 percent of new hospital employees within 1 month of their hire date
- To reduce the number of hospital staff by five by the end of next March
- To reduce the amount of discharge not final billed (DNFB) report to $500,000 within six months
- To reduce the number of duplicate tests by 25 percent by the end of the fiscal year

Goals will be determined by the type of IS and the needs of the healthcare facility. Once established, goals should be used to identify which information best meets the desired outcomes.

Once the IS is implemented, it should be evaluated regularly thereafter as to whether it met and will continue to meet or exceed the stated goals and objectives. For example, the support and evaluation will identify whether the duplicate tests were reduced by 25 percent or whether staffing was reduced by five.

Identifying the Project Manager and Project Team

The project manager and project teams are an important part of project management. **Project management** is a formal set of principles and procedures that help control the activities associated with implementing a usually large undertaking to achieve a specific goal, such as an IS project. Project leadership including the project manager and the **project team** members should be identified before the project begins. A **project team** is a collection of individuals representing various disciplines, such as billing, clinician, administration, or information technology assigned to work on a project. Their role is important because they are responsible for ensuring that the system implementation plan is carried out according to the project manager's specifications. The project team members' skills will vary according to the needs of the project. For example, implementation of an EHR will require information technology staff, health information management (HIM), physicians, nursing staff, and other clinical users of the IS. A project team is composed of people who are assigned to work on the project either part time or full time. The project team will be discussed in detail later in this chapter.

The **project manager** is in charge of leading the project and therefore must have an understanding of the IS being implemented. The project manager must have strong skills in a multitude of areas, such as project management, leadership, organizational skills, and conflict management. The project manager is responsible for ensuring that the project plan stays within the designated timeline, issues are resolved, desired outcomes are met, and customer satisfaction is achieved.

Obtaining Buy-in from Management and Users

It is critical that the healthcare facility's upper management support the project from the very beginning of the process. If management shows support for the IS, the employees will follow suit and support it. However, if management displays discontent or lack of support, the employees will most likely resist the change. Support can be shown by attending meetings; talking about the IS's benefits to the healthcare facility, its employees, and customers; and generally demonstrating that the IS is valued. Communication is critical at this stage. Staff and everyone to be affected by the IS should receive ongoing updates on the decisions, changes, and expectations. The more staff members are informed about the EHR or other projects, the less likely they will be to resist because they will know what to expect. If staff who will use the system are asked for their feedback they will feel valued and will be more likely to support the IS.

Change management is the formal process of introducing change, getting it adopted, and diffusing it throughout the healthcare facility. Although some people welcome change, most have a natural aversion to it. A great deal of change management involves reducing these fears and preparing them for what is to come. For example, if people are afraid they will lose their jobs with the implementation of new technology, these issues must be addressed. Administration must be open and honest about layoffs, changes in job roles, and other related changes.

Administration should be seen as a strong supporter of the IS. If administration does not publicly support the IS, then the employees may follow the administrator's lead and not see its value. It is important to the success of the IS that both administration and employees buy into the IS.

Employees should be kept current on the implementation process: they want to know what the IS will do for them, when training will occur, and the overall progress of the implementation, including any issues. This can be done in a number of ways, such as employee newsletters, announcements at meetings, and so forth. Employees should be involved in the process whenever possible. Several ways of doing this are discussed later in the chapter. Employees should have realistic expectations about what the IS can and cannot do so that they will not be disappointed when the IS is implemented. Thus, user preparation will make them more comfortable with the system when it is implemented.

All processes related to the IS must be reviewed and modified to accommodate the new IS. This means changes to policies and procedures, possibly changes in organizational structure, and any other changes needed to support the new IS.

Organization of the Project

Once the decision is made to implement an IS, the project's formal organizational structure must be put in place. A **project** is a plan and course of action that will address a specific objective, made up of a series of activities and tasks with defined start and stop dates. The plan has targeted objectives and deliverables to be accomplished. The project will need specific resources assigned to it in order to be completed; a project frequently has a separate budget that sets limits on spending. Another resource assigned to a project is staff. As discussed previously, a project team is assigned to the project. Temporary employees may be hired to either assist in the implementation or assume the tasks of staff members who have been reassigned to the project. An example of a project is the implementation of the EHR. Members of the EHR project would involve many different types of professionals including physicians, nurses, other healthcare providers, HIM professionals, computer programmers, network technicians, and many more.

The level of organization for the project depends on the level of complexity of the IS being implemented. If it is a small department IS, it may only require two or three people to implement. Major ISs that impact the entire healthcare facility can take hundreds of people to select and implement the system. In large projects, frequently subcommittees are responsible for small areas of the project. The subcommittees meet and work on their segments of the project. The chair of the subcommittee then reports back to the full project committee. Table 4.1 shows examples of what is and what is not a project.

Project Team

Most, if not all, IS projects require a project team of individuals to successfully implement the IS. The number of individuals needed and the composition of this team vary from project to project, depending on the needs of the implementation. For example, if the healthcare facility is implementing a chart deficiency system for use only in the HIM department, the project team should include the appropriate people in HIM and the IS. The project team would not need to include physicians, nurses, risk managers, or laboratory staff.

Table 4.1.   Examples of what is and what is not a project

Not a Project	Project
Monthly reports	Implementation of IS
Routine software update	Creating a security plan
Backing up data	Creating a business continuity plan

If the healthcare facility is implementing a CPOE, the project team would need representatives from the physician staff as well as from the HIM, nursing, laboratory, pharmacy, and other departments who are impacted to ensure that the IS is properly planned and developed. The project team works with the project manager to implement and manage the project. This project team will meet periodically, based on project needs, to discuss progress of the project and any issues that arise.

An HIM professional should frequently sit on the project committee because the IS may impact the HIM department indirectly, and having an HIM professional involved in the process will help ensure that the department's needs are addressed. Additionally, the HIM professional serves as a consultant and source of information for compliance, privacy, security, legal, and other concerns. For example, the HIM professional can assist with retention, privacy, security, data quality, and documentation issues, among many other considerations of the IS, which may ultimately affect the HIM department.

The major participants in the project management team are the IS project steering committee, project team, the user task force, the vendor, the project manager, and possibly one or more consultants.

The information systems project steering committee is responsible for every IS acquisition project in the healthcare facility. Each project team will report back to the steering committee. The steering committee's role is to ensure that the strategic IS is being efficiently and effectively implemented and that the project stays on target. This committee is frequently led by the chief information officer (CIO). The CIO is generally at the executive level and is responsible for all information resource management functions at the healthcare facility. The IS department, HIM, and other information management–related departments frequently report to the CIO. The CIO must have strong management skills. Although the CIO is not always a technical role, the individual must understand enough about information technology to ensure the proper management of the systems. Other team members may be administrators, managers, project managers, and other leaders in the healthcare facility.

The user task force is a group of users, who will ultimately be using the IS, who test the IS and perform other project-related tasks for which the committee receives feedback. These users are generally on loan from various departments to assist in the project. Some members of the user task force may be deployed as needed for testing (performing an examination or evaluation) and other tasks, whereas others are pulled out of their departments for the duration of the project. This reassignment may last a year or more, depending on the project.

The vendor representative is the expert on the IS and so will be an extremely valuable team member. This individual will be the liaison between the healthcare facility and the leadership at the vendor's company. The vendor representative knows the product and can be a valuable resource with regard to how best to implement and use the IS. Additionally, the vendor representative can give the project team information on what has (and has not) worked for other healthcare facilities. This information can help the healthcare facility recognize and use best practices and help it avoid costly mistakes. If not scheduled to be on-site during a meeting, the vendor representative may need to attend via telephone conference in order to provide expertise.

If the healthcare facility decides to hire a consultant, the consultant will be a valuable member of the project team as well. The consultant should not have ties to a particular vendor's product, but rather be objective to help the healthcare facility obtain the product that best meets its needs. The consultant should have experience in system selection and implementation.

The project manager is responsible for coordinating the individual project, monitoring the budget, managing the resources, conducting negotiations, and keeping the project on schedule. These roles require the project manager to have technical, analytical, and people skills. The project manager should be skilled in conflict resolution, communication, and project management. Leadership skills are also important because the project manager must be able to develop a consensus and manage meetings for the project team. The project manager would have to handle any problems that arise during the implementation.

Defining Scope of Project

The healthcare facility must define what the accomplished project is. The project definition is determined during the project planning process to tell the healthcare facility exactly what it is trying to do with the IS being implemented and the expected outcomes. The healthcare facility must identify:

- The purpose of the IS
- How the system links to the healthcare facility's business strategy
- The goals for and scope of the project

The scope of the project determines exactly what work is—and is not—to be included in the project based on resources available. Identifying the project's definition is important to prevent scope creep. Scope creep happens when items not included in the original scope are added after the project has begun. For example, a project starts out to implement an EHR in a medical clinic and then the decision is made to add the EHR to the outpatient surgery area. The needs of these two areas are different, so more time and resources would be required. These additions to the project will increase the time needed for the project and the money and resources required to accomplish it. To help keep the project on target, a project plan should be created.

Project Plan

Once the healthcare facility knows what it plans to do, the project team can begin dividing the project into specific activities or tasks. The project team may start out with a basic skeleton of a project plan and continue to add substance to it as they go along. This project plan should describe each task to be completed, how it will be completed, who is responsible for its completion, when a task should begin, and when the task should be finished. The basic components of the plan are as follows:

- Feasibility study: This study defines the objectives and need for the project and justifies the plan.
- Resources: This component identifies the resources needed to meet the objectives of the plan. Resources include money, time, staff, and space.
- Design: In the design stage, the project team identifies the specific details required to implement the plan. For every task identified, the plan must provide the start and end dates and a person responsible. If the project requires programming, the team must establish the standards that will be used in writing the program.
- Hardware and software procurement: This stage ensures that the healthcare facility has all of the hardware and software needed and that any missing components arrive in a timely manner. For example, hardware delivery may take six weeks, so ordering needs to be done early in the process.
- Transition: The transition phase prepares the healthcare facility for the conversion from the old system to the new. This stage includes not only the actual conversion of data but also preparing staff for the change.
- Implementation: The implementation stage includes the steps to be taken to prepare for the implementation and the actual conversion to the new IS.
- Support and evaluation: The support and evaluation stage begins immediately after implementation is complete. The project team must evaluate itself to prepare for the next project. It should also include an evaluation process to determine if the objectives of the project were met and how the process could have been improved.

Project Management Tools

A number of tools can be used to control the project. These tools include Gantt charts, project evaluation and review technique (PERT) charts, project plans, trouble tickets, and status reports.

The project plan provides details for how to accomplish a project and guides the project team on activities, timing, costs, and the sequencing of activities. The project plan could include project tools such as the Gantt chart and the PERT chart.

The Gantt chart is a project management tool that records specific tasks, their start and end dates, the person responsible for the tasks, and any connections between tasks. The Gantt chart (see figure 4.2) can easily show which tasks are behind schedule, which are on target, and which are ahead of schedule. A PERT chart (see figure 4.3) is a management tool that evaluates the tasks, the dependencies on other activities, the activity sequence, and the time required to complete the task. Because the PERT chart shows interdependencies between tasks, it will help determine whether the implementation date is slipping because of delinquent tasks. This slippage is shown by review of the critical path, which shows the longest amount of time to complete the project. If key tasks along the critical path are delayed, the critical path itself lengthens, thus lengthening the duration of the project.

Status reports are periodic updates on the current state of the project, what has been accomplished, and what issues have been encountered. Solutions for the issues should be identified in the report. Status reports are typically directed to the information project steering committee to keep that group informed on

Figure 4.2.   Sample Gantt chart

		Task Name	Duration	Start	Finish
1		Identify project manager	1 day	Fri 8/8/08	Fri 8/8/08
2		Identify project team	1 wk	Mon 8/11/08	Fri 8/15/08
3		Conduct systems analysis	6 mons	Mon 8/18/08	Fri 1/30/09
4		Write RFP	6 wks	Mon 2/2/09	Fri 3/13/09
5		Distribute RFPs to vendors	2 days	Mon 3/16/09	Tue 3/17/09
6		Meet with vendors	1 day	Mon 4/6/09	Mon 4/6/09
7		Receive RFP submissions	1 mon	Tue 4/7/09	Mon 5/4/09
8		Review RFPs	1 mon	Tue 5/5/09	Mon 6/1/09
9		Site visits	1 mon	Tue 6/2/09	Mon 6/29/09
10		Check references	1 wk	Tue 6/30/09	Mon 7/6/09
11		Make decision on system	1 wk	Tue 7/7/09	Mon 7/13/09
12		Sign contract	1 wk	Tue 7/14/09	Mon 7/20/09
13		Order hardware for users and data center	1 wk	Tue 7/21/09	Mon 7/27/09
14		Site preparation (add outlet, shift existing computers)	3 days	Tue 7/21/09	Thu 7/23/09
15		Install hardware in computer room and units	18 days	Mon 9/7/09	Thu 9/24/09
16		Update network to accommodate increased traffic	18 days	Mon 9/7/09	Thu 9/24/09
17		Install software on file server	1 day	Fri 9/25/09	Fri 9/25/09
18		Configure settings in system	1 mon	Mon 9/28/09	Fri 10/23/09
19		Write routine reports	3 mons	Mon 9/28/09	Fri 12/18/09
20		Develop new screens	3 mons	Mon 9/28/09	Fri 12/18/09
21		Develop training plan	2 mons	Mon 9/7/09	Fri 10/30/09
22		Identify data conversion needs	5 days	Mon 9/29/08	Fri 10/3/08
23		Write interfaces	2 mons	Mon 9/28/09	Fri 11/20/09
24		Write program required for data conversion	1 mon	Mon 10/6/08	Fri 10/31/08
25		Write user manual, training materials and policies and procedures	6 mons	Mon 10/26/09	Fri 4/9/10
26		Test software	2 mons	Tue 12/1/09	Mon 1/25/10
27		Correct errors identified in testing	1 mon	Tue 1/26/10	Mon 2/22/10
28		Train the trainers	2 wks	Mon 4/12/10	Fri 4/23/10
29		Conduct training	2 mons	Mon 4/26/10	Fri 6/18/10
30		Go-live	3 days	Mon 6/21/10	Wed 6/23/10
31		Acceptance testing	2 mons	Thu 6/24/10	Wed 8/18/10
32		Evaluation of implementation	2 wks	Thu 8/19/10	Wed 9/1/10

Project: chapter 5 gantt
Date: Fri 1/29/10

Task		Project Summary
Split		External Tasks
Progress		External Milestone
Milestone		Deadline
Summary		

Page 1

the project's progress. The status report is generally written by the project manager, but could be written by a designee.

Additionally, software applications can be used to help manage a project. Project management software can create the Gantt and PERT charts as well as other types of tools for the project team to review. It can also track how much of each task is complete (0 to 100 percent), who has been given the responsibility for each task, the beginning and ending dates, the sequencing of tasks, and more.

Figure 4.3.   Sample PERT chart

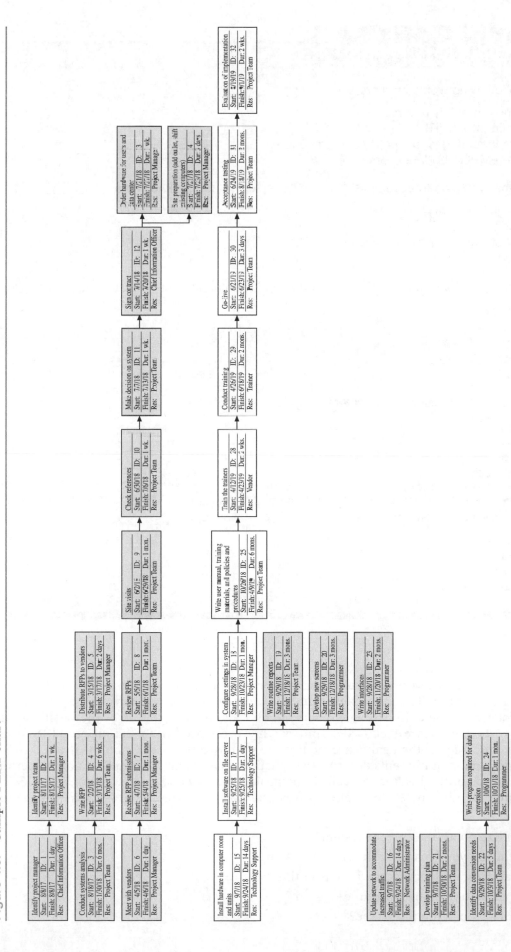

CHECK YOUR UNDERSTANDING 4.1

1. Which of the following would be a project?

   a. Completing a monthly report
   b. Implementing the EHR
   c. Making minor changes to a policy and procedure
   d. Utilizing the MPI to update information

2. Specifying what you plan to accomplish with an IS implementation is known as _____.

   a. Project definition
   b. Project plan
   c. Feasibility study
   d. Status report

3. The PERT chart shows if there is slippage in the implementation date. This slippage is shown by _____.

   a. Dependencies
   b. Gantt chart
   c. Project plan
   d. Critical path

4. Identifying the specific details in implementing an IS is found in the _____.

   a. Transition plan
   b. Design plan
   c. Project plan
   d. Feasibility study

5. The original plan was to create an EHR that will be used for the emergency department, but now the EHR must be used for all outpatient services. This is an example of _____.

   a. Scope creep.
   b. Project plan
   c. Project definition
   d. Project tool

Systems Analysis

Systems analysis is an important process of collecting, organizing, and evaluating data on the healthcare facility and the information that it needs. Systems analysis should be performed early in the project as it helps the project team determine the data, storage, reporting, and functionality needs of the healthcare facility. In systems analysis, the healthcare facility determines what users need from the proposed IS. This stage reviews the current processes of the healthcare facility, the proposed processes, and the desired functional requirements. Functional requirements describe the functionality that an IS should be able to perform.

To identify the needs of the healthcare facility, the project team would look at the existing ISs and the needs of the users and identify and evaluate alternatives. During systems analysis, users are asked questions such as:

- What do you like about the current system?
- What problems do you have with the current system?
- What changes do you foresee that will impact this system?
- What information do you need from the system?
- What functions would you like to see?

Answering these questions helps the project team understand the current IS and how it meets or does not meet the needs of the users. An IS will be used by the healthcare facility for many years and therefore must be adequate both at the time of go-live and in the foreseeable future. Go-live is the official time and date that the healthcare facility begins using the new IS.

To identify the needs of the healthcare facility for the foreseeable future, the project team needs to understand the environment in which the system will operate. No one can see into the future with certainty, but internal and external environmental scanning can identify some issues that must be addressed. Internal scanning entails identifying changes within the healthcare facility that will impact the IS, such as if new services or new clinics will be implemented. External scanning is identifying changes outside of the healthcare facility that will impact the healthcare facility. The healthcare facility may be aware of pending legislation, trends, or other issues that may impact the IS under consideration. Understanding the environment helps ensure that the IS will work today and for the expected future.

Questionnaires, interviews, observations, flowcharts, and other data collection tools may be used to obtain the data needed to answer these questions. The planning team should collect data from all levels and types of users. The needs of the clerical staff will be very different from the needs of management staff. Many managers believe they know the needs of their staff, but many of them know what the policy states, not what is actually happening. The information gathered should include all aspects of the system such as data elements, reports, privacy, security, and overall functionality.

Questionnaires allow for a large number of users to provide input about the needs of the IS as the results are easy to collect and analyze. This is especially true if closed-ended questions are used so that the responses can be tabulated quickly and easily. Closed-ended questions can be answered with yes or no, Likert scales, and other limited choice responses. Likert-scales are great for obtaining the users' beliefs regarding a statement. An example of a Likert scale begins with a statement such as: "On a scale of 1 to 5, with 1 being 'strongly agree' and 5 being 'strongly disagree,' rate the following statement." An example of a belief could be, "The new EHR will improve the efficiency of the healthcare facility." An example of a typical closed-ended question could be, "Do you generate reports as a part of your job?" Obviously, the response to this question is limited to yes or no. Computerized tools make the aggregation and analysis of the responses quicker. The downside of questionnaires is that the correct questions may not be asked, so there may be gaps in the data collected and the information needed. The use of open-ended questions may help fill some of these gaps, but they slow down the aggregation of data and data analysis. Open-ended questions are designed to get more information from the participants as they can expand on their response; however, the project team must collect, read, and analyze each statement individually. An example of an open-ended question is "How does the current information system help you in your job?"

Interviews are powerful tools for obtaining information. There are three types of interviews: structured, unstructured, and semistructured. In the structured interview, everyone is asked the same questions. This improves analysis of the findings but does not encourage the interviewee to talk openly about pertinent issues, thus taking the risk that important data will be overlooked. In the unstructured interview, the interviewer does not have a list of questions but rather gets the interviewees talking about their jobs, their data needs, and other issues related to the IS. The semistructured interview is a combination of the structured and unstructured formats. There are questions that interviewees are asked, but they are also encouraged to discuss in detail their jobs, data needs, and other issues related to their IS needs. The unstructured and semistructured formats make it harder to identify trends and to analyze data, but major issues that could have been overlooked otherwise may be identified.

Typically, two members of the project team are needed to conduct interviews because one person interacts with the interviewee and the other person takes notes. Because of the increased staffing needs, the amount of time required to collect and analyze the data, and the need to meet with users individually, interviews are very time-consuming, which makes them costly. This means that the planning team may interview fewer individuals than would be involved with questionnaires.

Observation is watching an action being performed. It is useful in determining what employees are actually doing. This is important because supervisors or others frequently tell the interviewers what they think is happening but in reality something very different is occurring. The use of observation is a way to validate what the interviewee has been told. If using observations, each observation session should be short because the observer can be disruptive to the work environment. Also, observation sessions should be scheduled throughout the day because different tasks may be performed at different times.

Flowcharts may be used to illustrate the flow of information within the healthcare facility (see figure 4.4). The flowchart uses standardized symbols to demonstrate the steps performed. Problems and inconsistencies

Figure 4.4.   Sample flowchart

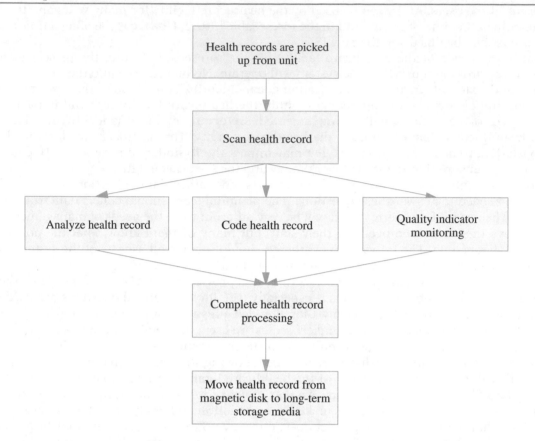

may be identified through the development and analysis of the flowchart. The process on the flowchart would depend on the type of IS being developed but could represent the flow of the health record in the HIM department, the flow of a physician query, or the steps in denial management. The flowchart would identify critical points in the process as well as problem areas. This information can be used to improve new processes implemented along with the new IS.

Many healthcare facilities use a combination of questionnaires, interviews, observations, and other data collection tools to obtain the best information. The use of multiple tools also allows the project team to involve more users and at the same time obtain detailed, validated information. The large number of participants helps to foster buy-in from the users. Buy-in refers to the acceptance of the system and recognizing its value to the user and to the healthcare facility. Users who buy in to the system are more supportive and less likely to resist the changes that the system brings to their jobs.

It is a mistake to ignore or give only minimal attention to systems analysis during the system implementation process. Systems analysis is critical because it forces the healthcare facility to evaluate itself and to look at how it does business. This understanding will help select the IS that will best meet the needs of the healthcare facility.

Design Phase

After the project itself has been decided on and the formal structure has been created, a number of decisions have to be made. The design should reflect IS objectives, output specifications, input specifications, database design, and expected costs. The requirements identified in systems analysis are used to create specifications for the IS. The specifications will be used for programming the IS if developed in-house or for evaluating vendor systems. The design should specify what data are collected, from where the data will originate, and in what format the data should be stored as well as the size of the database and amount of activity expected. Once the specifications are developed, they should be presented to administration for approval. The design phase includes determining who will build and maintain the system, choosing between integrated and interfaced ISs, and making the decision on which IS will be selected.

Determining Who Will Build and Maintain the System

One of the critical decisions to be made during the planning process is whether a healthcare facility should build the system itself, purchase it from a vendor, or use vendor services such as cloud computing. Cloud computing is when the system operates on a computer that is owned and maintained by a vendor. This IS is at the vendor's location, not the healthcare facility's, so the IS and its data must be accessed remotely. To do this, a user logs into and accesses the IS exactly as if the data center were located in-house. The data center is the area where the computers and other hardware that run the various IS operations are kept. Advantages to cloud computing are as follows:

- Collaboration—Physicians and others can share information such as the health record at the same time from two different locations.
- Speed—This advantage is evident in two ways: the speed at which the IS is updated and speed at which information is accessed.
- Mobility—With cloud computing, information is available from anywhere, making health information very mobile.
- Privacy and security—Laws and regulations must be met by the cloud providers just like healthcare providers.
- Decreased costs—Healthcare providers do not have to purchase hardware and pay for maintenance of the system (Blaisdell 2013).

The cloud computing method is favored by healthcare facilities that do not have staff with the necessary skills to develop and maintain an IS. A disadvantage of cloud computing is that the user may not have as much control over the IS. For example, the scheduling of maintenance and upgrades is up to the host. Another disadvantage is that the healthcare facility is renting the IS. It is not investing in its own structure and therefore would have to make a large investment should it ever decide to bring the system in-house.

The second option would be for the healthcare facility to build the IS. If a healthcare facility decides to build an IS, it would be designed to meet the specific needs of that healthcare facility. Creating a prototype is a way to quickly design and develop an IS. With prototyping, programmers quickly develop an IS, show it to the users, obtain feedback, make revisions to the program, and continue this cycle until the IS is developed. Although this is an option for system design, most IS designs are much more formal and detailed. The IS would have the look and feel that is desired as well as the desired functionality. There are, however, disadvantages:

- It could take longer to develop.
- The planning must be more detailed than if purchasing an IS.
- If the healthcare facility loses the staff that developed the system, it may be difficult to upgrade the system to meet the needs of the healthcare facility over time or to troubleshoot any issues that arise.
- There could be high development costs.

The final option, which most healthcare facilities choose, would be to purchase a predeveloped software system from a vendor. The vendor has invested millions of dollars in research and development and has a support system to assist the healthcare facility in the implementation of the IS being purchased. As with other options, there are advantages and disadvantages. A system purchased from a vendor may not be exactly what the healthcare facility wants, but it would be faster to implement, and the healthcare facility would benefit from extensive research and development conducted by the vendor.

When working with a vendor, the healthcare facility may have the opportunity to be an alpha site. An alpha site is the first healthcare facility to implement the information. The healthcare facility generally receives a discount in exchange for participation in the development of the IS. Because the IS is still being developed, the healthcare facility may face problems with the implementation that would not be encountered with a more mature version of the same IS. It also takes more time than a typical implementation. The healthcare facility may also be asked to be a beta site. Beta sites are the next healthcare facilities who subsequently implement the IS. Many of the problems have been resolved with the alpha site, but these beta sites are likely to encounter numerous problems as well.

Choosing Between Integrated and Interfaced Information Systems

If the decision is made to purchase an IS from a vendor, the next decision is whether the product should be integrated or interfaced.

Integrated Information Systems

Integrated information systems separate applications that are designed to work together. Data are entered into one IS and then are accessible to the other ISs. Many healthcare IS vendors use this model to interface systems used by healthcare facilities. This type of IS is much easier to manage than an interfaced IS because of the lack of interfaces. Integrated ISs collect, store, and retrieve information from the same database. The ISs have a similar screen design, which makes moving from one IS to another easier for the user. The decision to purchase software from a single vendor is frequently called best of fit.

Interfaced Information Systems

In an interfaced IS, the products are not designed to work together, but rather are linked through an interface. An interface takes data from one system and plugs that data into another IS. In other words, an interface acts as a bridge between two ISs or databases to translate data into each IS's respective language. An interface has to know what data to retrieve, where the data are located in the first database, whether any data manipulation has to be performed (and, if so, what that manipulation is), and where the data will be entered into the second database. If the interface is not working, the ISs will not be able to share information until the problems with the interface are resolved. Another way of interfacing is to transfer a flat file from one system to another to share information.

Although an interfaced IS takes more effort to manage, many healthcare facilities choose this method because users can choose the various products that they want instead of choosing a single vendor's product that, for example, may have a wonderful encoder but an inadequate laboratory IS. Choosing the ISs based on functionality rather than by vendor is called choosing the best of breed.

System Selection

The healthcare facility must identify what they demand from an IS, such as specific functions and compatibility with existing ISs. This information is used to determine which IS best meets the needs of the healthcare facility. There are a number of steps in the system selection process:

1. Request for information and proposal
2. Evaluation of the proposed IS
3. Selection of an IS
4. Contract negotiation

Some of the steps in the SDLC are linear, but others can be performed concurrently. For example, the request for proposal can be begun during the earlier systems analysis process, but it would not be finalized until after the process has been completed. It is imperative to remember that throughout the project, the plan itself is a working document and will continuously change and evolve.

Request for Information and Proposal

The request for information (RFI) is a formal document requesting information on IS. The RFI asks the IS vendor for basic information about the product and how the IS would meet the requirements outlined in the RFI. The RFI can be used to select minor IS, or the information gathered in the RFI can be used to determine who will receive the more rigorous request for proposal (RFP), a type of business correspondence asking for very specific product and contract information that is often sent to a narrow list of vendors that have been preselected after a review of requests for information during the design phase of the SDLC.

The RFP is a much more detailed document than the RFI and is critical to the selection process. The purpose of the RFP is to give the vendor all the information needed to propose an IS that meets the needs of the healthcare facility. The RFP describes what IS is needed, the healthcare facility, and the desired functions. Common components of the RFP are:

- Letter of introduction
- Information for potential vendors
  - Information about bidders' conference
  - Description of healthcare facility
  - Patient (or other) volume statistics—historical and future or projected growth

- Description of the system
  - Technical requirements
  - Functional requirements
  - Interface requirements
- Required format of response
- Instructions for RFP
- Request for sample documentation
- Request for sample contract
- Request for vendor profile
- System testing requirements
- Request for sample resumes of implementation staff
- System selection criteria
- Training requirements
- References

Appendix A shows a detailed template for an RFP.

Letter of Introduction

The letter of introduction is a cover letter that is sent to the vendor along with the RFP. The letter introduces the vendor to the RFP and identifies who the vendor should contact at the healthcare facility. It may also provide some information that did not make it into the RFP. The letter also specifies the date, time, location, and other information of the bidders' conference.

The **bidders' conference** is a meeting for vendors to come to the healthcare facility to ask questions about the RFP, the healthcare facility, and other important points. This meeting enables all of the potential vendors to hear the same information and to get all of their questions answered so that they can completely respond to the RFP.

Information for Potential Vendors

The description of the healthcare facility section provides the vendor with enough information about the healthcare facility to enable the vendor to properly respond to the RFP. This information includes the size of healthcare facility, number of employees, number of employees who would use the system, and number of locations that would use the IS. This section also should describe the healthcare facility's existing ISs so that the vendor can respond concerning how it can work with the existing system.

It should also include patient (or other) volume statistics that would be related to the IS (see table 4.2). The statistics may include number of discharges, number of surgeries, number of emergency department visits, and the number of outpatient visits—whatever is needed for the proposed IS.

Table 4.2. Sample of requested volume

Healthcare Facility Volume Statistics	Number
Average number of discharges per day	45
Average number of emergency department visits per day	60
Average number of outpatient surgeries per day	25
Average number of outpatient visits per day	125
Average number of pages—inpatient discharge	100
Number of synchronous users	75
Number of locations software is to be used	12

Description of the Proposed System

In the proposed system section, the vendor describes the IS that it is proposing to meet the needs of the healthcare facility. The vendor should describe the infrastructure required, licensing, the capabilities of the IS, the benefits that would be realized, and all pertinent information.

As stated earlier, the functional requirements identify the desired functions of the IS, which makes this a significant part of the proposal. This document is developed during the systems analysis process and outlines all of the functions expected of the system. The functions should include all aspects of the information, including but not limited to, individual data elements, data entry methods, reporting, management of the system, functionality, and technical issues. Technical issues can include topics such as the type of database used and the ability to work with a certain operating system or interface with existing products.

Each functional requirement is listed. The vendor indicates whether the function is available, is available with customization, will be available in the future, or is not available. The healthcare facility will take this same list of functional requirements and use it to evaluate the proposal. There are at least two ways to classify each functional requirement. The first way is to designate each functional requirement as mandatory or desirable. Some proposals use three categories: mandatory, desirable, and luxury. Another option is to develop a numeric rating system in which each function is scored based on its importance. For example, each function is rated on a scale of 1 to 5 (1 = unimportant, 5 = highly important). The functional requirements qualifying the availability of each function are part of the RFP, but the evaluation rating is not. The functional requirements are used in the system evaluation to determine if a vendor has all of the functionality and to determine if the missing functionality is important. For example, if there is a functional requirement to combine duplicate health record numbers, and it is missing from one of the products under review, the rating would help the reviewer determine whether this is a serious gap.

Other RFP Requirements

The required format of response tells the vendor what the healthcare facility requires regarding the proposal. For instance, the healthcare facility might require a specified number of paper copies and an electronic copy in a specified format; it may limit the number of pages or the design of the document; it may even provide an electronic template for the vendor to complete. The instructions for proposal may include rules regarding whom the vendor can talk to at the healthcare facility, the deadline for submission, and a statement that the vendor must assume responsibilities for the expenses to complete the proposal as well as the expenses for any on-site demonstrations, along with expenses for proposal preparation.

The request for sample documentation and for a sample contract is simply a request for a copy of the documents. The vendor profile is a description of the vendor and is designed to ensure that the company is financially sound. This is important because the vendor needs to be around for many years to provide technical support and any updates needed. The RFP asks for information on the number of installations of similar ISs the vendor has performed, financial viability of vendor, and the number of years the product has been available.

IS testing requirements would outline the expectations the healthcare facility has regarding testing. The proposal would provide the types of testing to be performed and the role of the vendor in that testing.

Many healthcare facilities request sample résumés from the vendor's staff, which provide details of the experience and qualifications of the staff who could be assigned as consultants to that particular project. These sample résumés are used to ensure the vendor has experienced staff members who can support the healthcare facility throughout an implementation. It is not a guarantee that any of the individuals represented would be assigned to the project, but rather a representation of the experience that the vendor's employees have.

The RFP should specify the system selection criteria. These criteria would include major evaluation methods, such as findings from the demonstration, findings from site visits (visiting a healthcare facility that has already implemented the system), review of the RFP, costs, expected benefits, and reliability of vendor's products. It would not include rankings of importance and other details that the project team will utilize to make the final decisions.

Finally, the RFP should request the training recommendations for the IS, including the number of people trained by the vendor, cost of training, the estimated time it should take to train each user, types of training required, and other recommendations regarding the training process.

CHECK YOUR UNDERSTANDING 4.2

1. A report is sent to the state each month on the services provided. This needs to be listed as part of the _____.

   a. Functional requirements
   b. Gantt chart
   c. Project definition
   d. PERT chart

2. Identify the tool that shows a work process.

   a. Observation
   b. Questionnaires
   c. Interviews
   d. Flowchart

3. The healthcare facility is trying to determine who they will send a RFP to. Identify the tool that can assist in this decision.

   a. RFI
   b. External scan
   c. Flowchart
   d. Vendor profile

4. The SDLC phase that identifies the functions that are needed in an IS is _____.

   a. Planning and analysis
   b. Design
   c. Implementation
   d. Maintenance and evaluation

5. Justify the decision to be an alpha site.

   a. All of the problems have been worked out of the IS at this point.
   b. Although the IS is new, many of the issues have been resolved by the beta sites.
   c. It will enable us to meet federal and state laws.
   d. It allows the healthcare facility to play a significant role in the design of the IS.

Evaluation of Proposed Systems

The evaluation process used to select an IS should be established during the planning process. The process should have multiple components, including:

- Onsite and online demonstrations
- Site visits
- Review of RFP
- Reference checks

Onsite Demonstrations

In an onsite demonstration, the vendor brings its product to the healthcare facility, either as a demonstration version or a full version of the product. Project team members and other users gather to view the IS and to ask questions of the sales team. The idea is to have as many users and members of the project team as possible watch the demonstration to see what the IS can and cannot do. All attendees should bring to the demonstration situations they encounter in their daily tasks and ask how the IS would handle it. Examples of situations are admitting Medicare patients, ordering medication, and merging duplicate health records.

The on-site demonstration allows for multiple user involvement and is an important opportunity to learn about the information. This may be the only chance for some team members or other users to see the IS before implementation; not everyone can go to site visits to see the IS in a live environment.

Site Visits

Site visits are a great way to view the products in a live environment. A site visit usually consists of a small group of team members visiting a healthcare facility, preferably similar in size and characteristics, that has the product implemented to observe the IS in use. During the visit, the project team asks the healthcare facility's staff questions about the IS. Often the salesperson for the product will attend the site visit to answer questions and ensure that the project team obtains the information needed to make a decision. Seeing the IS operating in a real environment is quite different from a demonstration environment and thus gives the project team a much more realistic view of the IS and how it works.

Reviewing RFP Responses

The vendor spends a lot of time responding to an RFP, so the RFP should only be sent to the vendors who are seriously being considered. Responding to the RFP is time consuming and therefore very expensive for the vendor. The number of RFPs submitted is typically limited to three to five vendors. The vendor's proposal should be received by a designated person, generally the project manager. The project manager then coordinates the review of the proposals. The healthcare facility also spends hours reviewing the RFP responses because for major IS purchases, the responses could fill a three- or four-inch binder. A spreadsheet is frequently developed to assist in the analysis of the RFPs, and this enables the decision makers to compare key information between products more easily when making their decision.

Some of the information that could be included in the spreadsheet includes cost, compatibility with existing system, the level to which the system meets functional requirements, and the reaction to site visits. A sample comparison is shown in table 4.3.

Table 4.3.   Sample of comparisons among vendors responding to RFP

System Capabilities	System A	System B	System C
Works with existing hospital IS	Yes	Yes	Yes
One-time costs	$654,000	$498,500	$576,000
Ongoing costs (3 years)	$65,000	$89,000	$79,000
Hardware needed	File server	File server	File server
Works with existing database	Yes	Yes	Yes
Number of years vendor in existence	31	12	6
Number of installations	123	26	2
RFP shows financial viability	Yes	Yes	Yes

Reference Checks

The healthcare facility should contact several other healthcare facilities where the product is currently in use. These reference checks are a great way to learn if other facilities are satisfied with the product without the expense and time it takes to go to on-site visits. The vendor will provide a list of references, and the evaluating healthcare facility should try to obtain a complete list of client sites from the vendor or independently identify client facilities that are not on the reference list. Best practices recommend that the evaluating project team contact healthcare facilities from the vendor's reference list, as well as healthcare facilities that are clients of the vendor but are not included on the reference list, including any site visit personnel. The reference list may contain only customers who are satisfied with the product and leave off the unsatisfied ones. Healthcare facilities not on the list may be identified through the corporate offices, networking, or cold calls. Notes from these reference checks should be collected and used as part of the decision-making process.

Selection of an Information System

It is the responsibility of the project team to review the responses to the RFP and other evaluation tools to determine which IS will best meet the needs of the healthcare facility. To prevent disagreements over which system to choose, there should be a quantifiable means of evaluating the ISs. One way is to assign points to the RFP review, site visits, observations, and other evaluation methods. If a point system is used during the evaluation process, then the system with the highest number of points should theoretically be the best IS and therefore the one that is chosen. However, this is not always the case, because a vendor may have the overall highest score but have low scores in some important functions; the selection team should not only consider the total points but each individual task as well.

A useful method of ascertaining the best EHR product and vendor is a weighted decision matrix, a method used to help select an IS based on what features are the most important to the healthcare facility. For example, compliance with privacy and security requirements is more important and deserves a higher weight than the ability to change the color of the screen. Points are typically awarded and the system with the highest number of points is the frontrunner for selection. The project team is responsible for determining the criteria to rate the EHR systems chosen. It is best to limit the number of EHRs in the weighted decision matrix; otherwise, it would become unwieldy. Three comparisons are usually sufficient. The objectives of the EHR system RFPs are an excellent beginning for choosing the criteria used in the decision matrix. Additional measurable and demonstrable criteria can be formulated by the project team with input from stakeholders.

The project team should perform the following steps to create the weighted decision matrix:

1. Determine objective, measurable, and quantifiable criteria against which the EHR system can be evaluated. Most of these criteria should come from the objectives of the RFP.

2. Rate each criterion in terms of its importance based upon the objectives and input from the project team members. The rating system of 1 = lowest to 5 = highest is a good start, but it can be modified depending on input from the project members. However, it must be consistent throughout the matrix.

3. Rate each EHR system to the degree it achieves or meets each of the criteria. Again, the rating system of 1 = lowest to 5 = highest is a good start, but it can be modified depending on input from the project members. Again, it must be consistent throughout the matrix.

4. Multiply each criterion rating by the EHR rating. This numeric product is the score for that criterion and EHR system. It is a partial score.

5. Total the numeric products for the EHR system for all the criteria. This numeric result is the complete score for the EHR system based on the assigned criteria and the respective partial scores.

6. The EHR system with the highest complete score is the one that best meets the healthcare entity's preferred criteria better than the other EHR systems evaluated from their RFPs (Swenson 2013, 696).

As shown in table 4.4, EHR System Vendor #2 has scored the highest and therefore best meets the criteria established by the project team for selecting an EHR for the healthcare entity.

Table 4.4.   EHR system vendors decision matrix example

Criteria	Criteria Rating of Importance (1 = low, 5 = high)	EHR System Vendor #1 Rating : Product	EHR System Vendor #2 Rating : Product	EHR System Vendor #3 Rating : Product
Criteria #1: System price	4	3:12	5:20	1:4
Criteria #2: EHR certification	5	4:20	3:15	4:20
Criteria #3: Vendor stability	3	5:15	4:12	4:12
Additional criteria	1–5	Additional ratings	Additional ratings	Additional ratings
Total product rating	—	47	57	36

Step 4: Contract Negotiation

Once the decision of which IS to purchase has been made, the contract negotiation process begins. Some healthcare facilities start negotiations with more than one vendor. Based on the initial meetings, the healthcare facility chooses one vendor to continue with negotiations. Typically, a contract team, not the project team, negotiates the contract. The negotiating team should include at least the CIO and an attorney; however, with a minor implementation, the HIM director may work with a member of administration. A minor IS might be a chart location system that is used only by the HIM department, is quickly and easily implemented, and has a simple contract. A major implementation would involve multiple areas of the healthcare facility, a significant period of time to implement, and a complex contract. The goal of the contract negotiations is a win-win situation. The healthcare facility wants a good product at a reasonable cost that is implemented in a reasonable time period. The healthcare facility should not try to secure the product under such strict requirements that the relationship with the vendor is negatively impacted from the beginning. With many of these installations, the healthcare facility will be working with the vendor for 10 years or longer; therefore, it is in the healthcare facility's best interest to create a good working relationship. The healthcare facility should not accept the sample contract provided by the vendor because this contract is written in favor of the vendor. The negotiation team is responsible for working with the vendor to develop a contract that works for both parties.

Some of the clauses covered by the contract include:

- Software license
- Delivery dates
- Warranties and guarantees
- Responsibilities of each party
- The state whose laws govern the contract
- Cost
- Milestones for payment
- Force majeure
- Software in escrow
- Cancellation of contract
- Version of software to be installed
- Penalties
- Acceptance testing
- Maintenance and updates
- Training
- Documentation

A software license describes what the healthcare facility can do with the software. It controls the locations that can use it, who can use it, and how it can be used. It may also include how many users can access the IS and if the IS is used solely by one department or the entire healthcare facility. The healthcare facility is prevented from using the IS in a way outside the license.

Delivery dates are the dates that the software and hardware will be delivered to the healthcare facility. The inclusion of these dates in the contract is important because nothing can be done until the software is available and installed at the healthcare facility. Warranties and guarantees are affirmations the vendor makes for which they are held accountable. Samples of warranties are:

- Vendor has the legal right to sell software.
- If it is found that the vendor does not have the right to sell the software, then the vendor is legally responsible.
- IS will be available 99.9 percent of the time.
- IS will perform query within 3 seconds.
- Technical support will respond within 30 minutes.

Contract law varies by state; therefore, the contract must specify which state's laws cover the terms of the contract. The vendor generally asks for the laws of its state and the healthcare facility asks for its state, so negotiation is required.

It is important to detail the responsibility of each party in the contract (see table 4.5). This helps ensure that no problems will arise later over who is responsible for what. This information will be used in the negotiation of the price. The more participatory a vendor is during implementation, the more the vendor should be paid.

Table 4.5. Sample allocation of responsibility list

Task	Responsible Party
Train the trainer(s)	Vendor
Train end users	Healthcare facility
Develop interfaces	Healthcare facility and vendor
Design screens	Healthcare facility
Testing	Healthcare facility and vendor

The cost of the IS is one of the last clauses negotiated. The amount of money paid to the vendor will be based on the responsibilities of the vendor, the number of users specified in the contract, and other clauses. The healthcare facility should require a fixed price so it knows exactly what the cost of the IS will be. Healthcare facilities should never pay the entire negotiated amount or a large percentage of the cost up front; rather, the contract should then establish payment milestones (see table 4.6). A payment milestone is an action that triggers payment to the vendor. This payment is a specified percentage of the total cost of the IS. This must be negotiated and spelled out in the contract. Typical milestones include delivery of software, go-live, and acceptance testing. A significant percentage of the payment should be held until acceptance testing is complete. Failure to do so could result in the vendor moving to the next installation and not responding in a timely manner to any outstanding issues. If there is a significant amount of money involved, the vendor is more likely to be responsive to the needs of the healthcare facility.

Table 4.6. Sample milestones for payment

Milestone	Percentage of Vendor's Payment
Signing of contract	20 percent
Delivery of software	10 percent
Commencement of testing	10 percent
Go-live	30 percent
Completion of acceptance testing	30 percent

Force majeure is a legal term that refers to "an event or effect that cannot be reasonably anticipated or controlled" (Merriam-Webster 2017). This contract clause is designed so that the parties of the contract cannot be held accountable to a deadline if there was an "act of God" that prevented compliance. For example, if an IS is being implemented and a tornado hits the hospital two days before the implementation date so that the date is delayed, the vendor would not be held accountable for any penalties as specified in the contract.

Healthcare facilities have the need to protect themselves in the event the vendor goes bankrupt. One way to do this is to place a clause in the contract that requires the vendor to place the source code in escrow. Source code is the programming code that was used to develop the system. Escrow is a situation in which a third party holds a copy of the software in case the vendor goes bankrupt. This means that if the vendor goes out of business, the healthcare facility can obtain access to the code behind the software so that they can maintain the IS themselves or hire someone else to do so. The vendor prefers this method as well because it does not want its trade secrets to be widely available.

Cancellation of the contract becomes important if the product or vendor does not meet the needs of the healthcare facility. This clause allows the vendor or healthcare facility to void the contract with appropriate notice. There should also be a period of time in which the contract is in force unless canceled earlier by either party. This clause may require a 30- or 60-day notice to the other party in the event of a cancellation.

The version of software that will be delivered to the healthcare facility should be specified in the contract. The vendor will know when the next version is scheduled for release. Depending on the time frame of implementation, the healthcare facility may receive the current version or the new version. The contract may also state that the healthcare facility will install the current version but will receive the upgrade to the new IS as part of the contract or at a reduced cost.

The contract should specify penalties for both the vendor and the healthcare facility for failure to meet the dates specified in the contract. Penalties vary widely and can be monetary or in the form of free training, free software modules, or other forms. The penalties should be serious enough to keep the parties on target, but not so punitive they would seriously risk the financial stability of either party. For example, one healthcare facility had negotiated such a tight time frame with major penalties that the IS department essentially did not do anything other than implement the new IS and keep the current ISs operational for an entire year. If departments needed assistance with the IS, they were told to hire someone to do it for them. Placing this amount of pressure on the vendor or the project team is not the purpose behind the penalties in the contract. The purpose is to keep everyone on task and on target.

Acceptance testing is a type of testing that occurs after the go-live date. It tests the IS to confirm that it is working as expected as per the contract, RFP response, and any other documentation. It is a critical part of the IS implementation because it establishes whether the terms of the contract have been met regarding performance and functionality. For more information on testing see chapter 5. The contract must spell out what outcomes are acceptable. These outcomes will be used to determine when the acceptance testing is complete and the vendor can receive payment. ISs are constantly changing. Maintenance must be an ongoing responsibility for both the vendor and the healthcare facility. The contract should spell out the responsibilities of both parties. The contract should also specify if upgrades to the IS are included in the contract and the costs for those upgrades. These upgrades will assist the healthcare facility in remaining compliant with accreditation, regulations, and other mandates. The system updates also repair any issues found in the IS and keeps the system operational.

Training responsibilities of the vendor, including issues such as the number of people to be trained, where they will be trained, the cost of the training, and the length of the training, should be specified in the contract. The contract should also spell out the ongoing training needed after implementation and the associated expenses.

The contract should include the type of documentation provided by the vendor to the healthcare facility. This documentation generally includes technical manuals for technical support as well as user manuals.

CHECK YOUR UNDERSTANDING 4.3

1. In order to analyze the RFPs that have been submitted, what tool could be used?
   a. Trouble ticket
   b. Spreadsheet
   c. Gantt chart
   d. Weighted decision matrix

2. The vendor was scheduled to implement the EHR yesterday but a tornado hit the area and it was unable to. Identify the section of the contract that addresses this.
   a. Warranty
   b. Force majeure
   c. Escrow
   d. Payment milestone

3. A healthcare facility should strive for what in contract negotiation?

   a. A contract that completely benefits the healthcare facility
   b. A contract that benefits the vendor
   c. A contract that is a win-win for both parties
   d. A contract that is based on the laws of the vendor's state

4. Which of the following can assist protecting the company's interest in case the vendor goes out of business?

   a. Escrow
   b. Warranty
   c. Prototype
   d. Force majeure

5. A weighted decision matrix is used to _____.

   a. Identify the functional requirements needed
   b. Select the IS to be purchased
   c. Identify the structure of the project
   d. Negotiate the contract

Real-World Case

Floribama Hospital just learned that their current EHR will no longer be supported by the IS vendor starting in two years. In the hospital's rush to select an IS, it decided to take some short cuts. These short cuts included:

- Creating a committee of only three people to select the system
- Not going on a site visit
- Not performing systems analysis
- Deferring planning until after the contract is signed

This was the recommendation of the chief executive officer of the healthcare facility. The logic behind his recommendation to defer planning was that there will be some time after the contract is signed but before the software is available, so the planning can fill in this time period. The contact was signed yesterday so the planning is ready to commence.

CHAPTER REVIEW

1. Identify the step that would allow the healthcare facility to learn of a new legislation.

   a. Internal scanning
   b. Request for proposal
   c. Request for information
   d. External scanning

2. One of the goals of the IS under consideration is to improve patient care. This is an example of a(n) _____.

   a. Project definition
   b. SMART goal
   c. Intangible benefit
   d. Tangible benefit

(Continued)

3. In a SMART goal, a goal that is challenging but can be accomplished given the time and other factors is known as _____.

   a. Measurable
   b. Realistic
   c. Attainable
   d. Timely

4. The hospital has gone into a partnership with an IS vendor. The hospital will be the first healthcare facility to utilize the EHR under development. The hospital is known as a(n) _____.

   a. Alpha site
   b. Beta site
   c. Project plan
   d. Critical path

5. Before the project began, the healthcare facility decided to implement an EHR that will be used at all three of the hospitals owed by the organization. This is an example of a(n) _____.

   a. Acceptance test
   b. Project definition
   c. Scope creep
   d. Feasibility study

6. The vendor's right to sell a product is an example of a(n) _____.

   a. Warranty
   b. Force majeure
   c. Acceptance test
   d. Source code

7. The healthcare facility has decided to purchase all of the ISs from one vendor. This strategy is known as _____.

   a. Best of the best
   b. Best of breed
   c. Best of fit
   d. Best of choice

8. Identify which of the following is a project.

   a. Change to screen formatting on three screens
   b. Developing the IS strategic plan
   c. Change setting related to number of days until a bill drops
   d. Write ad hoc report on number of patients who had a cholecystectomy

9. Which of the following evaluations would get the most users involved?

   a. On-site demonstration
   b. Site visit
   c. Reference checks
   d. Reviewing RFP responses

10. Where would warranties be found?

   a. RFP
   b. RFI
   c. Contract
   d. IS strategic plan

References

Austin, C. J. and S. B. Boxerman. 2003. *Information Systems for Healthcare Management*. Chicago: AUPHA Health Administration Press.

Blaisdell, R. 2013. "Five Cloud Computing Advances for the Healthcare Industry." *CloudTweaks* (blog). Februry 5, 2013. http://www.cloudtweaks.com/2013/02/5-cloud-computing-advantages-for-the-healthcare-industry/.

Gulla, J. 2012. Seven reasons why IT projects fail. *IBM Systems Magazine*. http://www.ibmsystemsmag.com/mainframe/tipstechniques/applicationdevelopment/project_pitfalls/?page=1.

LaTour, K. M., S. Eichenwald Maki, and P. Oachs. 2013. *Health Information Management: Concepts, Principles, and Practice*. Chicago: AHIMA.

Merriam-Webster. 2017. Force majeure. Merriam-Webster Dictionary Online. http://www.merriam-webster.com/dictionary/force+majeure.

Swenson, D. X. 2013. Managing and Leading During Organization Change. Chapter 23 in *Health Information Management: Concepts, Principles, and Practice*, 4th ed. Edited by K. M. LaTour, S. Eichenwald Maki, and P. Oachs. Chicago: AHIMA.

Swenson, D. X. 2016. Managing and Leading During Organizational Change. Chapter 22 in *Health Information Management: Concepts, Principles, and Practice*, 5th ed. Edited by P. Oachs and A. Watters. Chicago: AHIMA.

Wager, K. A., F. W. Lee, and J. P. Glasier. 2013. *Health Care Information Systems: A Practical Approach for Health Care Management*. San Francisco, CA: Jossey-Bass.

System Implementation

Learning Objectives

- Identify the steps in system implementation.
- Make recommendations for the testing and implementation of the information system.
- Develop training materials and conduct training classes for users.
- Recommend conversion needed for data being transferred from existing system.

Key Terms

Computer-assisted instruction (CAI)
Data conversion
Graphical user interface (GUI)
Reengineering

Screen design
Setting configuration
Site preparation
System evaluation
System implementation

Test environment
Train the trainer
Trouble ticket
User preparation

In chapter 4, the system development life cycle (SDLC) was introduced and the first two stages were discussed. In this chapter, the last two stages, implementation, and maintenance and evaluation, will be covered. System implementation is the process of preparing and launching the information system (IS) that has been selected for use. The system selection process continues until the IS is in use and has been evaluated as to whether or not it meets the objectives established at the beginning of the process.

Steps included in the implementation process are as follows:

1. Site and space preparation
2. User preparation
3. Installing hardware and software
4. Programming and customization
5. User configurations and settings
6. Screen design
7. Reengineering processes
8. Policy and procedure development and documentation
9. Testing plan

10. Training

11. Conversion

12. Go-live

13. System evaluation

First, the impact that the decisions made during the design phase have on the implementation of the IS will be covered.

System Design

Many tasks are involved in implementation of an IS. Some of these steps can be completed concurrently, whereas others must have one or more of the steps preceding them completed before proceeding. If any of these tasks are omitted or given too little attention, the project will fail. The strategy used to implement the IS should have the least impact on the healthcare facility. For example, the healthcare facility can switch over to the new IS at midnight when the activity in the hospital is low, or a clinic can be switched overnight.

Because it may take several weeks to receive hardware (computers, monitors, servers, and so on), staff needs to plan accordingly and place the order early. The most critical piece of hardware is the file server or other computer storage component that will house the application software. System implementation may be delayed if the file server or other hardware is not available according to the project plan.

The application software will be provided to the healthcare facility by the computer vendor based on the date specified in the contract. The version of the software provided will also be controlled by the contract. If the vendor is late in sending the software for installation, the implementation of the IS will be delayed.

Site and Space Preparation

Site preparation requires making any needed changes to the physical location where the computer, workstations, printers, or other hardware will be installed. The needs of site preparation vary widely, from construction of a new building, to renovation of an old one, to use of existing structures and upgrades to the infrastructure. Modifications needed may require the installation of special air conditioning or floors designed to run cables under it, added security measures, or more electrical outlets, to name a few. However, site preparation may be as simple as moving existing hardware around to make room for the new. The nursing units, the health information management (HIM) department, and other locations may need to be renovated to add space for computer terminals, barcode printers, network printers, and other hardware. The data center, where computers will run the IS, must be completed first because the nursing units and other departments will not use the IS until go-live. In addition to the physical plant, the healthcare facility network may need to be updated to accommodate the extra traffic resulting from the new system.

Failure to properly prepare the site and infrastructure will result in delays in the installation of hardware and software, which will in turn delay the entire implementation plan of the system. For example, a healthcare facility attempted to plug in the hardware and did not have an available electrical outlet.

User Preparation

User preparation involves providing the users with enough information about the IS being implemented so that they are prepared both psychologically and through training to use it. This part of the change management process is discussed in chapter 4 and continues throughout the project. It is important for IS users to be notified and updated throughout the system selection and implementation process. The users need to know that the IS is being implemented and should have an accurate understanding of what to expect from the IS and what is expected of them. Many people fear computers when new ISs are installed; therefore, these fears must be addressed. For example, they may have a fear of change because it takes them out of their comfort zone. Management must be open and honest with the users regarding expectations, downsizing, changes in job descriptions, and other concerns. The information must be accurate; otherwise, users will lose trust in the manager's word. Sometimes a new system is promoted so intensely that users expect more than the IS can provide. These unrealistic expectations lead to disappointment and, in turn, a lack of support from the users. There should be as many users involved in the IS selection and implementation as possible to obtain their support. Their involvement can be through the systems analysis function, being part of the implementation team, assisting in testing, and other ways. Even those users not involved in the selection and implementation need to have realistic expectations. Their expectations can be managed through training, articles in the healthcare facility newsletter, updates at department meetings, and other formal and informal means of communication. If the IS does not live up to the user's expectations, they may not use the IS to its fullest or take the time to use it properly; thus impacting the overall success of the implementation.

Installing Hardware and Software

Once the hardware arrives, it will need to be set up and installed in the data center. Computers will also need to be installed in the nursing units, training rooms, and other locations according to the project plan. The printers, network, scanners, and other hardware will also need to be installed.

The software will then need to be loaded onto the file server, mainframe, or other computer in the data center. Some applications require software to be used on an individual user's computer. If this is the case, the software will have to be installed on all authorized computers prior to implementation, especially for development and testing. Any failures in the site preparation will be identified in this stage.

Programming and Customization

Programming may or may not be required, depending on the type of IS, complexity of the IS, and whether the healthcare facility is purchasing an IS or programming one themselves. If the IS interfaces with other ISs to share information, such as patient demographics or other information, the interfaces will have to be programmed. If the healthcare facility is converting data from another IS, computer programming will have to be done to perform data conversion. Data conversion is the process whereby data are copied from the existing IS, manipulated into the format required by the new IS, and entered into the new IS. This mapping from one format to another is critical. For example, if a health record number is stored in the current system as a 10-digit number (0000123456) and the new IS requires a 12-digit number, then two more leading zeroes would need to be added to the number (000000123456).

The healthcare facility may want to have some changes made to the software to better meet its needs. This customization of the IS can be completed by either the healthcare facility or the vendor. Although customization may better prepare the IS to meet the needs of the healthcare facility, there are reasons why the healthcare facility should not customize the software beyond what is already built into the IS by the vendor:

- If the healthcare facility makes changes to the software and then has trouble with the IS, the vendor can blame the modifications. The vendor may then refuse to work on the system.
- The vendor may not give the healthcare facility a service agreement.
- Every time that the healthcare facility receives a software update from the IS vendor, the IS staff will have to check the modifications to see if they are affected by the new update. Because the healthcare facility may receive several updates a year, this can be an onerous task. (Rollins 2006)

User Configurations and Settings

Most computer software purchased by healthcare facility generally provides some flexibility in the implementation of the IS. This flexibility is allowed through setting configuration. Setting configuration is the entry of the desired behaviors of the IS into tables or setting fields. For example, if the IS will keep track of the patient type, the hospital determines if patients will be classified as inpatient, outpatient, emergency department, testing, outpatient surgery, or another patient type. The healthcare facility may even be able to determine that I means inpatient.

The project team sets up the specifications by filling in tables and other fields with the desired setup. They will also be able to update tables that provide their reimbursement rates, tax identification number, national provider identifier, or other appropriate values. Other settings may include time frame before bills drop, data and format of claims submitted to fiscal intermediary, and what fields are required. The settings will ensure that the IS works according to the needs of the healthcare facility.

It can take minutes or months to get all the specifications and tables updated, depending on the complexity of the specifications and the IS. An example of a table that must be uploaded is the user table. In this table, each user's information must be entered into the IS, including their username, initial password, location, type of access, and permissions as to what they can perform within the IS. For example, Mary Smith may have access to the laboratory results, but she can only view these results—not delete or modify them. Determining who has access to what information and what they can do with it is a time-consuming task.

Screen Design

The IS may allow the healthcare facility to make changes to the computer screen so that it works the best for the healthcare facility. **Screen design** means developing screens of an IS to meet the needs of the user and to promote job efficiency. To accomplish this goal, team members involved in this process must be aware of the needs of the users and the work they perform. Reasons why the healthcare facility may want to change the computer screen include the following:

- No single screen contains the data needed to make data entry or viewing efficient.
- The vendor's screens do not have data elements in a logical order for the workflow of the users.
- The existing screens are too cluttered for the users' preference.
- Changing the screen will improve the process workflow.

When designing screens used in the IS, the fields should be in a logical sequence to facilitate data entry. The title of the screen should be descriptive of the data contained on the screen such as "Lab Results." The logical flow of data helps the users to locate information. For example, if reviewing a screen containing basic patient demographic information, the address, city, and state would be located together in that order rather than address at the top and city beneath other data elements. The flow of data entry should be from left to right and top to bottom. Screens, like paper forms, should have a title and a control number to manage the screen. Screens should be simple to use and have a standardized terminology across screens to facilitate data entry, training, and data quality. For example, the health record number should be called the same name on all screens—not medical record number on one and health record number or patient identifier on another. Screens should also have the same look and feel so that the user can easily move from screen to screen. A standardized look and feel for a screen includes the same colors, location of key data elements such as patient name, and same location and terminology for key buttons such as "Next Screen." Instructions can be posted on the screen where necessary to assist users. Color, blinking, and reverse video can be used to draw the user's attention to important data such as allergies. In reverse video, the font is the normal color of the background and the background is the normal color of the font. These special features should be used sparingly so that the user's attention is drawn to the information displayed. The color of the screen and text should comfortable for users to view for long periods of time. For example, red and bright neon colors are typically used only sparingly. An example of good screen design is seen in figure 5.1 and an example of poor screen design is seen in figure 5.2. In figure 5.1, the data elements are listed in a logical order, there is a descriptive title for the screen, it has a screen number, and the buttons are clear in their function and are in a logical location. In figure 5.2, the data fields are not in a logical order nor are the buttons. There is neither a title nor a screen number.

Figure 5.1. Example of good screen design

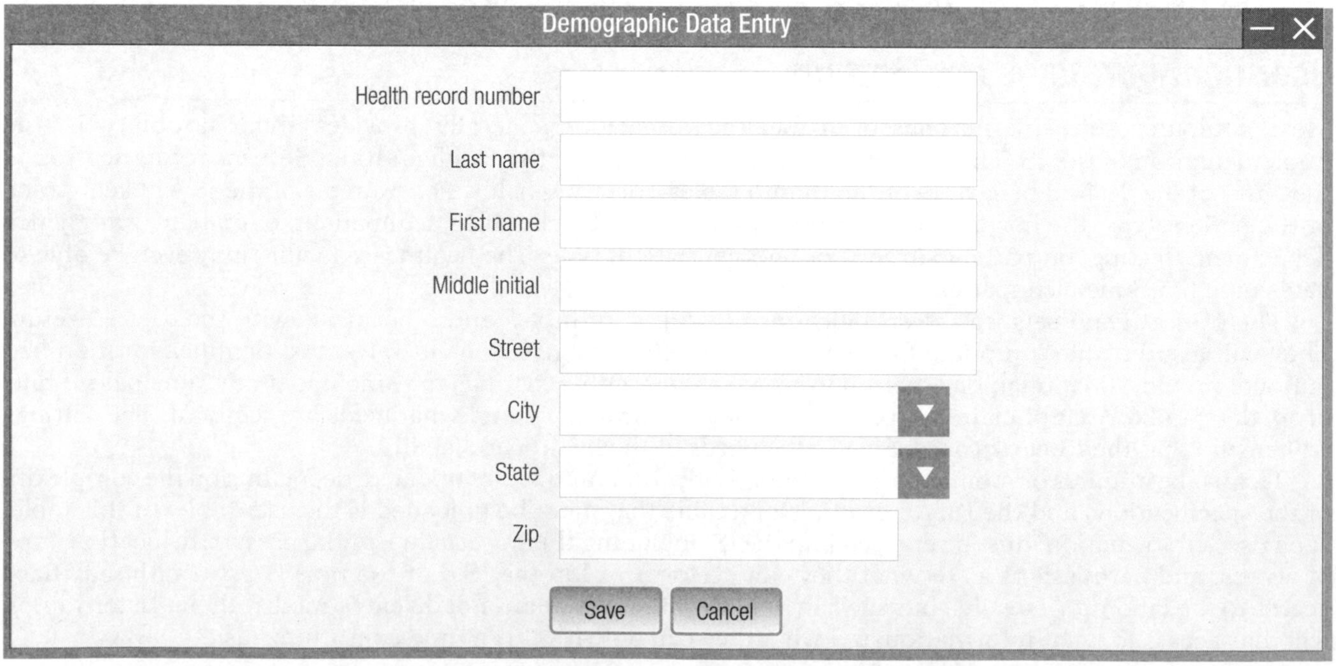

Figure 5.2.   Example of poor screen design

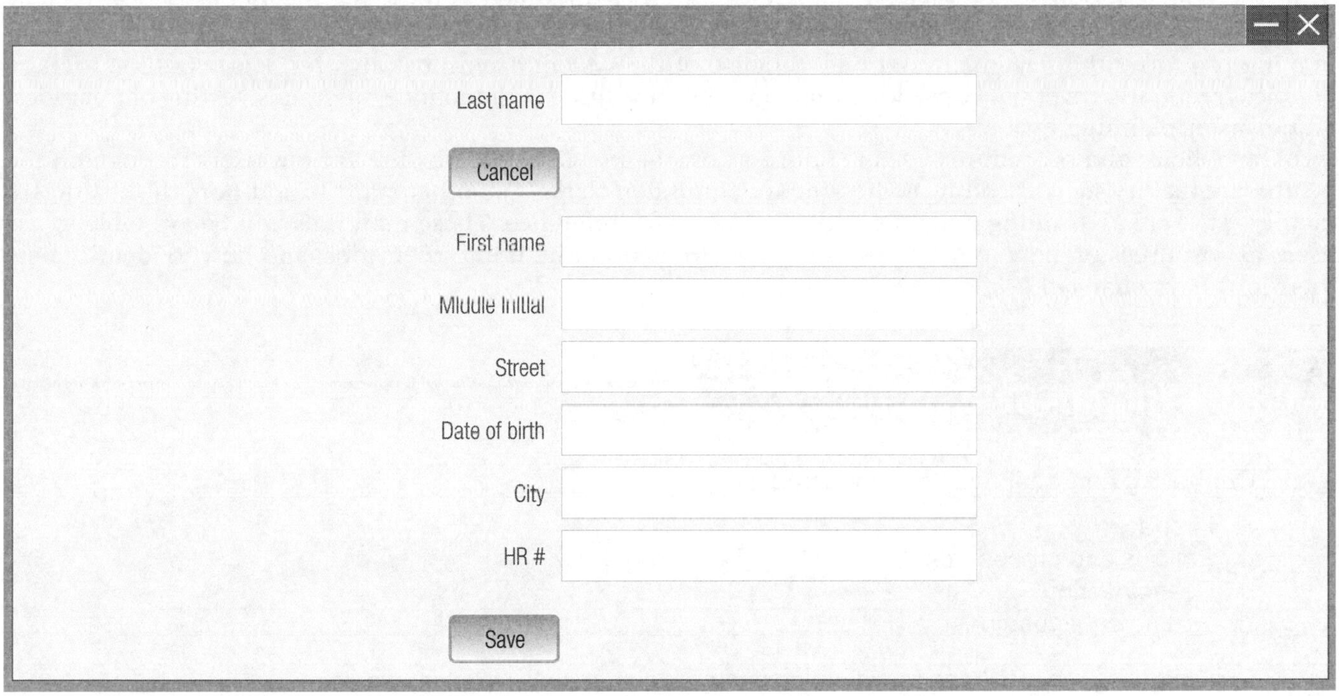

The screen design may include designing computer views for various types of users. This flexibility would allow nurses to see new orders, care plans, or other information first; the cardiologist and neurologist would have first access to cardiac and neurologic tests, respectively.

A graphical user interface (GUI) is a term used to describe the interaction of users and the computer whereby the user clicks on icons, menus, and other tools to assist in the use of the IS. Frequently, these icons are shown on a toolbar. Icons provide shortcuts to functionality within the system, along with buttons and menus, allowing the user to command the software to perform specific tasks.

The HIM professional must work with the information technology professionals to ensure the screens in the IS are designed to support quality data entry. Information technology is the field that includes hardware, software, and databases. Information systems (IS) is a broader term that includes information technology as well as the staff and processes needed to operate and manage them (Florida Institute of Technology 2017). One of the ways this can be done is through required fields. A required field does not allow the user to proceed until it is completed. Not all fields should be required because not all fields apply to all patients. For example, obstetrical data fields would not be required for male patients. If a field is identified as required inappropriately, the users would become frustrated and may resort to entering erroneous data to be able to proceed.

Reengineering Processes

Reengineering is evaluating the way the healthcare facility does business in order to improve efficiency. Reengineering is a task that is frequently overlooked in the efforts to implement the IS. Every task and preconceived notion must be challenged. The question "why" should be asked over and over. Everything is subject to evaluation and change, without exemption. This is challenging to employees who are comfortable with the status quo. Some of the tasks performed by the employees have been performed for years. The reason behind the task may be outdated, but the task continues because the employee is afraid to stop. The implementation of a new IS is a perfect time to critique the tasks performed to try and improve efficiency, costs, and effectiveness.

The employees may feel threatened and intimidated because of the changes impacting their jobs, but reengineering is a necessary part of the IS process. The healthcare facility cannot implement an IS and expect the work processes to remain the same. The healthcare facility will need to change procedures, update the policy and procedure manual, change workflow, eliminate unnecessary tasks, and add new tasks. Failure to do so can decrease efficiency rather than maximize the benefits the IS affords. The IS changes the way a healthcare facility conducts business and impacts the manual processes and workflow as well as their overall interaction with the computer. The policies and procedures tested during the testing phase should contain the revised processes.

Policy and Procedure Development and Documentation

After the reengineering is completed, the policy and procedure manual must be updated to reflect the new way of doing business. Policies and procedures should blend together the manual processes and decision-making processes. Management and maintenance of the system itself must also be clearly outlined. These policies frequently cover backups, downtime policies for routine maintenance, upgrades, testing of upgrades, and disaster planning.

The policies and procedures need to address how the IS will be used by the various users throughout the healthcare facility such as coding professionals, admission clerks, and other staff. In addition, the healthcare facility must create training manuals and user guides for reference. These materials will be available to the users as resources on how to use the system, how to incorporate it into their jobs, and how to identify how their jobs have changed.

CHECK YOUR UNDERSTANDING 5.1

1. Controlling how an IS works is impacted by _____.

   a. Interfaces
   b. Policies and procedures
   c. Reengineering
   d. Setting configurations

2. Implementing a new IS and reevaluating and changing processes is known as _____.

   a. Integration
   b. Updates
   c. Reengineering
   d. Adapting

3. Making room for new computers is part of which of the following?

   a. Site preparation
   b. System selection
   c. Flow charting
   d. Reengineering

4. IS A's health record number field allows 8 characters. The same field in IS B allows 12 characters. How is this handled?

   a. Data conversion
   b. Site preparation
   c. Policies and procedures
   d. Setting configuration

5. What is used to interact with the computer?

   a. GUI
   b. Policies and procedures
   c. Conversion
   d. Reengineering

Testing Plan

All components of the IS will need testing before the go-live. Testing helps the implementation team identify any problems with the system so that they can be corrected. This is a cyclical process, so the team will test the IS, identify problems, fix problems, and test the system again. The test cycle will continue until all problems have been resolved. Testing requires careful and detailed planning to ensure that complete and accurate testing is carried out in a timely manner.

Types of Testing

Many types of testing must be performed in preparation for an IS implementation. The types of testing include the following:

- Interface testing: Ensures that the interfaces function properly. The healthcare facility must test to confirm that data from the source system are transferred into the new IS in the correct field and in the right format. Data to be transferred vary by IS, but commonly include the patient's name, health record number, date of birth, and other demographic information. Other types of data that may be transferred include laboratory tests, radiology results, and any other data that are collected.

- Integration testing: Ensures that all hardware, including computers, printers, and scanners, work together as they should. Examples of testing to be performed include the ability to scan documents, print a report, or scan a barcode. Some computers may have limitations placed on their abilities for privacy, security, or other reasons. For example, the healthcare facility may choose not to print laboratory results on the nursing units to protect confidentiality, thus forcing users to look up the most current results available.

- Application testing: Ensures that every function of the new IS works. Application testing also ensures that the IS meets the functional requirements and other required specifications in the request for proposal (RFP) or contract. Application testing should also ensure that every conceivable situation that the computer will be used to address can be handled. The project team must also test the reports to ensure that the data and statistics contained therein are correct.

- Documentation testing: During the implementation process, a number of documents, including user guides, policies and procedures, and training materials, are created. These documents should be followed during the testing process to ensure that the instructions in the documents are accurate. In testing the documentation, the tester follows and tests the IS documentation that will be provided to the users. Errors in the documentation will be identified and corrected so that the user will have the proper instructions.

- Conversion testing: Ensures that the project team is able to transfer data from the old IS to the new IS. Conversion testing will confirm that the data conversion is performed correctly. Testing usually begins with a small amount of real data that have been copied. After the initial test has been run, the project team would fix any problems, rerun the test, and then continue to add larger and larger amounts of data. This testing will continue until the project team is certain that the problems have been resolved prior to the actual data conversion.

- Training testing: The project team should train a group to see how well the training materials, agenda, format of training, time allotted for training, and other attributes work. Changes are made to the training process as needed before real training begins.

- Volume testing: Most of the testing performed on the application is done with a handful of people sitting at an IS trying to identify problems. The IS may work fine with a small group of people, but most ISs are used by large groups of people simultaneously. To test the IS in as real an environment as possible, volume testing should be performed. Volume testing gets as many people to use the IS at one time as possible. Volume testing confirms that the IS and the network can handle the large volume of users and data. The user task force as well as other users throughout the healthcare facility can be brought in for volume testing. The project team will need to recruit as many users as possible to use the IS at the same time.

- Parallel testing: Running parallel tests is used for both testing and facilitating the transition of data and business processes. Unlike most other testing, parallel testing occurs when the new IS is operational. This is not a required test, but can be a valuable one. In parallel testing, the healthcare facility runs the old and the new ISs simultaneously and compares the reports and data from the two systems to validate both performance and synchronization. For example, the healthcare facility could compare the number of admissions for a specific date, the number of tests ordered, or the number of times that a test was ordered. Because of the extra resources needed to operate both ISs, this test is frequently omitted. The benefit to parallel testing is that if the new IS does not work as expected and the healthcare facility has to shut it down, then the existing IS is current, thus not impacting the operations of the healthcare facility.

- Acceptance testing: Like parallel testing, acceptance testing occurs after go-live. It is a time to verify that the IS is working as expected in a live environment. It gives the healthcare facility time to confirm that the new IS meets response time, functional requirements, and other standards guaranteed in the contract. (Amatayakul 2017, 267)

Test Plan

The testing plan is a document that covers areas such as what is to be tested, who will be involved in the testing, dates of testing, documentation of testing results, and types of testing. The testing must continue until all problems have been fixed. The testing must include the documentation created for use with the IS as well.

The testing plan should create a realistic **test environment**, which is an exact duplicate of the IS in use, excluding data. In this test environment, changes can be made to the IS and then tested to see what happens. For example, the settings in the test system environment should be the ones that the healthcare facility will utilize during operation. The testing plan will identify a "laundry list" of functions that must be tested before the IS is implemented. One way to test the functions is scenario or use-case testing, during which users bring real-life situations to be addressed by the IS. These scenarios should be documented in the plan. The use of scenarios allows the user to think through how a situation will be handled by actually using the IS. Scenario testing thoroughly tests the system because it addresses entries into the IS, tasks, and output.

Testing Documentation

Many healthcare facilities use what is frequently called a trouble ticket to report problems encountered during the testing phase. The **trouble ticket** is a form that is used to give specific information on problems encountered. The information provided may include the screen where the problem occurred, function being performed, error message received, data entered, report with incorrect data, or other problems encountered. The information provided must be as detailed as possible so that the problem can be replicated by the project team. The trouble ticket is logged into some type of tracking system when received, assigned a tracking number, and assigned to the appropriate project team member to solve. Once the problem has been resolved, the resolution is recorded, and the IS testing begins again. The project team cannot just test the part that was broken because the change that was made to fix the problem may have broken something else.

Training

Training is crucial to the success of the implementation process. There needs to be a well-designed training plan that addresses the timing and methods used to train the users. The plan must be properly executed or negative repercussions can occur. Users may feel like they are reverting back to being a novice employee after being an expert in their position. Job security may be another concern. Individuals who are most concerned with the new ISs are often those who have little experience with computers. Communicating with employees and keeping them informed of changes, impact, and expectations of their position will help prepare them for training.

The learning curve is different with each employee. Learning ability is impacted by age, maturity level, and experience. People have different preferred learning styles—auditory, visual, and so forth. Because of these factors, instructors should use a variety of methods that will accommodate all learning styles.

Instructors and trainers should have a basic understanding of adult learning principles and practice them in the development and implementation of training. Some key adult learning principles are:

- Adults like being responsible for their own decisions: They resent not having control, so the instructor should let the learners have a say in the program. This can take the form of helping to set the agenda, deciding which of two or three activities to do, strategies to use, and so on.

- Adults are experienced: Adult learners come to the training session with a lot of experience and knowledge upon which they can draw. Not all adults have the same knowledge and experience. The instructor and students can learn from each other. The varied backgrounds and knowledge can make for an interesting discussion and an improved learning experience.

- Adults need to know why: Instructors should get into a habit of telling the adults why they need to do something or why they need to learn what they are being taught. They need to know why something is important just as much as they need to know how to do it.

- Adults need to see relevance: Adults do not want to waste their time. They want to learn what they need to know for the immediate future. The instructor will need to tie the class material to what the individuals in the course will be doing. In other words, do not teach nurses how to do something with the IS that only the HIM department will be doing in the future. The nurses need to know what they will be doing. If adult learners do not see relevance to themselves, they will not be motivated to learn.

- The adult needs to be ready to learn: Training sessions may be mandatory and the learners may show up physically to the session, but they cannot be forced to learn. The instructor must engage the learner and encourage the desire to learn.

- The learner has to be motivated to learn: Some healthcare facilities have motivated learners by making them take a competency test at the end of the training session. This test makes the learner use skills they learned in class. Learners are motivated because the healthcare facility sometimes ties employment to successfully completing this test. These tests are generally very easy, but occasionally some people cannot pass them. These users are usually given a second or third chance before they are terminated. The threat of termination is not the best motivation because motivation to learn should come from within; however, the healthcare facility must know that the users are competent to use the ISs.

Planning for Training

There should be someone on the project team who is responsible for planning the complete training process. This trainer has a wide range of responsibilities including developing objectives, developing the training plan, and implementing the training.

The trainer would attend project team meetings in order to keep up with the status of the project. The trainer needs to know when training will be needed, the type of training needed, and also be a superuser (or expert) on the new IS. With this knowledge, the trainer will be prepared to develop the training program necessary to teach others to use the IS. The trainer is responsible for sharing and providing the necessary knowledge needed to prepare other trainers to teach as well.

The trainer will also work with the training staff from the vendor. The vendor's staff knows the product well and will be able to offer the project team suggestions on different teaching methods directly related to the IS. The vendor should provide the trainers with resources that can be customized for the healthcare facility.

The trainer will be working with both administration and end-users during the training planning and training implementation stages. These interactions make the trainer an excellent liaison between the two groups. The trainer will be able to communicate expectations of administration to users as well as communicate the fears and concerns of the users back to administration.

Contents of the Plan

The project team should create a training schedule that allows everyone who needs training to participate. The schedule should include sessions for all work shifts, including day, evening, night, and weekend shifts. The training plan should contain learning objectives that show both trainer and trainees what will be accomplished throughout the training sessions. The training plan should also outline the agenda, which describes the functions of the IS that will be covered, how they will be covered, and how much time will be spent on each topic. Teaching tools such as presentations, hands-on training, demonstrations, and computer-assisted instruction (CAI) are to be used during training.

The training plan should also address the content that will be covered, such as rollout schedule, policies and procedures, confidentiality, and security. When planning content, trainers need to determine each trainee's level of computer literacy before deciding what training is needed. Based on how many students will attend each session, the number of trainers and training sessions can be determined. The planners will also have to determine the necessary resources, such as a training room, computers, Internet access, training database, data projector, and handouts.

Not all users need the same training, so the training will be designed in modules based on the areas of content. Two examples are by department (such as nursing) or by function (such as order entry). In other words, the planner needs to decide whether the session will teach all nurses together or will teach people how to look up test results and have everyone who needs to know how to do this included in the same session. The division of the training into modules will impact the number of teachers, the schedule, and the training materials.

Selecting the Training Location

Not every trainer is fortunate enough to have a dedicated training facility. Trainers may be forced to reserve computer classrooms throughout the healthcare facility. A room would not be necessary if online training is utilized.

Scheduling the Training

Scheduling can be a very complicated task because trainers have to conduct different training classes required by patient care providers, administrative office staff, and other groups of users. Follow-up sessions after go-live should be offered as well to answer any questions that the users have once they start using the IS.

Many healthcare facilities are open 24 hours a day, 7 days a week, and thus, employees work a variety of shifts. Because of this, training must be offered on all shifts, including weekends, to accommodate all employees needing training. The following issues should be considered:

- Breaking modules down into separate classes helps to avoid confusion. If there is more than one class required, the team must make sure that they are offered in a logical format. For example, employees would need to know how to retrieve a patient file before they can learn how to place an order for a patient.
- This is further complicated by the fact that the trainers need to schedule the classes as close as possible to go-live while starting training early enough to get everyone trained in time. Completing training too early is also problematic because the users can forget what they learned before the IS is implemented, thus making the transition difficult for the user and the healthcare facility.
- Length of a session matters. Short sessions tend to work better because users are less likely to become overwhelmed. Also, if they are unaccustomed to sitting down, they may become frustrated by inactivity.
- The training sessions should not be scheduled during holidays because many people take time off, which causes scheduling problems with getting everyone trained.
- Physicians should be scheduled for one-on-one training sessions to accommodate their schedules. It could be early in the morning, at lunch, late in afternoon, in the evening, or on weekends in order to avoid interfering with physicians' office schedules.

Resources Needed

Each user should be provided a handout at the training session. Training materials are excellent resources to remind users how to do some task that may have been forgotten. Several days, weeks, or even months may pass between the initial training session and the implementation of the IS. During that time, users are likely to forget much of the material learned. To help them retain the knowledge acquired in training, the healthcare facility may also want to make the IS available (in test mode) to users for practice throughout this interim period.

Content suggestions for the development of educational materials provided to the students are as follows:

- The objectives should be clearly outlined.
- The agenda for the course should be sent to the scheduled attendees ahead of time. The agenda is subject to change, but acts as a guide to help keep trainers on track.
- Providing information about the IS prior to training offers a useful preview.

Train the Trainer

Train the trainer is a method of training certain individuals who, in turn, will be responsible for training others on a task or skill such as how to use the new IS. These people are generally called superusers. Superusers return to the healthcare facility and train other trainers who will in turn help conduct training sessions.

The user identifies the trainer as an expert on the system and its uses and who is likely to be a go-to resource. This visibility will make the trainer a key player in the hours and days following go-live. Users turn to the trainer with questions and fears.

Conducting the Training

Now that all of the work planning the training is finished, it is time to conduct the class. Instructors should be prepared and check the classroom to make sure it is ready for training—software has been installed, all computers are working, and so on. The trainer should make sure the room is physically comfortable. This means that the room is at a comfortable temperature, has appropriate lighting, and the workstations are ergonomically sound.

Evaluating the Training

Trainers must be evaluated on their delivery, impact, and knowledge of the application to make sure objectives of the training are being met. The following four outcomes of training should be critiqued:

1. Reaction: Evaluate what the trainees thought about the training
2. Learning: Determine whether the trainees have learned what was expected
3. Behavior: Determine how behavior has changed
4. Results: Determine impact on performance (Patena 2016, 754)

A valuable method for obtaining feedback is to have each trainee complete a written evaluation at the end of the session, answering questions about the overall training and the ability of the trainer. These evaluations can help to identify what is and is not working. Findings may identify needed improvements such as in the handouts, poor instructors, or not enough time for hands-on activities. Findings from the trainee evaluations should be shared with the instructors anonymously to identify any needed modifications and to evaluate the overall training plan performance. Evaluation results should be used to improve the quality and method of training where needed. There is always room for improvement.

The overall training program should also be evaluated on a continuing basis to ensure that goals of training are met. A formal plan for evaluation should be developed prior to the start of the training sessions.

Additional and Ongoing Training

After the training phase and before go-live, the healthcare facility eventually will not need the same number of trainers or frequency of class sessions. Training needs should be reassessed to determine frequency and specific needs. Training may be reorganized in conjunction with the healthcare facility's human resources department new employee orientation program or it may be separate. Training may be required before an employee is issued a user identification and password.

In a perfect world, the IS on which users are trained would remain the same as the one implemented. However, changes to the IS will be made and are necessary for technology advances, resolving glitches, and other issues. Therefore, training does not end with go-live of the IS. When significant changes are made, training may be needed to update and prepare users for the changes. Also, existing employees may need additional training to learn advanced capabilities, reinforce what they have already learned, or acquire new skills if they transfer to other jobs or their job changes over time.

Computer-Assisted Instruction

Computer-assisted instruction (CAI) is a software program designed to use multimedia and interactive technology to teach a topic. Multimedia can use audio, video, simulation, self-quizzes, and other tools to engage the learner. Drill and practice CAI reinforce material that the learner already knows, whereas problem solving addresses issues that the learner may face in his or her discipline.

The benefit of CAI is that learners are able to work at their own pace and on their own schedule. They are able to receive immediate feedback on whether or not they do something right. CAI also reduces costs, provides standardized training, and is designed to use multiple learning styles.

The downside is the start-up costs and the amount of time required to develop the training. Also, CAI should not be used when the content changes frequently because the CAI software will require updating with every change.

Documenting the Training

Documentation of all training provided is critical. Attendees should sign into each training session to provide proof of attendance for both employee's and employer's benefit. If a competency test is given, documentation of the results also should be maintained. Copies of all training materials and objectives for the training also should be retained.

Conversion

With most new ISs, a healthcare facility is converting from one IS to another—even if the first system is paper. The healthcare facility cannot ignore the historical data but, rather, must bring some (if not all of it) to the new IS. In a paper system, the historical data must be captured through abstracting, scanning, or other data entry methods. In an IS implementation, conversion is transferring data from one IS to another while simultaneously making any necessary changes in format or content. A conversion is more difficult than it sounds because systems frequently store data very differently or the healthcare facility may be making changes to how it wants data to be collected. For example, the health record number may be 10 digits in one IS and 12 in the other, or Medicare may be entered as M in one system and MCR in another. During conversion planning, the project team has to determine how much data are being converted and what data fields will need to be converted from one format to another. The amount of data transferred is a decision that must be made by the healthcare facility. The decision will be influenced by the type of IS, laws and regulations, whether or not the old IS will remain operational, and other issues. Sometimes healthcare facilities decide to transfer data from a specified time period only into the new IS. For example, they may decide to convert only the last two years. Other conversions require all data be transferred. The healthcare facility may also choose to enter data for all time periods, but only selected data elements rather than all data collected.

Once the conversion planning is finished, a program needs to be written that will make the necessary changes. A formal testing plan is required to determine how the project team will test the conversion to work out any problems before go-live. Once the IS is ready for use and the healthcare facility is ready for the IS, the data conversion plan must be implemented to move the existing data into the new system in the appropriate format. If data conversion is successful, the healthcare facility is then ready to start using the new IS. Healthcare facilities frequently capture the information available in the IS at midnight so that they can determine what data are in the old IS and what data are in the new. A specific time period of transition is useful in case the healthcare facility has to go back to the old IS because the new system did not work.

Go-Live

As stated in chapter 4, go-live is the official time and date that the healthcare facility begins using the new IS. The go-live is generally scheduled for a time when the healthcare facility is the least busy. For example, a hospital will generally go-live during the night shift because there is less activity at that time.

Go-Live Models

Go-live strategy generally refers to how an application will be implemented throughout a healthcare facility (such as departmental sequencing). There are three types of go-live strategies: phased, pilot, and big bang. There are two turnover strategies: straight turnover and parallel processing. These strategies are discussed in the following sections.

Phased Approach

One go-live strategy is the phased approach. In this method, the implementation starts with one module of the IS and then gradually other modules are added. A module is a subset of an IS, such as pharmacy orders in a CPOE system. All units, departments, and other entities utilize the system, but they only use it one module at a time. For example, a hospital could start using their order entry system by ordering medications only. After the medication ordering is successful, then laboratory will be added, and so on. With an electronic document management system, hospitals frequently start scanning emergency department records, then outpatient surgery, and then other record types until they work their way up to inpatient records. The advantage of this method is that staff is not overwhelmed by trying to do everything at once and the impact on the staff is lessened. The disadvantage is that it takes an extended period of time to finish the start-up process, which disrupts the operations of the healthcare facility.

Pilot Method

The next approach is the pilot method in which only one nursing unit, department, or other entity starts using the new IS at a time. Once consistently successful, the next group is implemented. For example, the 3W nursing unit starts ordering everything using the new IS, but nobody else uses the system. The next unit scheduled would be unit 3E. Again, this method is designed to limit the impact on the healthcare facility.

Big Bang Method

The last method, the big bang method (also called the cutover method), is the riskiest. With this method, the healthcare facility stops using the old IS and starts using the new system. It is the riskiest because the healthcare facility may not have the old system as a backup and the new IS is being used all over the hospital.

Parallel Processing

Parallel processing is similar to parallel testing, as described in the testing section. Although parallel start-up works well, it is labor intensive and therefore expensive. Because the old IS is in place and current, this approach provides a safety net and has the least amount of risk involved.

Straight Turnover

With straight turnover, the former system and processes cease with the implementation of the new IS. There is a risk here if the new IS has to be aborted; however, it is more cost effective and reduces the work load significantly because there is no duplication of efforts.

Planning for Go-Live

Whichever method is chosen, planning is critical because IS implementation cannot interfere with patient care. Certain steps should be taken no matter which plan is selected.

Initial Support

There should be a member of the project team in every unit or department when the IS goes live. These project team members should be highly visible to one another; for example, they could wear matching shirts. Project team members are needed to answer questions and generally ensure that the IS start-up runs as smoothly as possible. Trainers play an important role not only in the training but also during go-live, which means they are a key part of the implementation presence throughout the healthcare facility.

Ongoing Support

Initially, someone must be available 24 hours a day, 7 days a week to assist users. The length of time that this intensive support is needed will depend on the magnitude of the IS and how well the implementation is going. Generally, this intensive support is needed for only a few days. There should be a help desk that users can call when help is needed. The amount of coverage will eventually be reduced to the regular help desk support. The project team must be prepared to go back to the old IS if the new one does not work.

System Evaluation

After the new IS is implemented and functioning properly, the project team will need to evaluate how well the implementation went. System evaluation is how the healthcare facility determines whether or not the IS functions as expected. The project team needs to learn what did and did not work during the implementation process and determine how they can improve the next implementation. For example, the team may not have started system testing early enough, or maybe there were expenses that were not budgeted for. The project team will also want to know if the healthcare facility met the goals that were established for the project and if the project came in on budget. This evaluation allows the project team to learn from mistakes and from the experience.

After a predetermined time period, the project team will need to determine if the healthcare facility has realized all expected benefits and all of the goals that were established during the planning and analysis phase. For example, did the healthcare facility save the money that was expected, or did it reduce the turnaround time on obtaining test results?

In the immediate support and evaluation period, problems may be found that were not revealed during the system testing and will need to be resolved. Changes may be needed to correct the problems and more testing will be done. Even after the system is working well, periodic updates will ensure that the IS is current. There will also be routine maintenance and upgrades, such as backing up data, increasing storage capacity, and upgrading hardware and software. As discussed earlier, major computer systems have what is called a test system or a test environment.

It is in the test environment, and not the production environment, that the software changes can be tested without worrying about problems resulting from the changes. This will enable support staff to solve problems before the update is live; once the IS is working appropriately in the test environment, it can be implemented into the live one.

Also in this stage, there will come a time when the IS is no longer meeting the needs of the healthcare facility. The vendor may stop supporting it, the healthcare facility may need more functionality or users than the current system will accommodate, and other needs may arise. When this obsolescence occurs the process begins again.

CHECK YOUR UNDERSTANDING 5.2

1. Where is an update to software loaded first, before the users start using it, to ensure it works as expected?

   a. Production environment
   b. Test environment
   c. Training environment
   d. Pilot implementation

2. Which of the following denotes the go-live model in which the old system and the new system are used at the same time?

   a. Phased
   b. Pilot
   c. Cutover
   d. Parallel

3. Which of the following is an adult learning principle?

   a. Adults need to see relevance.
   b. Adults like to be told what to do.
   c. Adults learn well even if not motivated.
   d. Adults have the same knowledge and experience.

4. The type of testing that ensures that all components of the IS work together is known as
   _____.

   a. Volume testing
   b. Integration testing
   c. Parallel testing
   d. Application testing

5. The implementation stage when the team determines what they could have done better is known as

   a. Training
   b. Testing
   c. Support and evaluation
   d. Systems analysis

Real-World Case

Home Health of America is about to implement the new EHR. This EHR will be used by all of the nurses, nursing aides, therapists, and other staff members who work with patients in the patient's home. It will also be accessed in the home office for billing and other administrative purposes. The chief executive officer mandated the big bang go-live strategy. He also mandated that the go-live begin on Monday, which is their busiest day. His thoughts were that if the EHR could handle Monday, then it could handle anything. The users ran into several problems on the first day. Some of the functionality did not work, the cellular connections used to connect to the IS did not work at some of the homes, and the documentation was slow, which prevented them from seeing the patients in a timely manner. They had planned for some overtime as they knew that documenting in the new EHR would be slower. The overtime ended up being twice what was expected and they still did not see three of the patients. The decision was made to go back to the paper system while the problems were worked out.

CHAPTER REVIEW

1. Installing an update to the information is performed in which SDLC stage?

   a. Planning and analysis
   b. Design
   c. Implomontation
   d. Support and evaluation

2. If the healthcare facility wants to avoid risk during go-live, which go-live strategy should be used?

   a. Straight turnover
   b. Big bang
   c. Pilot
   d. Parallel processing

3. The type of testing that addresses the sharing of data from a source system to the new IS is known as _____.

   a. Interface testing
   b. Integration testing
   c. Application testing
   d. Conversion testing

4. Identify the adult learning principle.

   a. Adults do not need content to be relevant to their position.
   b. Adults like to be told what to do.
   c. Adults need to know why.
   d. Adults do not have to be prepared to learn.

5. Identify the true statement about conversion of data.

   a. Conversion of data is only needed in rare instances.
   b. Conversion of data requires interfaces to be programmed.
   c. Conversion of data is only needed in integrated systems.
   d. Conversion of data is only needed when multiple ISs are connected together.

6. The training evaluation outcome that identifies how performance has changed is known as _____.

   a. Reaction
   b. Learning
   c. Behavior
   d. Results

7. Select the policy that should be adopted regarding screen design.

   a. Bright colors should be used for text on computer screens.
   b. Color should be used throughout the screen to draw attention to the different fields.
   c. Fields should be in logical order.
   d. All fields on a screen should use the same field type.

8. Which of the following denotes the go-live model in which the implementation of the new system is first used in one department or nursing unit?

   a. Phased
   b. Pilot
   c. Cutover
   d. Parallel

(Continued)

CHAPTER REVIEW (*Continued*)

9. The type of testing that ensures that the information system can handle a large number of transactions at the same time is known as _____.

   a. Volume testing
   b. Integration testing
   c. Parallel testing
   d. Application testing

10. When conducting reengineering what question should be constantly asked?

    a. When?
    b. How?
    c. Why?
    d. Where?

References

Amatayakul, M. K. 2017. *Health IT and EHRS: Principles and Practice.* Chicago: AHIMA.

Florida Institute of Technology. 2017. Information Systems vs. Information Technology. https://www.floridatechonline.com/blog/information-technology/information-systems-vs-information-technology/.

Patena, K. R. 2016. Employee Training and Development. Chapter 24 in *Health Information Management: Concepts, Principles, and Practice*, 5th ed. Edited by P. Oachs and A. Watters. Chicago: AHIMA.

Rollins, G. 2006. The perils of customization. http://library.ahima.org/doc?oid=64283#.Wn-NJuRy5jo

Computers in HIM

Learning Objectives

- Identify the information systems needed to support efficient operations in the health information management (HIM) department.
- Differentiate between the various software products used in the HIM department.
- Improve the quality of the data within the HIM systems.

Key Terms

Automated codebook encoder
Birth certificate information
  system
Cancer registry information system
Chart deficiency system
Chart locator system
Chart tracking system
Clinical documentation
  improvement (CDI) system

Computer-assisted coding (CAC)
  system
Dictation system
Disclosure management
  system
Encoder
Expander
Grouper
Health informatics

Healthcare quality indicator
  system
Natural language processing
  (NLP)
Release of information (ROI)
  system
Rules-based encoder
Trauma registry software
Transcription system

The entire culture of health information management (HIM) is changing to accommodate the increasing use of technology, changing avenues of patient care, and consumer demands upon the healthcare field. Informatics is a term that has been added to many HIM educational programs to indicate this change and to reflect the growing change that is occurring within HIM. Health informatics is the scientific discipline that is concerned with the cognitive, information-processing, and communication tasks of healthcare practice, education, and research, including the information science and technology to support these tasks.

HIM professionals in all settings must be acutely aware of technological evolution and the impact it has on their profession. These professionals engage in designing software for HIM and patient care, develop and implement information systems for clinical and administrative research, conduct and analyze research in many areas of healthcare, and manage and improve training and education on new technology and processes for all levels of healthcare professionals, among many other duties (ONC 2016).

Information systems are critical to the HIM department. Many of the department's processes depend on information systems to function efficiently and effectively. Some of the information systems used by the

HIM department staff, such as the master patient index and the financial information system, are available to authorized users throughout the organization.

Other information systems are designed specifically for HIM functions, which may limit the usage to the HIM department only or for other departments to use to support the HIM department or the health record. Healthcare facilities vary in their organizational structure; as a result, some of these information systems may be used by staff in other departments but in support of HIM. For example, the birth certificate software may be solely used by the HIM department to create and report births occurring in the healthcare facility, whereas the dictation system may be purchased and managed by the HIM department but is used by physicians. All of these HIM systems greatly improve the efficiency and effectiveness of the HIM department. The HIM systems include the following:

- Release of information (ROI) and disclosure management systems
- Encoder and grouper system
- Cancer and other registry systems
- Chart locator system
- Birth certificate system
- Chart deficiency system
- Transcription system
- Healthcare quality indicators system
- Dictation system
- Computer-assisted coding (CAC) system
- Clinical documentation improvement (CDI) system

This chapter presents an overview of the information systems that support the HIM functions and their functionality, common data elements found in these systems, and reports.

Release of Information and Disclosure Management Systems

The HIM department receives requests for copies of health records on a daily basis. These requests for copies of health records must be logged into the information system to allow for tracking on the status of the request. The release of information (ROI) system is designed to manage the processing of requests for protected health information (PHI) received and processed by the HIM department. For more on PHI, refer to chapter 13. Use of the information system begins when a new request is entered into it. It continues to track the request as it is processed and acts as a historical database of all requests processed and ultimately used to generate reports.

A disclosure management system tracks the disclosures made throughout the healthcare facility for reporting purposes. Disclosure is the release, transfer, provision of access to, or divulging in any manner of information outside the healthcare facility holding the information. This tracking is required by the Health Insurance Portability and Accountability Act (HIPAA). The covered entities (discussed in chapter 13) must provide the patient with an accounting of disclosures upon request. The disclosure management system may be part of the ROI system or it may be a separate information system used by HIM and non-HIM departments. In addition to disclosures, a disclosure management system may also track requests for amendments to PHI as well as restrictions to disclosures. If a separate disclosure management system is used, it would also have a link to the hospital information system to populate basic patient demographic information. It would keep up with who received information, what information was provided, date of release, any charge for accounting of disclosures, and more.

ROI System Functionality

The ROI system is a valuable tool for the ROI staff. Once the requests for copies of records are entered into the ROI system, the data can be used for many different purposes to support the workflow.

The ROI staff also can use the system to check on the status of requests. The staff will be able to determine where in the process the request is and to whom the request has been assigned. The patient's name or health record number can be entered and the appropriate request opened to identify status and the personnel responsible.

Throughout the release process, the status of a request must be updated and kept current by ROI staff at all times. The status can include details about issues encountered, a need for review by risk management, a need for a health record or microfilm to be pulled, or other action required. Once the health record has been copied (in hard-copy or electronically) or reports printed, the request should be marked as complete. Completed requests generally include an indicator showing that the request is in the complete status, the date processed, and specifically what has been sent. Individual reports and dates of reports would also be entered. Based on the number of copies and other activities, the ROI staff would also record any changes that were applied. See figure 6.1 for a workflow diagram of a typical ROI process.

Figure 6.1.   ROI process

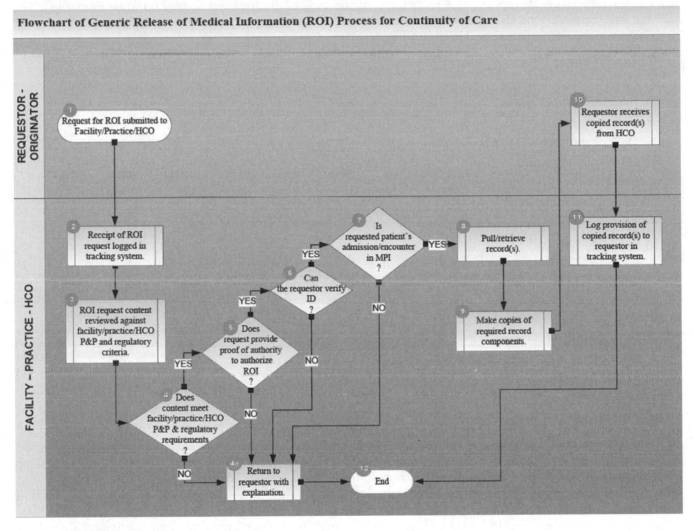

Source: Betz et al. 2013.

The ROI system provides a number of reports and statistics for the HIM management team. Some of the data provided to the management team include the following:

- Requests that have not been processed
- Requests that have been processed
- Turnaround time of requests
- Revenue collected
- Accounts receivable
- Productivity by individual staff members
- Overall productivity
- List of frequent requesters
- Multiple customized letters

If the supervisor receives a complaint from a requester regarding the inability to obtain copies of health records, the ROI system would be the first place to start investigating the situation. The ROI system also can be used toward the healthcare facility's **HIPAA** compliance because it provides some of the information needed to respond to an accounting of disclosure request. This accounting report includes by whom and when request was made; the specific information requested; the process to release; when, how, and to whom information was transmitted; and more. The ROI system and the disclosure management system work together. Management may periodically archive old requests in the ROI system, but the completed requests should not be deleted until after retention requirements are met so that the disclosure management system can use the data to create reports. HIPAA requires accounting of disclosure information to be available to the patient for three years, so that is the minimum amount of time for the requests to be maintained.

Common data elements found in an ROI system are:

- Patient name
- Health record number
- Patient type
- Date request received
- Type of requester
- Name of requester
- Name of contact at requester
- Address of requester
- Type of request (for example, insurance, patient, attorney, or patient care)
- Assigned to
- Action taken (request completed, type of letter sent, records requested, valid authorization needed, and more)
- Date action taken
- Date request completed
- Information sent (specific documents and dates of reports)
- Charges
- Amount paid
- Amount due
- Comments

The basic patient information, such as name and health record number, are frequently populated in the ROI system by an interface from the admission, discharge, or transfer information system, thus eliminating the need to enter this information. An interface is the zone between different information systems across which users want to pass information (for example, a computer program written to exchange information between the information systems or the graphic display of an application program designed to make the program easier to use). This link between the two information systems improves data quality because there is consistency in the data and reduced risk of typographical error. Typically, the requests can be retrieved by items such as patient name, health record number, or requester name.

Tables are an important part of the ROI system. Some tables are the default within the information system while others can be set up and customized by the healthcare facility. For example, the user only has to enter the name and address of a requester once, thus managing time wisely. After the initial entry, the user is able to select the requester from a drop-down box or other graphical user interface tool. This customization function improves the efficiency of the processes making it easier and faster for the employee to complete the task. If the requester is from a large organization, there can be a table listing individuals in that organization so that the copies are forwarded to the correct person. Tables also may be used to record charge information, such as charge per copy, microfilm, certification, and other chargeable actions.

Another use of tables is identifying all of the individual forms or groups of forms that may be released. The table may list discharge summary, history and physical examination, operative report, pathology report, laboratory report, and other forms individually. The ROI system may feature requests for common groupings of reports, such as the entire health record or the discharge summary and history and physical examination. Tables help to save the user a significant amount of time because the user does not have to individually type each document released. Drop-down boxes or check boxes containing the individual documents or sets of documents also allow for consistent data entry.

The ROI system will allow ROI staff to pull up a work queue showing the requests that need to be processed. With the use of the electronic health record (EHR), more of the requests can be fulfilled without the need for the paper health record. ROI staff members just need to print, fax, or generate a CD (or other portable electronic storage media) of the requested documents from the appropriate information system. Once the number of pages and other chargeable actions are known, the ROI coordinator can post the charges into the information system and, once received, post payment.

The ROI software can perform many other tasks. For instance, the ROI system reminds the ROI staff of the need to perform maintenance tasks on the information system, which can include backups, deletion of old requests, or archiving of completed requests to speed processing.

Reporting

Reporting is an important part of an ROI system. Reports are used by ROI or HIM staff and to communicate with requesters. In a paper environment, the ROI coordinators can generate a list of health records to be pulled so that the appropriate contents of the record can be copied. This list can be sorted into terminal digit or other numeric or alphabetic order to facilitate the retrieval process. Depending on the structure of the department, the ROI or file area staff can use this list to retrieve the paper records.

Customized letters are critical to the ROI system. Customized letters and forms may be used to communicate with the requester for many purposes, including to:

- Notify requester that the healthcare facility does not have a record of the patient being treated at the healthcare facility or on that date
- Remind requesters that they have an outstanding balance for copies of health records
- Request that copies of health records be paid prior to their release
- Provide cover letter for health records being sent
- Notify requester that the authorization is invalid
- Notify requester that an authorization is needed
- Notify requester that there will be a delay in the release of the information
- Notify requester that the health records will be released as soon as the healthcare facility has received prepayment for copies
- Generate invoices for the copies of the health record
- Generate reminder invoices when payment is not received in a timely manner

HIM department managers monitor the efficiency of the ROI staff through a multitude of management reports. These reports provide information on various functions including turnaround times, productivity, backlogs, revenue, and accounts receivable, to name a few. Depending on the information contained in the report, the report can include requests by employee, by requester type, by specific requester, or all requests. For example, a report on the average turnaround time for all requests or for BlueCross BlueShield requests can be obtained. The manager also can track the turnaround times by employee, which can be used in performance evaluations and other management monitoring. Many of these reports come prepackaged with the software, but many information systems allow users to develop and customize their own routine and ad hoc reports.

Encoder and Grouper

Healthcare facilities must assign diagnosis and procedure codes to every patient encounter. These codes are submitted to the insurance company on the bill. The encoder is specialty software used by coders to select the appropriate code for the diagnosis(es) and procedure(s) supported by the health record. There are two types of encoders. A rules-based encoder requires the user to type in the name or portion of the name of the diagnosis or procedure. This entry into the encoder generates a list of suggestions from which the coder selects. For example, if the coder types in pneu-, the encoder may suggest pneumonia and pneumonitis. From there the coder scrolls down until the proper code is selected. The automated codebook encoder lists diagnoses and procedures in alphabetic order much like the alphabetic index located in the *International Classification of Diseases, Tenth Revision, Clinical Modification* (ICD-10-CM) and *Current Procedural Terminology* (CPT) codebooks. This similarity eases the transition from the book to the encoder.

The grouper is a computer program that uses specific data elements to assign the diagnostic and procedural codes entered into the encoder into the appropriate Medicare severity diagnosis-related group (MS-DRG) or other diagnosis-related group (DRG). The grouper uses the appropriate grouping software for the insurer assigned to the patient. The most common groupers are the MS-DRG grouper and ambulatory payment classification (APC) grouper; however, other insurers, including some Medicaid programs, have developed their own groupers for use in determining payment to the healthcare facility. The MS-DRG or other DRG indicates the amount of reimbursement owed to the healthcare organization from the insurer. The grouper software is connected to the billing system so it is important that the HIM staff have a strong relationship with the billing and finance personnel.

Coding quality and MS-DRG assignment are not ensured using an encoder because the code selected is only as good as the data entered into the information system. It is the responsibility of the coder to identify the correct diagnoses and procedures to be coded and entered into the encoder appropriately.

Encoder and Grouper System Functionality

One of the biggest advantages in the use of an encoder or grouper is prompts. For example, if a higher-paying MS-DRG can be assigned with the addition of a specific diagnosis, specific procedure, complication and comorbidity, or major complication and comorbidity, then the computer will ask the coder if any of them are present. The grouper allows the coder to resequence the principal diagnosis when more than one diagnosis meets the definition of the principal diagnosis. The coding guidelines allow the healthcare facility to choose any of the diagnoses as the principal as long as it qualifies. The encoder can assign the ICD-10-CM, ICD-10-PCS, CPT, and Healthcare Common Procedural Coding System (HCPCS) codes required on the patient claim. These assigned codes must be validated through the Medicare Code Editor, the National Correct Coding Initiative, and other edits. These edits will look for invalid codes, illogical codes, nonspecific codes, and other possible errors. For example, the coder cannot give a newborn code to an adult and cannot assign a hysterectomy code to a male. These edits are designed to catch errors before they can be submitted on a claim improperly and to improve the quality of the code assignment.

Coders are also permitted to manually enter codes into the information system rather than looking them up each time. For the more frequent diagnoses, such as diabetes or dehydration, this is a more efficient method. Once entered, the information system will then confirm and validate the code.

Common data elements in an encoder or grouper are:

- Admitting diagnosis
- Principal diagnosis
- Secondary diagnoses
- Principal procedure
- Secondary procedure
- Age of patient (or date of birth)
- Discharge disposition
- Gender
- Patient name
- Health record number
- Account number

The encoder and grouper are usually linked to the hospital's financial information system so that the codes can be automatically transferred to that information system for billing. Without this link, the coder would have to reenter codes into the financial information system. This double entry leaves room for data entry errors, which would in turn cause problems with billing and reimbursement.

Encoder and Grouper System Reporting

The encoder or grouper does not contribute heavily to reporting. Rather, the encoder is more about assigning codes and MS-DRGs using edits to assist the coder in proper assignment of codes and other information transferred to the hospital financial system. However, if needed, the information system may be used to generate a report listing all of the codes and respective MS-DRGs or APCs assigned.

CHECK YOUR UNDERSTANDING 6.1

1. Which of the following software programs should one use to assign the diagnosis and procedure codes?

   a. Registry
   b. Release of information
   c. Encoder
   d. Grouper

2. Which of the following is the type of encoder that mimics a codebook?

   a. Rules-based encoder
   b. Release of information
   c. Automated codebook encoder
   d. Disclosure management

3. A software program designed to place similar diagnoses codes into organized categories and calculate reimbursement depending on diagnoses and procedural codes is a(n) _____.

   a. Grouper
   b. Release of information
   c. Disclosure management
   d. Encoder

4. The information system used to notify requesters of invalid authorization is called a(n) _____.

   a. Grouper
   b. Release of information
   c. Registry
   d. Encoder

5. Which information system would keep track of what health information was sent to authorized requesters?

   a. Grouper
   b. Release of information
   c. Disclosure management
   d. Encoder

Cancer and Other Registries

There are many types of registries currently found in healthcare. A registry is a collection of care information related to a specific disease, condition, or procedure that makes health record information available for analysis and comparison. These registries track conditions such as cancer, diabetes, trauma, and transplants. Although registry software across these different diseases and situations has similarities, each has its own unique characteristics. All registries are designed to record data on patients who meet criteria for inclusion in the registry. These registries would generally require basic demographic information, reporting, treatment, description of condition, and frequently long-term patient tracking. Commonly found data elements across registries include:

- Patient name
- Health record number
- Dates of service
- Physician

- Date of birth
- Date of diagnosis

Two common registries will be discussed in more detail—cancer (tumor) and trauma registries.

Cancer (Tumor) Registry

The **cancer registry information system** tracks information about the patient's cancer from the time of diagnosis to the patient's death. The cancer registry information systems are extremely complex and track very detailed information regarding diagnosis and treatment. Some of the common data elements unique to the cancer registry include:

- Site of cancer
- Type of cancer
- Treatment received
- Date of last contact
- TNM (tumor, node, metastasis) stage
- Number of lymph nodes involved
- Behavior type
- Date of death
- Grade of neoplasm
- Size of mass
- Physician name
- Accession number
- *International Classification of Diseases for Oncology* (ICD-O) code (CDC 2017)

Cancer Registry Functionality

The cancer registry can electronically submit a file containing the data required for state cancer reporting. Once data on all the identified cancer cases for a designated time period are verified by the cancer registrar (or designee) of the healthcare facility, a programmed report is automatically generated and transmitted to the respective state-wide cancer registry normally housed in the state's Department of Health. As the patient's treatment and clinical follow-up progress, this information is entered into the registry so that it reflects the patient's current treatment and status of the cancer. Figure 6.2 shows an information system that supports pathology analysis for staging the cancer to determine the severity of a diagnosis for a particular case.

Edits assist the cancer registrar in the data entry and cancer staging. These edits, which vary widely, are key to ensuring the quality of the data in the registry. For example, an edit can notify the user that data, such as the discharge date, has been entered in an inappropriate format. It should be entered in MMDDYYYY format rather than MMDDYY. An edit may also verify that a code number is valid. Cancer registry software can also assist the registrar in the patient follow-up process. The software tracks the last contact date and manages letters and other activities related to the follow-up process.

Cancer registry software typically provides many functions for the registry staff. Some examples of this functionality are:

- Checking the Social Security Death Index to see if the patient died
- Transferring data to the state registry
- Performing edit checks on data entered
- Performing various cancer staging methods to determine severity of the illness
- Providing links to SEER (surveillance epidemiology and end results) manuals
- Referencing previous versions of staging systems such as Facility Oncology Registry Data Standards (FORDS)
- Assigning an accession number
- Suspending records for abstracting when the documentation is incomplete
- Providing a list of disclosures made for compliance with the HIPAA accounting of disclosure
- Validating the ICD-O code

Figure 6.2. Information system used for cancer staging

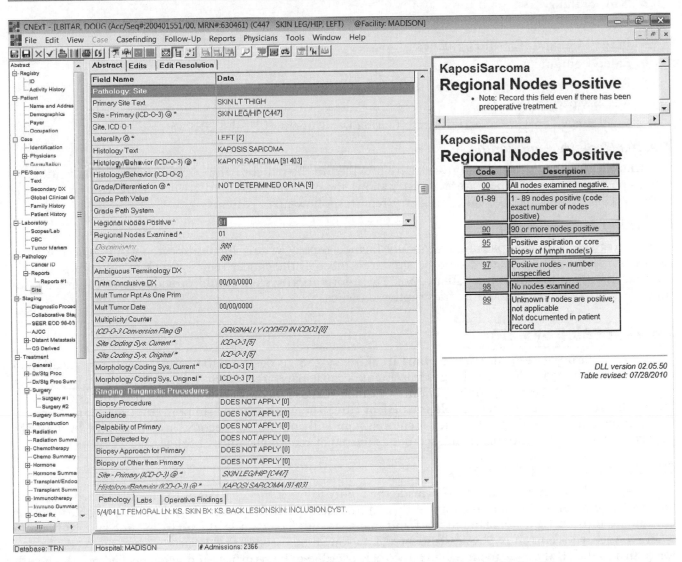

Source: CNet 2018. Reprinted with permission from CNET, a program of the Public Health Institute.

Cancer Registry Reporting

Reporting is a key function of the cancer registry system. The information system can provide management reports such as productivity as well as reports on the content of the registry. Common reports include life expectancy, follow-up rate, list of patients due for follow-up, patients lost to follow-up, and follow-up letters to patients and physicians. The registry will also allow the reporting of patient-specific information such as patient abstracts and accounting of disclosures.

Ad hoc reporting is an important part of a registry. These reports would be designed specifically for a research project or other purpose for which the report is being run. For example, these reports could be based on site of cancer, cell type of cancer, life expectancy, or treatment modalities.

Trauma Registry

Trauma registry software tracks patients with traumatic injuries from initial trauma treatment to death. Data elements in this system include:

- Site of injury
- Type of injury
- How injury occurred

- Date of injury
- Time of injury
- Work-related injury
- ICD-10-CM and ICD-10-PCS codes
- Safety equipment
- Registry number
- Autopsy performed
- Emergency department arrival time (Florida Department of Health 2017a)

Trauma Registry Functionality

The trauma registry software also tracks care provided to the patient before and during hospitalization, as well as posthospital care. The trauma registry allows the registrar to code ICD-10-CM diagnosis codes to the injuries. This registry, like the cancer registry, requires follow-up of patients.

Reporting

Trauma registry software packages generally include report writers for ad hoc reporting. The common reports for the trauma registry would be similar to those of the cancer registry, such as outcomes, follow-up rates, and best practices for patient care. The information system would provide statistics on cause of injuries, types of injuries, and other descriptive statistics.

Chart Locator System

The **chart locator system**, also called **chart tracking system**, is designed to identify the current location of the paper health record. This tracking is important because paper records are moved from place to place for patient care, quality reviews, coding, and many other purposes. The Joint Commission regulations require health records to be readily accessible for patient care. The chart locator supports that mandate. Because of the transition to the EHR, the chart locator system will continue to become less important to the HIM department and will eventually be phased out as the paper record becomes obsolete.

Chart Locator Functionality

The purpose of the chart locator is to provide the ability to track the location of the health record from one location to another. All of the functions of this information system support this objective. The chart locator is valuable to both HIM department staff and management. The data in the chart locator system identify where the record is currently physically located, how long it has been in that location, when the record is due for return to the HIM department, when a record is overdue to be returned, and who checked out the health record. These data are used to generate a list of records checked out to a location for auditing to ensure that the data in the chart locator system is accurate.

The emergency department and other locations may need 1 record or 50 records. When checking out multiple records to one location, the user only has to enter the location once and then enter all of the records being relocated. This entry of health records into the chart locator system is frequently supported by barcodes, which, at a minimum, contain the patient's health record number and volume number of the record. Barcodes speed the data entry process and improve the quality of the data entered, thus improving the efficiency and effectiveness of checking in and out records.

Common data elements in the chart locator are:

- Patient name
- Health record number
- Volume
- Location to which the record is checked out
- Date record checked out
- Date record returned
- Who checked out/checked in the record

The information system may provide the previous locations of the record. This may be helpful in locating lost health records because it can help the user determine where in the process the health record has been and where it may have gone. Past locations may also be useful in privacy incident investigation or other risk management investigations to know who has had access to the record. For example, if an employee has been accused of improperly disclosing a patient's PHI, it would be important to know if the record has been in a location to which that employee would have had access.

Data quality is important because a significant amount of time can be wasted looking for records when the paper health record is not where the chart locator indicates. Tables, which are preprogrammed lists and options for a user to select from, can be used to save time and improve data quality. For example, only approved locations would be programmed into the "Locations" table. As a result, the user would choose the location desired from a drop-down box.

These tables are generally user defined during the implementation. The user can update the tables as needed to keep the content of the data current. To keep the chart location system accurate, routine audits should be conducted. These audits would confirm that records checked out to a location are actually at that location. It would also identify health records located outside the permanent file that had not been checked out at all.

Chart Locator Reporting

Management uses the chart locator reporting for multiple purposes, including identification of most user requests of health records, productivity tracking, identification of trends in the volume of health record retrievals, and identification of areas of the healthcare facility for which records are not returned in a timely manner.

Chart Deficiency

Physicians and other clinicians have certain documentation requirements mandated by healthcare facility policy and medical staff rules and regulations. Documentation requirements are based on the accreditation regulations, state licensure regulations, federal requirements, and other standards or regulations that the healthcare facility is subject to. The specific documentation requirements mandate when reports such as the history and physical examination should be dictated or written. It should also mandate the content of the various reports analyzed and the deadline by which the entire health record should be complete. This deadline would include the presence of all required documents and the authentication of these documents. If the health record comes to the HIM department with a deficiency, then the documentation omission is recorded and tracked in the chart deficiency system. Deficiencies can be in paper, imaged, or electronic records depending on the information system used. With imaged or electronic records, the physician can complete the deficiency from his or her office, home, or other location. With paper records, the physician must come to the designated area in the healthcare facility. The chart deficiency system should be linked to the hospital information system so that patient name, discharge date, and other demographic information are maintained and automatically populated. With the implementation of the EHR, the need for a separate chart deficiency system is reduced or eliminated. The limited deficiency analysis needed in the future will be built into the EHR.

Functionality

The chart deficiency system is utilized by both staff and management. The chart deficiency system is used by staff to record what deficiencies a physician, or other clinician, has on specific health records. When these deficiencies are completed by the physician, the chart deficiency system is updated to reflect the change. The chart deficiency system will identify the incomplete records by physician so that the physician can be notified for completion. The following data elements are common:

- Patient name
- Health record number
- Discharge date
- Physician needing to complete deficiency
- Type of document with deficiency (for example, history and physical examination, discharge summary, or progress note)
- Type of deficiency (for example, sign or dictate)
- Date of surgery

- Comments
- Date physician last worked on records

When a patient is discharged from the hospital, the health record is automatically reviewed for deficiencies. When a deficiency is identified, the analyst is generally able to retrieve basic demographic information of the patient from the chart deficiency system. The analyst then enters other pertinent information, such as discharge date, physician, document type, type of deficiency, date of surgery, and any other information needed into the chart deficiency system. In a paper environment, sticky tabs or flags are frequently posted on the health record to indicate to the physician where a signature is needed. In an electronic environment, a work queue would route the deficiencies automatically to the assigned physician. The physician could then automatically complete all needed deficiencies from home, the office, or anywhere in the hospital.

When the physician dictates, signs, or completes the deficiency, the analyst is able to delete or update the status of the deficiency. An example of updating the deficiency would be to change the deficiency from dictated to transcribed or from transcribed to signed. Frequently there is an interface between the chart deficiency system and the transcription system to automatically update the transcription deficiency. There may also be a link between the dictation system and the chart deficiency system to automatically update the status when a report had been dictated or transcribed. This link would also help staff locate paper records for completion.

Data quality is critical to the chart deficiency system. Records inappropriately entered into the system can also have a negative impact on the accreditation or state/federal regulatory statistics as well as customer service. To improve data quality, routine audits of the records should be conducted to ensure that records are still incomplete and available to the physician.

Chart Deficiency System Reporting

Management uses the chart deficiency system to age the deficiencies for the Joint Commission tracking. The chart deficiency system can generate a report listing all physicians suspended for delinquent health records (an incomplete record not finished or made complete within the time frame determined by the medical staff of the facility), track when physicians are suspended (for use in medical staff credentialing), and monitor the volume of deficiencies by physician and service. A list of all health records in the information system can be printed out for use in auditing the quality of the data in the chart deficiency system.

The chart deficiency system also has customizable letters. These letters can be used for many purposes including notifying physicians that they have a deadline to complete health records, that they have been suspended for delinquent health records (or other penalty for noncompliance with medical staff rules and regulations), or to thank physicians for completing their health record(s).

CHECK YOUR UNDERSTANDING 6.2

1. Diagnostic codes assigned from the ICD-O to the patient record and abstract are found in which software program?

    a. Trauma registry
    b. Chart locator
    c. Release of information
    d. Cancer registry

2. Which type of software tracks patients who meet criteria for inclusion such as a specific disease or treatment?

    a. Registry
    b. Chart deficiency
    c. Chart locator
    d. Release of information

3. Which information system tracks the location of the paper health record?

    a. Chart deficiency
    b. Chart locator
    c. Release of information
    d. Disclosure management

4. Which information system collects the TNM stage?

    a. Chart locator
    b. Disclosure management
    c. Release of information
    d. Cancer registry software

5. What software can identify all patients admitted in 20XX due to injuries resulting from motor vehicle accidents (MVAs)?

    a. Trauma registry
    b. Disclosure management
    c. Release of information
    d. Cancer registry software

Birth Certificate System

For years, birth certificates were typed on a typewriter and manually sent to the local health department. Now, after the HIM staff interviews the mother or other parents or guardians and reviews the health record, the birth certificate data are entered into a state-approved **birth certificate information system**. This software reports births occurring in the healthcare facility to the state health agency. Birth certificate software will capture the minimum data set established by the National Center for Health Statistics (NCHS) and any state-required data. Figure 6.3 shows the standard content of a US birth certificate.

Functionality

Functionality common in birth certificate information systems includes:

- Collecting data mandated by NCHS
- Reporting standard information such as name of healthcare facility automatically
- Allowing users to choose from obstetrical physicians table
- Capturing demographic information from hospital information system to improve efficiency
- Preventing omissions of required data before birth certificate is sent to the state using mandatory fields and edit checks
- Submitting birth certificate data to the state or local health department
- Submitting parent's request for social security number to the Social Security Administration
- Printing out data captured for parent(s) to proof
- Creating birth log, eliminating need for paper log in labor and delivery
- Using drop-down boxes to improve data consistency
- Using edits to improve data quality
- Allowing parent(s) to order copy of birth certificate (Florida Department of Health 2017b)

Some electronic birth registration systems have incorporated the preparation of fetal death reports as well. Additionally, most information systems allow the healthcare facility to download the data on their births to a spreadsheet so that they can create their own reports.

Many birth certificate fields have check boxes for completion. For example, the field for infections present or treated during pregnancy lists gonorrhea, syphilis, chlamydia, hepatitis B, hepatitis C, and none of these.

Figure 6.3. Content of US birth certificate of live birth

U.S. STANDARD CERTIFICATE OF LIVE BIRTH

LOCAL FILE NO.   BIRTH NUMBER:

C H I L D
1. CHILD'S NAME (First, Middle, Last, Suffix) | 2. TIME OF BIRTH (24 hr) | 3. SEX | 4. DATE OF BIRTH (Mo/Day/Yr)

5. FACILITY NAME (If not institution, give street and number) | 6. CITY, TOWN, OR LOCATION OF BIRTH | 7. COUNTY OF BIRTH

M O T H E R
8a. MOTHER'S CURRENT LEGAL NAME (First, Middle, Last, Suffix) | 8b. DATE OF BIRTH (Mo/Day/Yr)

8c. MOTHER'S NAME PRIOR TO FIRST MARRIAGE (First, Middle, Last, Suffix) | 8d. BIRTHPLACE (State, Territory, or Foreign Country)

9a. RESIDENCE OF MOTHER-STATE | 9b. COUNTY | 9c. CITY, TOWN, OR LOCATION

9d. STREET AND NUMBER | 9e. APT. NO. | 9f. ZIP CODE | 9g. INSIDE CITY LIMITS? □ Yes □ No

F A T H E R
10a. FATHER'S CURRENT LEGAL NAME (First, Middle, Last, Suffix) | 10b. DATE OF BIRTH (Mo/Day/Yr) | 10c. BIRTHPLACE (State, Territory, or Foreign Country)

CERTIFIER
11. CERTIFIER'S NAME: _____
TITLE: □ MD □ DO □ HOSPITAL ADMIN. □ CNM/CM □ OTHER MIDWIFE
□ OTHER (Specify)_____
| 12. DATE CERTIFIED ____ / ____ / ____ MM DD YYYY | 13. DATE FILED BY REGISTRAR ____ / ____ / ____ MM DD YYYY

INFORMATION FOR ADMINISTRATIVE USE

M O T H E R
14. MOTHER'S MAILING ADDRESS: □ Same as residence, or: State: ____ City, Town, or Location: ____
Street & Number: ____ Apartment No.: ____ Zip Code: ____

15. MOTHER MARRIED? (At birth, conception, or any time between) □ Yes □ No
IF NO, HAS PATERNITY ACKNOWLEDGEMENT BEEN SIGNED IN THE HOSPITAL? □ Yes □ No | 16. SOCIAL SECURITY NUMBER REQUESTED FOR CHILD? □ Yes □ No | 17. FACILITY ID. (NPI)

18. MOTHER'S SOCIAL SECURITY NUMBER: | 19. FATHER'S SOCIAL SECURITY NUMBER:

INFORMATION FOR MEDICAL AND HEALTH PURPOSES ONLY

M O T H E R

20. MOTHER'S EDUCATION (Check the box that best describes the highest degree or level of school completed at the time of delivery)
- □ 8th grade or less
- □ 9th - 12th grade, no diploma
- □ High school graduate or GED completed
- □ Some college credit but no degree
- □ Associate degree (e.g., AA, AS)
- □ Bachelor's degree (e.g., BA, AB, BS)
- □ Master's degree (e.g., MA, MS, MEng, MEd, MSW, MBA)
- □ Doctorate (e.g., PhD, EdD) or Professional degree (e.g., MD, DDS, DVM, LLB, JD)

21. MOTHER OF HISPANIC ORIGIN? (Check the box that best describes whether the mother is Spanish/Hispanic/Latina. Check the "No" box if mother is not Spanish/Hispanic/Latina)
- □ No, not Spanish/Hispanic/Latina
- □ Yes, Mexican, Mexican American, Chicana
- □ Yes, Puerto Rican
- □ Yes, Cuban
- □ Yes, other Spanish/Hispanic/Latina
(Specify)_____

22. MOTHER'S RACE (Check one or more races to indicate what the mother considers herself to be)
- □ White
- □ Black or African American
- □ American Indian or Alaska Native (Name of the enrolled or principal tribe)_____
- □ Asian Indian
- □ Chinese
- □ Filipino
- □ Japanese
- □ Korean
- □ Vietnamese
- □ Other Asian (Specify)_____
- □ Native Hawaiian
- □ Guamanian or Chamorro
- □ Samoan
- □ Other Pacific Islander (Specify)_____
- □ Other (Specify)_____

F A T H E R

23. FATHER'S EDUCATION (Check the box that best describes the highest degree or level of school completed at the time of delivery)
- □ 8th grade or less
- □ 9th - 12th grade, no diploma
- □ High school graduate or GED completed
- □ Some college credit but no degree
- □ Associate degree (e.g., AA, AS)
- □ Bachelor's degree (e.g., BA, AB, BS)
- □ Master's degree (e.g., MA, MS, MEng, MEd, MSW, MBA)
- □ Doctorate (e.g., PhD, EdD) or Professional degree (e.g., MD, DDS, DVM, LLB, JD)

24. FATHER OF HISPANIC ORIGIN? (Check the box that best describes whether the father is Spanish/Hispanic/Latino. Check the "No" box if father is not Spanish/Hispanic/Latino)
- □ No, not Spanish/Hispanic/Latino
- □ Yes, Mexican, Mexican American, Chicano
- □ Yes, Puerto Rican
- □ Yes, Cuban
- □ Yes, other Spanish/Hispanic/Latino
(Specify)_____

25. FATHER'S RACE (Check one or more races to indicate what the father considers himself to be)
- □ White
- □ Black or African American
- □ American Indian or Alaska Native (Name of the enrolled or principal tribe)_____
- □ Asian Indian
- □ Chinese
- □ Filipino
- □ Japanese
- □ Korean
- □ Vietnamese
- □ Other Asian (Specify)_____
- □ Native Hawaiian
- □ Guamanian or Chamorro
- □ Samoan
- □ Other Pacific Islander (Specify)_____
- □ Other (Specify)_____

Mother's Name | Mother's Medical Record No.

26. PLACE WHERE BIRTH OCCURRED (Check one)
- □ Hospital
- □ Freestanding birthing center
- □ Home Birth: Planned to deliver at home? □ Yes □ No
- □ Clinic/Doctor's office
- □ Other (Specify)_____

27. ATTENDANT'S NAME, TITLE, AND NPI
NAME: _____ NPI:_____
TITLE: □ MD □ DO □ CNM/CM □ OTHER MIDWIFE
□ OTHER (Specify)_____

28. MOTHER TRANSFERRED FOR MATERNAL MEDICAL OR FETAL INDICATIONS FOR DELIVERY? □ Yes □ No
IF YES, ENTER NAME OF FACILITY MOTHER TRANSFERRED FROM:
_____

REV. 11/2003

MOTHER

29a. DATE OF FIRST PRENATAL CARE VISIT	29b. DATE OF LAST PRENATAL CARE VISIT	30. TOTAL NUMBER OF PRENATAL VISITS FOR THIS PREGNANCY
___/___/___ □ No Prenatal Care MM DD YYYY	___/___/___ MM DD YYYY	_____ (If none, enter "0".)

31. MOTHER'S HEIGHT ____ (feet/inches)	32. MOTHER'S PREPREGNANCY WEIGHT ____ (pounds)	33. MOTHER'S WEIGHT AT DELIVERY ____ (pounds)	34. DID MOTHER GET WIC FOOD FOR HERSELF DURING THIS PREGNANCY? □ Yes □ No

35. NUMBER OF PREVIOUS LIVE BIRTHS (Do not include this child)		36. NUMBER OF OTHER PREGNANCY OUTCOMES (spontaneous or induced losses or ectopic pregnancies)	37. CIGARETTE SMOKING BEFORE AND DURING PREGNANCY For each time period, enter either the number of cigarettes or the number of packs of cigarettes smoked. IF NONE, ENTER "0".	38. PRINCIPAL SOURCE OF PAYMENT FOR THIS DELIVERY

35a. Now Living — Number ____ □ None
35b. Now Dead — Number ____ □ None
36a. Other Outcomes — Number ____ □ None

37. Average number of cigarettes or packs of cigarettes smoked per day.

	# of cigarettes		# of packs
Three Months Before Pregnancy	_____	OR	_____
First Three Months of Pregnancy	_____	OR	_____
Second Three Months of Pregnancy	_____	OR	_____
Third Trimester of Pregnancy	_____	OR	_____

38. PRINCIPAL SOURCE OF PAYMENT FOR THIS DELIVERY
□ Private Insurance
□ Medicaid
□ Self-pay
□ Other (Specify)_____

35c. DATE OF LAST LIVE BIRTH ___/___ MM YYYY	36b. DATE OF LAST OTHER PREGNANCY OUTCOME ___/___ MM YYYY	39. DATE LAST NORMAL MENSES BEGAN ___/___/___ MM DD YYYY	40. MOTHER'S MEDICAL RECORD NUMBER

MEDICAL AND HEALTH INFORMATION

41. RISK FACTORS IN THIS PREGNANCY (Check all that apply)

Diabetes
□ Prepregnancy (Diagnosis prior to this pregnancy)
□ Gestational (Diagnosis in this pregnancy)

Hypertension
□ Prepregnancy (Chronic)
□ Gestational (PIH, preeclampsia)
□ Eclampsia

□ Previous preterm birth

□ Other previous poor pregnancy outcome (Includes perinatal death, small-for-gestational age/intrauterine growth restricted birth)

□ Pregnancy resulted from infertility treatment-If yes, check all that apply:
□ Fertility-enhancing drugs, Artificial insemination or Intrauterine Insemination
□ Assisted reproductive technology (e.g., in vitro fertilization (IVF), gamete intrafallopian transfer (GIFT))

□ Mother had a previous cesarean delivery
If yes, how many _____

□ None of the above

42. INFECTIONS PRESENT AND/OR TREATED DURING THIS PREGNANCY (Check all that apply)
□ Gonorrhea
□ Syphilis
□ Chlamydia
□ Hepatitis B
□ Hepatitis C
□ None of the above

43. OBSTETRIC PROCEDURES (Check all that apply)
□ Cervical cerclage
□ Tocolysis

External cephalic version:
□ Successful
□ Failed

□ None of the above

44. ONSET OF LABOR (Check all that apply)
□ Premature Rupture of the Membranes (prolonged, ≥12 hrs.)
□ Precipitous Labor (<3 hrs.)
□ Prolonged Labor (≥ 20 hrs.)
□ None of the above

45. CHARACTERISTICS OF LABOR AND DELIVERY (Check all that apply)
□ Induction of labor
□ Augmentation of labor
□ Non-vertex presentation
□ Steroids (glucocorticoids) for fetal lung maturation received by the mother prior to delivery
□ Antibiotics received by the mother during labor
□ Clinical chorioamnionitis diagnosed during labor or maternal temperature ≥38°C (100.4°F)
□ Moderate/heavy meconium staining of the amniotic fluid
□ Fetal intolerance of labor such that one or more of the following actions was taken: in-utero resuscitative measures, further fetal assessment, or operative delivery
□ Epidural or spinal anesthesia during labor
□ None of the above

46. METHOD OF DELIVERY

A. Was delivery with forceps attempted but unsuccessful?
□ Yes □ No

B. Was delivery with vacuum extraction attempted but unsuccessful?
□ Yes □ No

C. Fetal presentation at birth
□ Cephalic
□ Breech
□ Other

D. Final route and method of delivery (Check one)
□ Vaginal/Spontaneous
□ Vaginal/Forceps
□ Vaginal/Vacuum
□ Cesarean
If cesarean, was a trial of labor attempted?
□ Yes
□ No

47. MATERNAL MORBIDITY (Check all that apply) (Complications associated with labor and delivery)
□ Maternal transfusion
□ Third or fourth degree perineal laceration
□ Ruptured uterus
□ Unplanned hysterectomy
□ Admission to intensive care unit
□ Unplanned operating room procedure following delivery
□ None of the above

NEWBORN INFORMATION

NEWBORN

48. NEWBORN MEDICAL RECORD NUMBER

49. BIRTHWEIGHT (grams preferred, specify unit)
____ grams ____ lb/oz

50. OBSTETRIC ESTIMATE OF GESTATION:
_____ (completed weeks)

51. APGAR SCORE:
Score at 5 minutes:_____
If 5 minute score is less than 6,
Score at 10 minutes: _____

52. PLURALITY - Single, Twin, Triplet, etc.
(Specify)_____

53. IF NOT SINGLE BIRTH - Born First, Second, Third, etc. (Specify) _____

54. ABNORMAL CONDITIONS OF THE NEWBORN (Check all that apply)
□ Assisted ventilation required immediately following delivery
□ Assisted ventilation required for more than six hours
□ NICU admission
□ Newborn given surfactant replacement therapy
□ Antibiotics received by the newborn for suspected neonatal sepsis
□ Seizure or serious neurologic dysfunction
□ Significant birth injury (skeletal fracture(s), peripheral nerve injury, and/or soft tissue/solid organ hemorrhage which requires intervention)
□ None of the above

55. CONGENITAL ANOMALIES OF THE NEWBORN (Check all that apply)
□ Anencephaly
□ Meningomyelocele/Spina bifida
□ Cyanotic congenital heart disease
□ Congenital diaphragmatic hernia
□ Omphalocele
□ Gastroschisis
□ Limb reduction defect (excluding congenital amputation and dwarfing syndromes)
□ Cleft Lip with or without Cleft Palate
□ Cleft Palate alone
□ Down Syndrome
□ Karyotype confirmed
□ Karyotype pending
□ Suspected chromosomal disorder
□ Karyotype confirmed
□ Karyotype pending
□ Hypospadias
□ None of the anomalies listed above

56. WAS INFANT TRANSFERRED WITHIN 24 HOURS OF DELIVERY? □ Yes □ No
IF YES, NAME OF FACILITY INFANT TRANSFERRED TO:_____

57. IS INFANT LIVING AT TIME OF REPORT?
□ Yes □ No □ Infant transferred, status unknown

58. IS THE INFANT BEING BREASTFED AT DISCHARGE?
□ Yes □ No

Mother's Name
Mother's Medical Record No.

Rev. 11/2003
NOTE: This recommended standard birth certificate is the result of an extensive evaluation process. Information on the process and resulting recommendations as well as plans for future activities is available on the Internet at: http://www.cdc.gov/nchs/vital_certs_rev.htm.

Source: National Center for Health Statistics 2003.

The birth certificate coordinator would document all infections that apply. See figure 6.4 for an example of an intake screen for the information required for a birth certificate.

Figure 6.4.   Intake screen for necessary information for a birth certificate

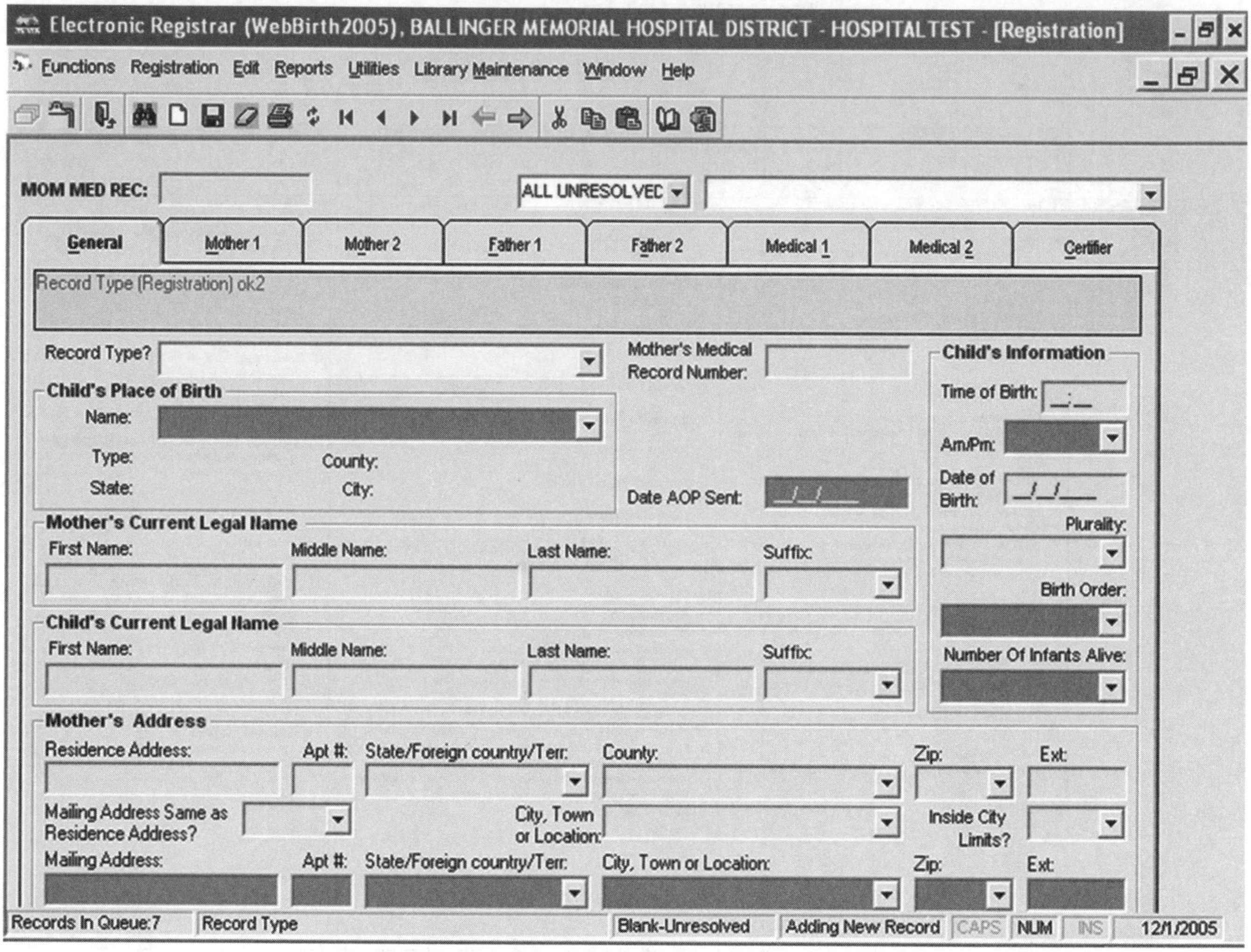

Source: Texas Department of State Health Services 2013. Reprinted with permission.

Birth Certificate System Reporting

The birth certificate systems used may be developed and provided to the healthcare facilities by the state or may be purchased from a vendor. State facility information systems are designed to focus on capturing and reporting birth certificate data. Vendor products may have more management and reporting tools than the state systems. These management tools may include reports such as productivity and turnaround times.

The birth certificate system may also generate statistical reports such as cesarean section rate or trending births rates. The key reporting capability, however, is the ability to report the births to the state in the approved format. The state may use the birth certificate data reported via the birth certificate system to feed other databases, such as immunization registry to enhance tracking of childhood immunizations.

Dictation and Transcription Systems

The dictation system is used by physicians to dictate various medical reports, such as history and physical examinations, discharge summaries, radiology reports, autopsy reports, catheterization reports, and other designated reports into the dictation system. The HIM department uses the dictation system to manage the dictated reports and to monitor the amount of transcription that is pending.

Dictating is the process of recording a physician's voice as he or she verbally describes a scenario, problem note, or some other type of report that is recorded electronically. The physician uses the dictation system to dictate, and the HIM department uses the system to transcribe the report.

Physicians and other appropriate clinical staff dictate into the healthcare facility's dictation system. The transcriptionist then types the actual report using the transcription system. Transcription is the process of deciphering the provider's recorded dictation and typing the medical document. The transcription system should be interfaced with the hospital information system so that the patient name, health record, and date of service are already populated within the information system. As voice recognition and the EHR are implemented throughout the healthcare facility, the dependence on this transcription system is reduced.

Most health information or EHR systems allow physicians to use dedicated dictation units or any telephone. However, voice and speech recognition technology is becoming more prevalent in EHR systems. Voice and speech recognition software translates the spoken word from the dictation to the written word or text in an electronic document. If the healthcare facility uses voice recognition, then the information system would be used by an editor, typically an HIM professional with transcription experience, to verify what has been translated into the written format rather than a transcriptionist to manually type what was dictated. The transcriptionist utilizes the transcription system to type the document. A document editor would use the appropriate documentation or transcription software to correct any errors that the system made in the translation of voice to text. However, the physician or provider is ultimately responsible for the content of the transcribed report and must make corrections or changes accordingly, if necessary.

Dictation System Functionality and Reporting

When dictating the report, the physician is expected to enter the patient's health record number or encounter number as well as the document type. The physician also may indicate that the dictation should be transcribed immediately. The date and time of dictation is automatically captured by the dictation system. The transcriptionists utilize the dictation system to listen to the dictation for transcription. The dictation system will route priority reports to the transcriptionists ahead of other dictated reports in the work queue. Priority status may be assigned to the report by the physician because of patient transfer or other reasons. HIM managers use the dictation system to route dictated reports to the various transcriptionists. For example, the transcription supervisor may need to assign another transcriptionist to type history and physical examination information to meet a specific turnaround time (such as "within 24 hours of dictation"). The HIM manager also uses the dictation system to monitor backlogs and trends on volume.

The key reporting focus for the dictation system is on workload. The system is able to track the volume of work dictated and how much is remaining to be transcribed. This information can be used to determine transcription staffing levels, overtime workload justifications, and trends and patterns in dictation usage.

Transcription System Functionality and Reporting

The transcription system works much like any word processor in that the transcriptionist is able to type, edit, and spell-check a document, but there are many features in the transcription systems that are not found in the word processor. Basic information is collected about every document. This information can include:

- Patient name
- Health record number
- Date of admission
- Date of discharge
- Date of surgery
- Dictating physician
- Date of dictation
- Date of transcription
- Report type
- Name of transcriptionist

The transcription system typically has user-defined templates for each report type. The template prevents the transcriptionist from having to type headings (such as history of present illness or review of systems) every time a history and physical examination is dictated. The information system typically uses expanders, which may also be called macros. An expander allows transcriptionists to type an acronym such as "CHF" and the full phrase "congestive heart failure" will automatically be spelled out, thus saving keystrokes and time. The expanders can typically be controlled by the healthcare facility.

The spell-checking capabilities are able to handle both the common language as well as medical terminology. Medical terminology includes not only terms, such as esophagogastroduodenoscopy, but also surgical instruments, medications, and other terms specific to healthcare and medicine.

In the event of a request for information or error, the document may need to be retrieved. The transcription system allows the transcriptionist to search for the document by patient name, health record number, date of dictation, dictator, document type, document number, and transcriptionist.

The transcription software products in use today are designed to work seamlessly with dictation systems and voice recognition systems to promote efficiency in the entire process. These products also are designed for transcriptionists to work from home as appropriate.

Once a document is transcribed, the transcription system is able to route reports to a departmental printer, fax, or other location. The routing of the report is based on settings established in the transcription system. This routing enables reports to reach the physician or patient care area faster. The report may also be available in the EHR.

The transcription system is used by management for various purposes. One purpose is to track productivity, which is critical because transcriptionists usually are paid based on it. Another purpose would be for incentive pay. Many information systems can calculate incentive pay automatically based on criteria established by the healthcare facility. Incentive pay is a system of bonuses and rewards based on employee productivity and is often used in transcription areas of healthcare facilities. Management may also use reports to monitor overall volume by report type to help identify trends and needs.

Healthcare Quality Indicator

The **healthcare quality indicator system** is an abstracting system that records information about the patient, the care provided to the patient, and the healthcare practitioner(s) involved in the care delivered. Abstracting is the process of extracting information from a document or data elements from a database to create a brief summary of a patient's illness, treatment, and outcome and entering the summary into an automated system. A quality indicator is a standard against which actual care may be measured to identify a level of performance for that standard. This software may be used by the HIM department or another department performing this function. HIM staff or nurses are the typical users of the healthcare quality indicator system; however, its use is limited. Users in the HIM department may be the coders or a separate group of employees with the necessary skills and qualifications to read, understand, and abstract information from the health record into the quality indicator system.

Abstracting and reporting are two critical aspects of the quality indicator systems. Information on the patient's care is entered into the information system to be in the healthcare facility quality improvement program. The data are then turned into information to evaluate the quality of care provided to the patient, patient safety, utilization review, and more. For example, the hospital could use information from the information system in the physician credentialing process. Problem areas would be identified and resources assigned in order to investigate and resolve the quality problems.

Healthcare Quality Indicator System Functionality

The healthcare quality indicator information system may be interfaced to the hospital information system to obtain demographic information. Data abstracting is the key functionality to the healthcare quality indicator system. Examples of data collected include:

- Units of blood
- Nosocomial infections
- Physician(s)
- Nursing unit
- Apgar score

The information abstracted can be used in reports and can be trended. The information can then be used to make changes in how care is provided. Some basic data are collected on all patients. Other fields required for data entry may change based on data entered previously. For example, the user may be required to enter estimated blood loss for a surgical patient, but would not be asked for this information when abstracting health patient data. Another example would be that an Apgar score is required for a newborn, but not for other patients.

Some of the data in the healthcare quality indicator system may be downloaded from other information systems used in the healthcare facility, saving time and improving data quality. These quality indicator systems could be the hospital information system's demographic information, the laboratory information system's laboratory results, and other clinical systems.

Healthcare Quality Indicator System Reporting

Because the data from this information system will be used in performance improvement, reporting is a key part of this information system. Reporting must be flexible so that the user is able to create the report needed for the study being conducted. The reports will include statistics and graphs to facilitate the identification of trends. Reports may include monitoring healthcare facility infection rate, number of deaths by physician, blood incompatibility, surgical errors, maternal deaths, and outcomes.

Computer-Assisted Coding System

The computer-assisted coding (CAC) system analyzes the clinical data found in an electronic health record. CAC is the process of extracting and translating dictated and then transcribed free-text data (or dictated and then computer-generated discrete data) into ICD-10-CM, ICD-10-PCS, and CPT procedural codes and evaluation and management codes for billing and coding purposes. It utilizes natural language processing (NLP) to analyze clinical data to identify diagnoses and procedures and to assign the appropriate ICD-10-CM, ICD-10-PCS, and CPT code to the CAC system. NLP is a technology that converts human language (structured or unstructured) into data that can be translated then manipulated by information systems.

CAC may be done while the patient is still in the hospital and then updated after discharge. Doing so speeds up the coding turnaround time and improves efficiency because coding rules are applied consistently and error rates are reduced. Despite this, the coder must review the health record documentation to confirm the accuracy of the code.

CAC System Functionality

The CAC suggests codes to be assigned. The coder reviews the codes and either accepts or rejects them. There is a work queue of records that the coder needs to review. This work queue can be prioritized depending on the healthcare facility's needs such as highest dollar or oldest unbilled claims.

CAC System Reporting

The CAC system generates productivity reports. It can also generate reports on the number of health records where the codes were changed from what the software originally recommended. These reports are important to evaluate the quality, accuracy, and completeness of the codes generated by the CAC system. This evaluation or review can be combined with the financial information to determine what impact this may be having on reimbursement claims and revenue cycle functions.

Clinical Documentation Improvement

The clinical documentation improvement (CDI) system assists in identifying ways to improve clinical documentation in the health record. CDI is the process a healthcare entity undertakes that will improve clinical specificity and documentation that will allow coders to assign more concise disease and procedural classification codes. When documentation improves, the code assignment will be improved because codes can be more specific. Another benefit of improved clinical documentation is more accurate reimbursement.

CDI Software Functionality

The CDI information system assists HIM and CDI staff in the physician query process by facilitating communication between the coding professional and the physician (see figure 6.5). The software looks for missing information that is needed to improve documentation. For example, if a laboratory test identifies the organism causing pneumonia, but the organism is not documented by the physician, then the information system can notify the CDI coordinator and a physician query can be created using a query template that is programmed within the EHR. A work queue identifies what health records need to be reviewed by the CDI coordinator. The information system can also monitor what queries are pending so that the coder can work with the physician to receive a response to the query.

Figure 6.5.   Sample physician query

Dear   (add provider(s) name)

Identify the opportunity   was documented within the   Reference document location(s)

Clinical Indicators: Signs and Symptoms: ·   Signs and Symptoms: ·   Risk Factors: ·

Treatment: ·   Treatment: ·   Other Indicators:

Based on the clinical indicators and your professional judgment Choose an item: ·
Please complete by selecting one of the options below.

- Click here to enter text:

- Click here to enter text:

- Other explanation of clinical findings Other Indicators:

- Unable to determine

- No further clarification needed

Source: Arrowood et al. 2016.

CDI Information System Reports

Reports will provide the hospital with information on MS-DRG assignment, statistics on the number of queries written, productivity statistics, turnaround times, and more. These reports will help the HIM and performance improvement staff determine areas in need of upgrading and enhancements, correction processes, and best practices for populating the health record with thorough and complete information to better evaluate patient care and reimbursement protocols. Research regarding clinical or administrative functions and outcomes will improve as a result of more comprehensive and complete documentation available for analysis.

CHECK YOUR UNDERSTANDING 6.3

1. What information system helps build data granularity, precision, clarity, and more detail in health information?

   a. Transcription
   b. Templates
   c. CDI
   d. Quality indicator monitoring

2. A physician speaks into a phone and gives a summary of the patient's care, which is later transcribed. What type of information system is the physician using?

   a. Dictation
   b. Chart locator
   c. Chart deficiency
   d. Quality indicator monitoring

3. To enter the number of units of blood that a patient received during a recent hospitalization, one would use the _____.

   a. Dictation
   b. Chart locator
   c. Chart deficiency
   d. Healthcare quality indicator

4. What information system would one use to enter data required by the NCHS?

   a. Birth certificate software
   b. Transcription
   c. Chart deficiency
   d. Quality indicator monitoring

5. Which information system would one be using if one typed out the abbreviation CABG and the phrase coronary artery bypass graft was spelled out?

   a. Abstract
   b. Bar code
   c. Expander
   d. Template

Real-World Case

Certain members of the executive management team at ABC Hospital are interested in adding voice recognition software to their current EHR. As director of HIM, Cynthia is preparing an extensive report on the impact this would have on the department. She is proposing that a feasibility study and subsequent request for proposal be completed.

The report includes information on voice recognition such as the projected workload of voice recognition software and how it would be implemented in the daily EHR operations. This includes its usage for the standard transcribed reports, such as discharge summaries; histories and physical exams; operative, autopsy, and consultation reports; physician progress notes; nursing care documentation; and other therapy documentation. A review of historic and current transcription workload, number of staff with respective salary and benefits, supplies, and equipment is completed.

Costs of implementing voice recognition software are a major concern. The cost of the software, including maintenance and upgrades, and hardware such as additional microphones and monitors are identified. Training costs for users and quality evaluators are determined. Staffing needs, including existing staff whose positions will be upgraded, for documentation quality and validation and technical support were also identified. Workload estimates for quality checks were figured into voice recognition projected costs. The human resources department was consulted regarding the process of lay-offs for some of the staff whose positions are not upgraded. Project management costs, including site visits, will be added to the proposal.

REVIEW QUESTIONS

1. What term describes the scientific discipline that is concerned with the cognitive, information-processing, and communication tasks of the healthcare practice, education, and research, including the information science and technology to support these tasks?

   a. Health informatics
   b. Health information management
   c. Data analytics
   d. Epidemiology

2. What legislation regulates the tracking of requests for and release of patient information?

   a. ARRA
   b. HIPAA
   c. HITECH
   d. TEFRA

(Continued)

3. What is the term used to indicate that reports and letters can be tailored and changed to meet the requirements of the request or the needs of the recipient within an ROI system?

   a. Manipulation
   b. Conversion
   c. Customization
   d. Renovation

4. In order to ensure an effective working environment to efficiently manage and produce MS-DRGs and the reimbursement claims, which two departments should have a strong relationship?

   a. Medical staff and billing
   b. Finance and billing
   c. ROI staff and coders
   d. HIM and billing staff

5. Which of the following is a method to determine how bad the cancer is by establishing the size of the tumor, the number of lymph nodes involved, and whether it has spread to other organs?

   a. TNM
   b. HIM
   c. SEER
   d. FORDS

6. Who typically completes the birth certificate when a baby is born in the hospital?

   a. Local health department personnel
   b. NCHS staff
   c. HIM staff
   d. Registration—admission, discharge, transfer staff

7. All of the following determine the requirements for the content of the hospital health record *except* _____.

   a. Joint Commission
   b. Medical staff rules and regulations
   c. State licensure and healthcare facility policies
   d. AHIMA

8. Which of the following allows transcriptionists to use abbreviations and acronyms while the software types out the complete words of the abbreviation or acronym?

   a. Expander
   b. Encoder
   c. Grouper
   d. Registry

9. What information system converts the spoken word into a documented word and may reduce the need to have human transcriptionists?

   a. Registries
   b. Voice recognition
   c. MS-DRGs
   d. CDI

10. What software improves the efficiency of the coding using the translated dictation reports and NLP to analyze clinical data?

    a. CDI
    b. TNM
    c. MS-DRGs
    d. CAC

References

Agency for Healthcare Research and Quality. 2015. Quality Indicators. http://www.qualityindicators.ahrq.gov/Downloads/Modules/IQI/V50/IQI_Brochure.pdf.

Arrowood, D., L. Bailey-Woods, E. Barnette, T. Combs, M. Endicott, and J. Miller. 2016. Clinical Documentation Improvement Toolkit. http://bok.ahima.org/PdfView?oid=301829.

Betz, R., L. Bouma, M. Brodnik, S. Burgess, J. Courteville, E. Delahoussaye, R. Dunn, et al. 2013. Release of Information Toolkit: A Practical Guide for the Access, Use, and Disclosure of Protected Health Information. bok.ahima.org/doc?oid=106371.

CNet. 2018. Cancer registry pathology severity rating. http://www.askcnet.org/software/features/

Centers for Disease Control and Prevention. 2017. Program Manual: National Program of Cancer Registries Version 1.0. http://www.cdc.gov/cancer/npcr/.

Florida Department of Health. 2017a. Florida Trauma Registry Minimum Data Set Requirements. http://www.floridahealth.gov/certificates/trauma-registry/_documents/ftr-mds-list.pdf.

Florida Department of Health. 2017b. Florida commemorative birth certificate. http://www.floridahealth.gov/certificates/certificates/birth/Commemorative/index.html.

National Center for Health Statistics (NCHS). 2003. U.S. Standard Certificate of Live Birth. https://www.cdc.gov/nchs/data/dvs/birth11-03final-ACC.pdf.

Office of the National Coordinator for Health Information Technology (ONC). 2016. Health IT Curriculum Resources for Educators: What Is Health Information Management? https://www.healthit.gov/providers-professionals/health-it-curriculum-resources-educators.

Texas Department od State Health Services. 2013. Texas Electronic Registrar Birth Registration Facility User Guide. https://www.dshs.texas.gov/vs/handbooks/birth/terbirthmanual.shtm.

Administrative Information Systems

Learning Objectives

- Determine what administrative information system is needed for a particular task.
- Differentiate among the administrative information systems.
- Differentiate between a decision support system and an executive information system.
- Describe how administrative systems impact health information management practices.

Key Terms

Administrative information
systems
Algorithm
Chargemaster
Clinical documentation
improvement (CDI)
Decision support system (DSS)
Enterprise master patient index
(EMPI)

Executive information system
(EIS)
Facilities management systems
Financial information system
Hospital information system
Human resources information
system (HRIS)
Master patient index (MPI)
Materials management system

Patient registration system
Practice management system
Registration-admission,
discharge, transfer (R-ADT)
Revenue cycle
Revenue cycle management
Scheduling system
Soundex

Administrative information systems, which manage the business of healthcare, were the first information systems to be used in healthcare. The data collected in administrative information systems are mainly financial or business-oriented in nature, rather than clinical. The administrative information systems perform many tasks throughout healthcare organizations. Some administrative systems, such as the master patient index (MPI), are used by many departments and employees throughout the organization. Other administrative information systems, like the decision support system, are utilized only by a select group of authorized users. The hospital information system, the major information system used by a healthcare facility, is made up of many administrative systems, such as the financial information system and the MPI. The main administrative information systems are summarized in the following list. Each of these components will be discussed separately:

- The financial information system monitors and controls the financial aspects of the healthcare facility.
- The human resources information system (HRIS) tracks and manages all employees and other contracted personnel within the organization.

- The **decision support system (DSS)** gathers data from a variety of sources to assist management and staff in decision-making tasks associated with the nonroutine and nonrepetitive problems.
- The **master patient index (MPI)** provides a permanent record of patients treated at the healthcare facility.
- The **patient registration system** collects information on patients receiving treatment.
- The **scheduling system** allows the facility to make efficient use of resources such as operating rooms.
- The **practice management system** combines a number of applications required to manage a physician practice.
- The **materials management system** manages the supplies and equipment within the facility.
- The **facilities management system** allows physical plant operations to control the automated systems within the facility for patient safety and comfort—that is, heating and air systems, automated key control, and preventive maintenance tasks such as testing fire extinguishers, elevator inspections, and the care of various equipment used in the healthcare facility.

Financial Information System

The financial information system is critical to the fiscal health of the healthcare facility. The healthcare facility must receive accurate financial information in a timely manner to monitor and manage the finances of the healthcare facility. This information can be used to plan and control the expenses of the day-to-day operations, as well as long-term investments.

The management of the accounts receivable and the accounts payable on a daily basis by the healthcare facility is known as **revenue cycle management**. The **revenue cycle** is a very complex process involving several departments and many employees who perform tasks of reviewing services provided for claims submitted as well as reviewing outstanding claims, returned claims, denials, missing accounts, bill holds, and other claims involving the revenue of the healthcare facility. Many health information management (HIM) professionals are involved in working with the revenue cycle in their facilities and some work for vendors who specialize in the area of revenue cycle management and clean-up as a business.

Financial Information System Functionality

The financial information system includes functions related to:

- Patient accounting
- Accounts receivable
- Accounts payable
- General ledger
- Investment management
- Contract management
- Payroll
- Billing and claims management

The patient accounting module collects all of the charges related to patient care. Some charges, such as the patient's room charge, are automatically generated, but others are created when nurses, respiratory therapists, and other staff enter charge information either through the financial information system or through a clinical information system that captures the information automatically and then shares it with the patient accounting system. These charges come from the chargemaster, shown in figure 7.1. A **chargemaster** is a financial management form or software that contains information about the healthcare facility's charges for the services it provides to patients (also called a charge description master [CDM]). The chargemaster automates the coding process for routine procedures such as laboratory tests and radiology examinations. Attached to each of these codes is the charge associated with the service. This amount and other charges recorded are used to determine the amount of money charged to the patient's account. For example, a healthcare facility may charge $100 for a chest x-ray. The information system then generates the bill and submits it to the third-party payer. The patient accounting system also generates the discharged not final billed report, which lists the patient accounts that have not been billed.

Figure 7.1. Example of a chargemaster

ITEM NUMBER	DEPT NUMBER	DESCRIPTION	PRICE	HCPCS CODE	REVENUE CODE	MEDICAID CODE	GL NUMBER
791002	761	CORONARY ARTERY DILATION	$1,550.00	92982	481	92982TC	0800.4601
791000	761	INJECTION, CARDIAC CATH	$ 220.00	93540	481	93540TC	0800.4601
761001	761	NURSING FAC CARE, SUBSEQ	$ 75.00	99307	636	7610	0800.4601
761002	761	HOME VISIT, NEW PATIENT	$ 80.00	99341	636	7610	0800.4601
761003	761	REPAIR EYELID DEFECT	$ 110.00	67915	636	7610	0800.4601
810003	761	REPAIR EYELID DEFECT	$ 550.00	67916	272	7610	0800.4601
810004	761	REMOVAL OF KIDNEY STONE	$ 390.00	50080	272	7610	0800.4601
810050	761	DECALCIFY TISSUE	$2,065.00	88311	272	7610	0800.4601
810061	761	CHROMOSOME COUNT, ADDITIONAL	$ 275.00	88285	272	7610	0800.4601
810072	761	ASSAY OF FREE THYROXINE	$ 159.00	84439	622	7610	0800.4601
810080	761	ASSAY OF THYROID ACTIVITY	$7,064.00	84442	272	7610	0800.4601
791004	761	ASSAY THYROID STIM HORMONE	$ 650.00	84443	272	7610	0800.4601

Source: Pilato 2013.

Because the chargemaster has such an impact on the healthcare facility, periodic updates are required. The classification system codes must be updated annually; HIM professionals must ensure that their respective chargemaster updates are completed annually by the healthcare facility's information systems (IS) department when the software updates are received. Otherwise, charges billed can mean a loss of revenue to the healthcare facility. Once the updates are performed on schedule, the healthcare facility is reimbursed the amount they are owed based on their particular geographic region of the country.

Accounts payable records what the healthcare facility owes to others. This amount may be a refund to a patient or an insurance company, or it may be payment to companies that provide supplies and equipment to the healthcare facility.

The general ledger records debits and credits to the various accounts managed by the financial information system. All of the financial transactions are recorded for the time frame. These transactions include receipt of payment, payroll, and disbursements.

Healthcare facilities invest their excess cash. The investment management features of the financial information system track the investment accounts and analyze the return on the investments. Changes to the investment portfolio can be made according to the findings.

Healthcare facilities sign many contracts, including those with software vendors, insurance companies, businesses that purchase healthcare services, and many other companies. The contract management portion of the financial information system can track particulars such as who the contract is with and expiration dates. The information that comes from the financial information system is used to negotiate managed care contracts and monitor the impact of the contract based on information such as the number of patients, amount of revenue, cost of care, and whether or not the facility is making money on the contract.

The last module of the financial information system to be discussed is the payroll functions. Payroll functions include tracking employees, salaries, taxes to be deducted, taxes to be paid, health insurance deductions, life insurance deductions, and direct deposits. The payroll functions would need to track salary increases and changes in deduction from one year to another.

The information is also used to generate financial reports that are needed by the healthcare facility's management staff. The financial information also provides the balance sheet, statement of revenue and expense, cost reports, and illustrates cash flow. These financial reports can assist in the pricing of services rendered, control inventory, analyses of productivity of staff, and other purposes.

Impact on HIM

The coding professional staff will populate the diagnosis and procedure codes either through direct data entry or from an interface to an encoder. HIM and coding staff have always played an integral part in the financial viability of the healthcare facility. This is particularly true with the completed transition to *International Classification of Diseases, Tenth Revision, Clinical Modification* (ICD-10-CM) and *International Classification of Diseases, Tenth Revision, Procedure Coding System* (ICD-10-PCS). Extensive and continuous training is required to maintain optimal skill in identifying the correct and appropriate diagnostic and procedural codes. With the massive increase in the number of codes due to increased specificity in ICD-10, coders must be thoroughly trained in anatomy and pathophysiology to assign the precise codes. However, codes can only be as accurate as the documentation allows. Clinical documentation improvement (CDI) is the process an organization undertakes that will improve clinical specificity and documentation that will allow coding professionals to assign more concise disease and procedural classification codes. The quality of this documentation is vital in order to properly evaluate patient care, meet all regulatory requirements, and obtain the appropriate amount of reimbursement. Because quality documentation, whether it be paper or electronic, is one of the cornerstones of the HIM profession, it is essential for the HIM and coding staff to be integral in all phases of CDI.

HIM professionals should also be involved in the development and management of the chargemaster. Services are added to and removed from the chargemaster as the services provided by the facility change. Both ICD-10 and current procedural terminology (CPT) classification codes are updated on a regular basis. These changes must be implemented and verified within the facility's chargemaster. In addition, the monetary value associated with each code must also be confirmed. Upwards of 700 new, revised, and deleted codes have been implemented for the 2018 fiscal year (CMS 2017).

Analysis of chargemaster data can indicate changes in billing time frames, productivity of coding submissions, reimbursement denials, diagnoses, and procedures that are most resource-intensive or cost-effective. The analysis of the billing and coding information and reports will help both HIM and finance departments to conduct performance improvement activities to become more efficient.

Human Resources Information System

A healthcare facility requires many staff members in order to operate. Many healthcare facilities operate 24 hours a day, 7 days a week. Because of staffing requirements, payroll expenses make up a large part of the operating budget. This large outlay of cash demands strong management of the human resources department within the organization.

Functionality

The HRIS tracks employees within the organization. This tracking includes promotions, transfers, terminations, performance appraisal due dates, and absenteeism. The individual data elements collected include:

- Employee name
- Employee number
- Department
- Title
- Salary
- Benefit information
- Hire date
- Results of performance appraisal
- Previous titles
- Termination date
- Certifications
- Disciplinary actions
- Eligibility for rehire

These elements and other data are used to create a permanent record for the healthcare facility. This information is used to manage current staff and to verify that past employees worked at the healthcare facility. The HRIS data will track the benefits that an employee has selected, such as family healthcare plan, dental insurance, long-term disability insurance, and retirement. The HRIS will be able to track the utilization of staff by department, job title, or other grouping. The human resources staff would have access to the records of all employees, whereas the various department directors should have access only to those employees reporting to that director.

Department managers may use an automated timekeeping system for their employees when staff members clock in and out. This HRIS tracks the hours per week worked by pay period. Human resources and managers can then use the HRIS to determine sick time, vacation time, and benefit time per employee.

The HRIS can also assist with the hiring process. For example, the HRIS can track résumés and applications submitted by potential employees. The information system can compare the skills and education of the candidate with those of the other applicants, thus speeding up the hiring process.

Reporting is important in the HRIS. Reporting features can be used to track items such as turnover rate, open positions, labor costs, benefits, budget, or overtime. The healthcare facility may also track employee satisfaction and report on the findings of the surveys. Many facilities offer in-house educational opportunities to employees and attendance at these events is tracked within the HRIS software. These might include optional educational seminars to advance managers with training and development skills. Other workshops might include cardiopulmonary resuscitation (CPR) training classes for staff. The HRIS software may also track mandated classes for all employees that require annual attendance such as fire and safety classes, OSHA standards, privacy and security training, and so forth. Department directors can then easily use the reporting function to assess the attendance within their own departments as well as results of these educational classes by their employees annually.

Impact on HIM

HIM department staff do not use the HRIS; however, the HIM director may use HRIS to generate reports, perform queries, review applications, and perform other tasks related to the HIM department staff.

CHECK YOUR UNDERSTANDING 7.1

1. Which part of an administrative information system would be able to identify which surgeries are most profitable for the healthcare facility?

   a. Encoder
   b. Decision support
   c. Financial management
   d. Practice management

2. Which information system assists the coding professional in selecting the appropriate code?

   a. Encoder
   b. Decision support
   c. Chargemaster
   d. Practice management

3. Which information system would be able to identify employee turnover rates in all departments within the healthcare facility?

   a. Decision support
   b. Revenue cycle
   c. Human resources information system
   d. Materials management

(Continued)

Decision Support System

The DSS, as defined earlier, is an information system that gathers data from a variety of sources and assists in providing structure to the data by using various analytical models and visual tools in order to facilitate and improve the ultimate outcome in decision-making tasks associated with the nonroutine and nonrepetitive problems. It is also used to solve structured problems. This means that the DSS is not used to schedule staff, determine inventory levels, or perform other routine decisions, but rather to make decisions about whether to open a new women's health center or a geriatric center. Other decisions that may be candidates for the DSS are whether or not to add new examination rooms in the emergency department or to open new operating rooms. To make these decisions, the DSS utilizes the data in the data repositories and data warehouses. The DSS uses models to run analyses such as "what if" to determine what would happen if certain decisions were made or to forecast the future. For example, the DSS would evaluate the profit or loss that would occur if a hospital added an extra patient room in the emergency department. It would take into consideration extra costs, extra patients, reduced wait times, extra staff, and more.

Executive Information System

The **executive information system (EIS)** is a type of decision support system that is designed to be used by healthcare administrators. As such, it must be easy to use and have access to a wide range of data. With the EIS, a lot of graphs and charts generally are used as part of the results. Advantages of the EIS include:

- Improved competitiveness of the healthcare facility
- Knowledge of the healthcare facility
- Making information available to authorized users throughout the healthcare facility
- Assistance in making strategic decisions about the healthcare facility

The EIS assists the administrator and other top administration staff in making quick decisions. To generate the data manually that the EIS generates with a few clicks of the mouse would take days.

A dashboard report gives administration-structured information to make intelligent decisions for the future. In this example, administration can view the dashboard report and see from the diagnostic-related groups (DRGs) and the length of stay (LOS) what the facility was actually reimbursed and what it actually cost the facility to treat the patient. The last columns give administration an idea of the profit that was expected versus the actual profit made. This type of report is useful to administration in planning for the future to make decisions.

Figure 7.2 shows an example of an EIS dashboard report. Administrators can view detailed data by types of graphs that are selected, depending on the software used. For this example, several bar charts and graphics are used. Administrators can easily view an EIS dashboard report and see the practice performance activity of the physician highlighted. In this case, performance is evaluated by identifying patient load, wait times for the patients, satisfaction survey results, and general patient demographic information. The same measures can be used to evaluate and compare all the other physicians listed across the top of the screen. Administrators must focus on the fluctuating monthly patient load and the differences in monthly wait times for various physicians. The data from this EIS planning tool is a visual representation to administration of where the problem is greatest and where the priority should be focused. The HIM department may or may not use the DSS depending on the type of DSS and the data stored within it.

Figure 7.2. EIS dashboard showing physician practice performance with bar charts

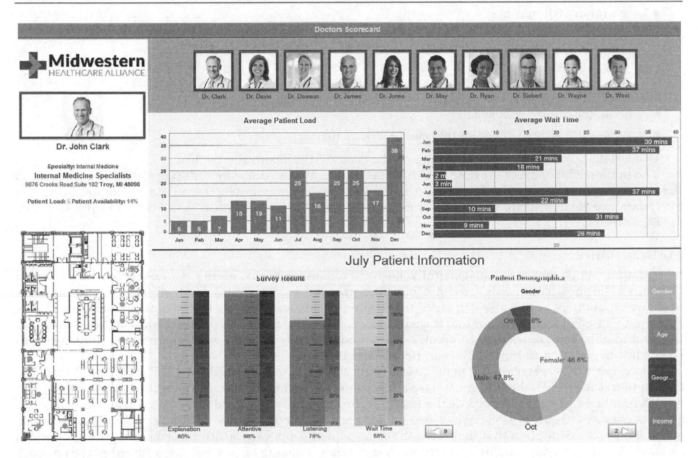

Source: iDashboards n.d. Reprinted with permission.

Master Patient Index

The MPI is part of the hospital information system. It is a patient-identifying directory, referencing all patients related to a healthcare facility, that also serves as a link to the patient health record or information, facilitates patient identification, and assists in maintaining a longitudinal patient record from birth to death. The MPI identifies every patient who has been admitted to the healthcare facility, and it is the key to locating all patient health records. The MPI lists patient names and health record numbers and cross-references them. An MPI is to be kept permanently as mandated by legal statutes. The information contained within the MPI was originally limited to demographics that could readily distinguish between any two patients as not having the same health record. These data include both demographic data and visit-specific information. The demographic information will include data such as the patient name. The visit information will include items such as discharge date. The data contained in the MPI include:

- Internal patient identification (that is, health record number)
- Person name (legal name with given name, surname, initial, suffixes, and prefixes)
- Date of birth
- Gender

- Race
- Ethnicity
- Address
- Telephone number (where patient can be reached)
- Alias, previous, or maiden names
- Social security number
- Universal patient identifier (not yet established)
- Account or visit number
- Admission, encounter, or visit date
- Discharge or departure date
- Encounter or service type
- Encounter or service location
- Encounter primary physician
- Patient disposition (Reynolds and Sharp 2016, 130)

Other data may be collected depending on the needs of the healthcare facility.

The person who collects the data in the MPI is frequently an admissions staff member who interviews the patient upon entering the facility at the time of the visit encounter. Once data are entered into the MPI, data are easily transferable into other screens and other information systems within the software for other users.

Functionality

Information about patients can generally be retrieved using many of the previously mentioned data elements. The most commonly used are patient name and health record number. The MPI usually has soundex capabilities, which allow the user to retrieve patients based on the sound of the name. Soundex is a phonetic-based indexing system that is easily incorporated into computer software for searching surnames that sound alike but are spelled differently. The soundex search is useful when there are multiple ways to spell a last name, such as Burger, Burgur, Berger, and Burgher.

There are times when a patient is issued one or more duplicate health record numbers. When the duplication is identified, the MPI must have the capability to combine these health records under one health record number and keep a record of the health record number eliminated. The MPI must also be able to address overlays. Overlays occur when two patients are assigned the same health record number because of the incorrect assumption that they were the same patient. Duplicate health record numbers and overlays cause problems with data quality and ultimately can create a quality of care risk because either the patient's information is fragmented or two patients' records are intertwined.

As mentioned earlier, the MPI is the data storehouse of patient information, which by legal statutes must be maintained permanently. The information stored in the MPI is also vital to the administrative functions of the healthcare facility's database system. When a patient is admitted, discharged, or transferred, the registration—admission, discharge, transfer (R-ADT) application is updated with the demographic information and serves as the foundation for the MPI.

Enterprise Master Patient Index

Integrated delivery systems (IDSs) typically have an enterprise master patient index (EMPI), which provides access to multiple repositories of information from overlapping patient populations that are maintained in separate information systems and databases. An IDS is an organizational arrangement of a network of health providers that may include hospitals, physicians, and health maintenance organizations (HMOs) that provide coordinated services along the continuum of care from ambulatory, acute, and long-term care and may extend across a geographical region.

An EMPI allows all of the components of the IDS to share information about the patient. The health record number assigned may be the same for all hospitals, ambulatory settings, and other components of the healthcare system. There may also be an enterprise health record number, with each component issuing its own health record number to the patient. The EMPI would identify all patient visits to the IDS and the data stored would include the facility that the patient visited.

Impact on HIM

The HIM department is a key user of the MPI. The HIM staff is responsible for the data quality of the MPI, so they perform the various tasks to maintain quality, such as combining duplicate health records and correcting overlays, along with other data quality issues. The HIM staff also uses the MPI to:

- Look up health record numbers
- Identify discharge dates
- Confirm that the health record contains all patient visits
- Look up when the patient was last seen in the healthcare facility
- Merge duplicate health record numbers
- Correct errors in data entry
- Unmerge overlays when one patient's record is overwritten by another patient record; these records must then be separated into their original files (Reynolds and Sharp 2016, 130)

Although this list of activities is not long, the amount of time HIM staff spend using the MPI is significant. For example, the release of information staff must look up the health record number on every authorization to release information that comes into the department. Depending on the number of requests, this could take hours.

An MPI can link to other databases within the facility and, as a result, duplicate health record numbers can easily be assigned by other departments such as admissions, clinics, and the emergency department. It is extremely important that the MPI be routinely maintained and updated for accuracy and data control.

Patient Registration (Registration—Admission, Discharge, Transfer)

Patient registration systems are frequently known as R-ADT. The R-ADT is defined as a type of administrative information system that stores demographic information and performs functionality related to registration, admission, discharge, and transfer of patients within the organization. The data collected include:

- Basic demographic information such as name, address, and gender
- Insurance information such as insurance company, policy number, and group number
- Information about the stay such as the admission date, discharge date, and attending physician

Functionality

The information collected in the R-ADT is transferred to other information systems. This transfer of data ensures that the demographic information is consistent and prevents data from being entered over and over again. If a patient needs multiple tests or services performed on the same day, such as laboratory, physical therapy, and x-ray, the registration system should be able to schedule all of these tests with one phone call. The R-ADT system issues the health record number assignment to the patient folder.

Because the MPI and R-ADT systems are both parts of the hospital information system, sophisticated algorithms can be used to help prevent duplicate health record numbers when admitting a patient. Algorithms are relatively short computer programs of rules or procedures containing conditional logic for solving a problem or accomplishing a task. When the user enters a patient's name and other identifying information into the R-ADT and there is a patient with the same or similar information, the R-ADT notifies the user. Essentially, the R-ADT asks the user if the patient being admitted is one of the patients listed. If so, duplication of the health record number can be avoided. Not only can algorithms identify exact matches based on name, social security number, and other identifying information, but they can also identify patients whose information is nearly identical, such as a patient whose social security number or date of birth is one digit off from an existing entry or whose last name has changed because of marriage or divorce since the last visit. Many MPIs utilize a ranking system to identify the amount of confidence that the MPI system has in the match. Exact information would receive the maximum score. A potential match with almost everything identical would be a high score but not a perfect score. A potential match with very little, if anything, matching will be a low score.

The R-ADT system generates some key reports used by many departments within the facility. These include the daily admission list, discharge list, census report, transfer list, and bed utilization reports. The facility may also generate monthly, quarterly, yearly, and ad hoc reports to show type of patient treated, number of discharges, number of admissions, occupancy rates, and other information needed. The R-ADT system may also print out routine documents, such as general consent form, notice of privacy practices acknowledgment, and advance directives that the patient needs to sign.

Impact on HIM

Although the HIM department does not generally register patients, the HIM department utilizes the reports that come from the R-ADT. For example, the discharge list is often used to confirm that all discharged health records arrive in the HIM department after discharge.

CHECK YOUR UNDERSTANDING 7.2

1. Which of the following would not be done with an MPI system?

   a. Merging duplicate health record numbers
   b. Identifying discharge dates
   c. Printing out patient general consent forms
   d. Looking up health record numbers

2. What type of report would give administrators structured information in a variety of graphs to better plan facility operations?

   a. EMPI
   b. IDS
   c. R-ADT
   d. EIS Dashboard

3. Algorithms are used to match duplicate patients in which of the following information systems?

   a. Decision support system
   b. Executive information system
   c. Master patient index
   d. Enterprise master patient index

4. What type of information system would be beneficial when developing 10- and 20-year strategic plans for the healthcare facility?

   a. Decision support system
   b. Executive information system
   c. Master patient index
   d. Enterprise master patient index

5. What is an IDS?

   a. A network of coordinated healthcare providers under the umbrella of a single HCO
   b. A database of all patients who have received services at an HCO
   c. A short computer program of rules and procedures to solve problems
   d. A type of decision support used by executive management in an HCO

Scheduling System

Scheduling systems are used to control the use of resources throughout the healthcare facility. These resources can include staff, equipment, rooms, and more. Scheduling systems may be centralized or independent. Centralized scheduling allows the scheduling of all services of the healthcare facility so that one call can make multiple appointments. The decentralized system utilizes the scheduling features of individual systems in use in each department, so calls would have to be made to more than one location to schedule multiple tests.

Functionality

Healthcare facilities need to keep expensive equipment and other resources generating revenue rather than allowing them to remain idle. The scheduling system can help with this by scheduling tests, beds, operating rooms, staff, and other resources wisely. For example, a subsystem of the main scheduler is used for scheduling surgeries. If Dr. Smith needs to perform an appendectomy on a patient, the scheduling system knows what operating rooms are available, how long the operating room will be needed, the staff required, and what equipment will be required. This scheduling of the patient and resources ensures that everything is available when needed, thus preventing unnecessary cancellation of surgeries.

To schedule a patient for admission, tests, or other services, the physician office may call the hospital or other healthcare facility to make the necessary reservations or the information system may be available for direct access by the healthcare provider.

In a typical appointment book scheduling system, a patient appointment can be made by the month and date by clicking on the month and date that is desired for the next appointment follow-up.

The patient's name is then entered into the timeline of the hour that the appointment time is made. Physician offices use these types of appointment books for routine patient visits in their offices. Clinics and ambulatory surgical facilities may also use these software applications. In some cases, the patient is able to log in and schedule routine tests, such as an annual mammogram.

The scheduling system can assist with many management functions. The reporting capabilities of the scheduling system can track cancellations, resource utilization, patient volume, and other topics important to management. The reservations can also be used as part of the preadmission process to collect data such as insurance information and precertification.

Impact on HIM

The HIM department does not use the scheduling system.

Practice Management

Practice management systems are used by physician practices. Scheduling, patient accounting, patient collections, claims submission, appointment scheduling, human resources, and other functions all are built into this single information system.

Functionality

The practice management system may be fully functional information systems, or the physician practices can select from a variety of modules as needed by the practice.

The practice management system can automate prescription renewals and other routine tasks. The practice management system may also connect to administrative information systems at the healthcare facility. One of the major functions of the practice management system is billing. The practice management system will capture the necessary data, review the claim to determine if all the necessary data are available, and then submit the data either to the insurance company or to a healthcare clearinghouse. The practice management system is able to generate reports. Sample reports include number of patients, profit or loss, most common services, and much more.

Impact on HIM

The HIM professional who works in the physician office manager role will utilize the practice management information system in many of the same ways as the financial information system, master patient index, and other administrative systems. These tasks include chargemaster management, entering codes for billing, reporting, and tracking patient visits.

Materials Management System

Healthcare facilities must manage a large amount of equipment and supplies. The typical materials management system automates the:

- Purchasing process

- Inventory control
- Menu planning
- Food service

Materials management personnel would work with the dietary or food service personnel to order and track various food stuffs and supplies for patients and staff. The materials management staff would work with clinical personnel to track and order bandages, blood pressure cuffs, thermometers, and other patient-centered resources.

Functionality

The materials management system can create requisitions, which use workflow in order to gain the necessary approvals for the purchases. Part of the process can be comparing the purchase to the budget to ensure that the necessary funds are available.

This functionality helps control costs in the healthcare facility. The materials management system can be set up to automatically order supplies and equipment based on predetermined thresholds for inventory supplies, allowing for just-in-time inventory controls. For example, if the healthcare facility wants to keep at least 200 suture kits in stock, the materials management system automatically triggers an order for suture kits with the preferred vendor when the inventory drops to 250 suture kits. The materials management system can notify the financial information system when the supplies arrive so that the vendor can be paid, thus increasing the efficiency of the healthcare facility.

The materials management system can generate bar codes to be applied toward supplies to be used and charged to the patient correctly. The use of materials management systems include cost savings through improved efficiencies, better knowledge of the supplies in stock, reductions in the amount of supplies retained in inventory, and reduced lost charges.

The dietary component of the materials management system tracks the patient's dietary needs, the healthcare facility's food inventory, and food costs. A number of menus can be entered into the information system from which the dietary management and dietitians can work. The materials management system should have a variety of menus available from which to choose.

Impact on HIM

The HIM department is not a frequent user of the materials management system. However, purchase requisitions may be used to order office supplies and other supplies for the HIM departments. This is dependent on the setup of the materials management and ordering system of each healthcare facility.

Facilities Management

The physical plant will require maintenance and upgrades over the years. The physical plant refers to the building structure, surrounding grounds, parking lots or decks, and various building equipment such as elevators. A facilities management system is used by a healthcare facility to manage the physical plant. A facilities management system will track routine maintenance such as elevator inspections, fire extinguisher inspections, and equipment preventive maintenance. Preventive maintenance will enable the equipment to last longer, so tasks such as filter changes, inspection of electrical cables, and other tasks will save the healthcare facility money. The facilities management system will track the preventive maintenance tasks and other inspections that can be used in risk management investigations as well as inspections from outside sources, such as accreditation and state licensing. With the focus by the Joint Commission on patient safety, the physical plant is focused on providing equipment and a healthcare environment that is vital to the well-being of the guests, staff, and ultimately the patients within the healthcare facility.

Functionality

The facilities management software can control various features of the healthcare facility, such as the thermostat, automatic locks, and key cards. For example, the temperature provided by the air conditioner and heating systems can be controlled, making the healthcare facility more energy efficient. Doors can be locked and unlocked automatically at a prescheduled time, and employees can be given access to or denied access to restricted areas.

Facilities management software can also track preventive management tasks, such as testing fire extinguishers, elevator inspections, and the care of various equipment used in the healthcare facility. It keeps track of when repairs and maintenance are performed, such as when a roof was put on a building or when filters are changed in the air conditioning system.

From time to time, major renovations or new construction is necessary. The facilities management system can track and plan the project through the use of project management tools such as project evaluation and review technique (PERT) charts and Gantt charts (refer to chapter 4).

Impact on HIM

The HIM department is not a direct user of the facility management information system. Indirectly, the HIM department may use key cards for entry into locked areas or doorways or use the automated HVAC (heating, ventilation, and air conditioning) system from the physical plant. The HVAC system is set by the physical plant staff, usually in zones for larger buildings, to run at set temperatures during various seasons to make operating costs of heating and cooling more economical.

CHECK YOUR UNDERSTANDING 7.3

1. Which of the following information systems would coordinate the schedules of five physicians and seven nurse practitioners based upon the needs of the patients within an internal medicine group practice?

   a. Materials management
   b. Practice management
   c. Facilities management
   d. Scheduling

2. Routine reports, such as number of admissions and discharges per month or per year, are generated by which information system?

   a. Materials management
   b. Registration
   c. Facilities management
   d. Scheduling

3. The scheduling system knows which of the following _____.

   a. Amount of time needed to perform colonoscopy
   b. Physicians who are up for reappointment to the medical staff
   c. Census report
   d. The latest version of the notice of privacy practice

4. The area most closely aligned with meeting the Joint Commission's focus on patient safety would be

   _____.

   a. Facilities management
   b. Practice management
   c. Registration
   d. Scheduling

5. Which information system typically assigns the patient's health record number to the patient?

   a. Scheduling
   b. Materials management
   c. Facilities management
   d. Registration

Real-World Case

The cardiology department of Smithville Community Hospital wants to expand the cardiovascular lab to include additional procedure rooms and equipment. Several cardiologists have mentioned that there seems to be an increase in the number of patients and number of cardiac procedures performed. The hospital CIO was asked to evaluate the request and provide an initial report to the Board of Directors. The CIO worked with the VP of clinical operations to write the report. Using the physician and procedure indices within EHR, the CIO and VP completed a 10-year historical analysis of all cardiac patients and procedures. They identified inpatient and outpatient procedures, documented the number of outpatients who were also cardiac inpatients at some point, and reviewed wait times for scheduling of procedures. Four years of historical data was available in the current EHR for wait-time analysis. The previous system was not able to track wait times for scheduling.

The CIO and VP identified financial data, including cost analysis of each procedure, how reimbursement of procedure varied by type of insurance, average length of stay (if inpatient), profit margins of each procedure, and MS-DRG analysis performed on inpatient cases. They performed physician profiles to identify which and how many procedures were performed by each cardiologist. Using external data provided by the city government and local economic development council, the CIO and VP made population projections for the next 20 years and found an increase in the local population of the over-50 age group. They generated anticipated cardiac services and procedures using predictive statistical modeling.

Based on the information the CIO and VP collected, they projected how many additional staff members and physicians might be needed and made space allocations for the increased number of procedure rooms. They are currently investigating the cost of additional equipment needed and completing a renovation budget and timeline. They expect to present their findings to the board by the end of the first quarter, and a final decision should be reached by the end of July.

REVIEW QUESTIONS

1. What term is used to describe the process of submitting claims for reimbursement, denials, billing matters, accounting, and any other issues or follow-up on claims?

    a. Deterministic algorithm
    b. Revenue cycle
    c. R-ADT
    d. Chargemaster

2. What is the name of the financial management software that contains information about the healthcare facility's charges for the services it provides to patients?

    a. Deterministic algorithm
    b. Revenue cycle
    c. R-ADT
    d. Chargemaster

3. The HRIS would track which of the following?

    a. Employee certification status
    b. Reimbursements received from CMS
    c. Inventory supplies
    d. R-ADT

4. Which information system can the HIM director use to determine salaries, assist in hiring new staff, evaluate turnover rates, and track training sessions?

    a. Practice management
    b. Materials management
    c. Facilities management
    d. Human resources

5. Dr. Smith treats highly unusual medical cases requiring many laboratory, radiology, and other diagnostic tests. Hospital administration wants to determine if additional facilities, personnel, and equipment are needed to meet current and future community demands. Which information system would be helpful in this scenario?

    a. DSS
    b. R-ADT
    c. HRIS
    d. EIS

6. Every October, the CEO and other members of the upper administrative staff have strategic planning meetings to address the upcoming year's goals and objectives. What information system would assist them in this process?

    a. DSS
    b. R-ADT
    c. HRIS
    d. EIS

7. During a disaster, which information system would help track the patients' movements through the hospital as they go through triage, surgery, intensive care unit (ICU), regular patient care floor, and finally discharge to a rehabilitation facility?

    a. DSS
    b. R-ADT
    c. HRIS
    d. EIS

8. Which information system is the gateway into a healthcare facility to identify if a patient has been treated there, contains demographic information to confirm patient identity, and shows if the patient has been treated at other facilities within an IDS?

    a. EMPI
    b. EIS
    c. HRIS
    d. R-ADT

9. If the CFO wanted to evaluate the supply shipping schedule, storage costs for supplies and equipment, timeframes for ordering supplies, and the distribution of equipment and supplies to the correct departments, which information system would facilitate this process?

    a. Materials management
    b. Practice management
    c. Facilities management
    d. EIS

10. If the medical office manager wanted to compare the amount of time it takes for a patient to be seen by a physician versus a nurse practitioner, which information system would be helpful in this analysis?

    a. Materials management
    b. Practice management
    c. Facilities management
    d. EIS

References

Centers for Medicare and Medicaid Services (CMS). 2017. 2018 ICD-10 CM and GEMs. https://www.cms.gov/Medicare/Coding/ICD10/2018-ICD-10-CM-and-GEMs.html.

iDashboards. n.d. Healthcare—Doctor's Scorecard. Accessed February 10, 2018. https://www.idashboards.com/dashboard-examples/healthcare-dashboards-doctors-scorecard/.

Reynolds, R. B. and M. Sharp. 2016. Health Record Content and Documentation. Chapter 4 in *Health Information Management: Concepts, Principles, and Practice*, 5th ed. Edited by P. Oachs and A. Watters. Chicago: AHIMA.

Pilato, J. 2013. Charging vs. coding: Untangling the relationship for ICD-10. *Journal of AHIMA* 84(2): 58–60. http://library.ahima.org/doc?oid=106071#.Wn271KinFRY.

Clinical Information Systems

Learning Objectives

- Differentiate between the various clinical information systems.
- Define clinical information system.
- Determine what clinical information system is needed to meet the needs of the healthcare facility.
- Make recommendations on the use and implementation of document management systems.

Key Terms

Anesthesia information system
Annotation
Backscanning
Barcode
Clinical documentation
Clinical information system (CISs)
Document management system (DMS)
Emergency department system (EDS)
Interdisciplinary charting system

Laboratory information system (LIS)
Nursing information system (NIS)
Optical character recognition (OCR)
Patient monitoring system
Pharmacy information system (PIS)
Picture archival communication system (PACS)

Radiology information system (RIS)
Scanner
Scanning workstation
Smart card
Symbiology
Target sheet
Telehealth
Telemedicine
Teleradiology
Telesurgery

A clinical information system (CIS) collects and stores medical, nursing, clinical ancillary areas (such as radiology and laboratory), and therapy department information related to patient care. Data contained within the various information systems are patient identifiable and are therefore protected by the Health Insurance Portability and Accountability Act (HIPAA). The clinical data stored in the CIS are used to diagnose a patient's condition, make treatment decisions, monitor the current condition, and manage overall care. The CISs discussed in this chapter are:

- Document management system (DMS)
- Radiology information system (RIS)
- Laboratory information system (LIS)
- Nursing information system (NIS)
- Pharmacy information system (PIS)

- Interdisciplinary charting system
- Emergency department system
- Anesthesia information system
- Patient monitoring system
- Telehealth
- Smart cards

Other CISs include computerized provider order entry (CPOE) and electronic medication administration system. These systems are discussed in chapter 9. CISs are frequently source systems for the electronic health record (EHR) because they populate the database that serves as the foundation for the EHR.

Demographic information is collected in the administrative or hospital information system which includes registration—admission, discharge, and transfer (R-ADT); see chapter 7 for more information on administrative information systems. The demographic information is passed on to the CIS, eliminating the need for duplicate data entry, which saves time and improves the quality of the data. Some of the data elements generally passed from the hospital information system to the CIS include:

- Last name
- First name
- Middle initial
- Date of birth
- Health record number
- Social security number

The CIS interface may be designed so that any changes to demographic information in the CIS are fed back to the hospital information system to keep demographic information in all information systems consistent. See figure 8.1 for an example of how individual departmental information systems feed into the main hospital information system.

Figure 8.1.   Health information systems

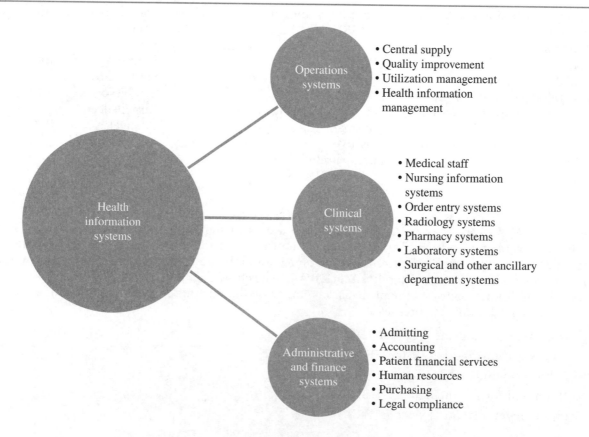

Clinical information systems are used to support patient care throughout the healthcare facility in many areas. The information provided within the system offers healthcare providers timely access to clinical data and complete data regarding the patient's care.

Document Management System

A document management system (DMS) is an electronic method of capturing and managing documents. The DMS is used primarily by health information management (HIM) departments and other departments to handle documents regarding patient care. These documents can be scanned or obtained electronically from other information systems. One of the advantages to the DMS is the use of workflow. The workflow processes identified with the DMS include health record completion, release of information, and routing documents for review. The DMS can be a standalone information system or a component of the EHR. A DMS can also be used in other areas of the healthcare facility besides the HIM department, such as human resources, patient financial services, purchasing, registration, and the business office.

Automated forms processing technology allows the user to type data directly into the computer, eliminating the need to manually complete a paper form and then scan it into the DMS. By entering the data directly into the information system, the data are available for manipulation. Electronic signature, document annotation, and editing are critical to the DMS because physicians and other users can electronically sign the documentation entered into the information system from anywhere. The user also should be able to add notes to existing documentation and to edit documents when errors are identified. Because the health record is a legal document, the original documentation must be retained so that the differences between the two documents are shown.

Document capture is much more than scanning paper images into the DMS. Voice, video, electronic transactions, and other forms of technology may be used to capture data. One example is optical character recognition (OCR). OCR is defined as a method of encoding text from analog paper into bitmapped images and translating the images into a form that is computer readable.

With OCR, a text can be scanned, and the content can be edited. Document indexing, barcoding, and character and form recognition are ways to link documents to a particular patient, thus allowing for retrieval. An index is an organized (usually alphabetical) list of specific data that serves to guide, indicate, or otherwise facilitate reference to the data. These indexing tools allow the user to locate and retrieve a specific patient's health record, a specific encounter, and even a specific document through the use of indexing by entering search criteria into one or more of the index fields. The user is then able to view the desired document as well as print, fax, or use another method of transmission. The purpose of the DMS is not to eliminate paper, but rather to manage documents. To manage these documents, the healthcare facility needs to use the DMS for more than document imaging. It should also use character recognition along with imaging to manage all documents for the healthcare facility and not just the health record. The DMS also uses workflow in order to facilitate the business process of the healthcare facility. The DMS includes multimedia technologies and moving documents from one information system to another without printing the document on paper.

Document Management System Versus Electronic Health Record

The DMS is not the same as the EHR. The EHR is an electronic record of health-related information on an individual that conforms to nationally recognized interoperability standards and that can be created, managed, and consulted by authorized clinicians and staff across more than one healthcare organization. Based on this definition, document imaging does not qualify as an EHR because the healthcare providers do not create the data within the DMS. If employees' expectations are not managed and they believe that a DMS is an EHR, they are often disappointed in the information system when it is implemented. Employees will soon recognize that the DMS will not be able to perform the functionality of the EHR. For example, unless OCR has been used, the DMS will not be able to perform searches on the content of the health records because the images are pictures of the paper documents. The DMS also will not assist in clinical decision support.

With the DMS, the image can be retrieved by any authorized user from any location. Multiple users can also view the same image at the same time, enhancing communication between care providers. The image of the scanned document cannot be searched, edited, or changed unless OCR is used. Although document imaging is not an EHR, it is a valuable tool to healthcare facilities that do not have the space needed to store paper records and that do not want to use microfilm. Many of the healthcare facilities that elect to implement a DMS use it as a component of the EHR.

Components of a Document Management System

A DMS is made of many components, including a scanner, magnetic storage, and file server. All of the components work together to scan, store, and retrieve the health record documents.

Scanner

The scanner is the hardware that is used to transform the paper document into a digital image. Scanners are rated based on the number of pages per minute (PPM) the scanner can process. High-powered scanners used to accomplish high-volume scanning, usually found in HIM departments, resemble a copier with an automatic document feeder. Departments with only light scanning needs may use a flatbed scanner. A flatbed scanner can only scan one page at a time because each page must be manually placed on the screen, scanned, and then manually removed before the next page is manually placed on the scanning bed. A high-powered scanner can scan a pile of documents in a short period of time because each page is automatically fed through the imaging bed of the scanner.

The scanner chosen should be fast enough to accommodate the volume of scanning that needs to be accomplished. Generally, the larger the healthcare facility, the faster the scanner needed. The scanner should be able to adjust the density and contrast of the scanning automatically based on the type of form being scanned. Contrast refers to the difference between the lightness or darkness of a letter, word, or diagram and the background color of the document. Density refers to how much content is on a document; a form that has many blank spaces is less dense than a full page of text. The need to adjust for density and contrast automatically comes from the fact that some forms or their documentation are lighter or darker than others; thus, they will need to be scanned darker or lighter accordingly—just as when a document is copied on a copy machine. The scanner is able to identify the type of form and make needed adjustments because of barcodes on either the form or the target sheets. Target sheets are pages that contain only a barcode that tells the scanner and, ultimately, the computer the content of the pages that follow. The barcode may contain the form name, the patient name, or some other piece of information. If the scanner cannot scan both sides of a two-sided document, the operator must scan the other side manually.

Because of the movement of the scanner and the dust that collects from the paper movement through the scanner, scanners must undergo frequent preventive maintenance. There will be times that even with preventive maintenance, the information system will become inoperable. This must be considered when selecting the number of scanners and PPM ratings needed.

Scanning Workstation

The scanning workstation is the desktop computer that controls the scanner. Once a document is scanned, the workstation compresses the file created by the scanner in order to save storage space. Another step performed by the scanning workstation is to give each document scanned an individual file name. The name is used to store the image and is ultimately used when the file is retrieved.

Abstracting and Quality Control Workstation

The abstracting and quality control workstation is also a personal computer (PC). Rather than scanning, this workstation is used for indexing and quality control. The healthcare facility determines the data elements to be indexed based on its needs. During the quality control process, the clerk views every image to check for the quality of the image and verifies that indexing is accurate and patient demographics are correct.

File Server

The file server is a large PC or other computer that is extremely powerful and has a large amount of memory and magnetic hard drive. When the user performs an inquiry on a PC to retrieve a patient's health record, the file server receives the request for the document images, retrieves the document images, and sends the document images back to the requester. When documents are scanned into the computer, the files created are stored on the file server's magnetic hard drive.

Retrieval Workstation

This is the workstation used by the physician, HIM staff, or other users to retrieve patient information and view document images. If the workstation is used to access few health records, a standard size monitor will work. With a standard size monitor (usually 22 to 24 inches, measured diagonally across the viewable screen), the entire image will not fit on the screen. The user will have to scroll to see the entire page. If the workstation is used heavily to view document images, it is easier on the user's eyes and for the display of the image to have an oversized monitor. It is important to evaluate what size monitor is needed because there is a significant cost difference between the two.

Printers

The healthcare facility will need to determine who has the rights to print reports from the DMS. The size of the printer will be based on the volume of printing performed by that area. For example, in the typical HIM department a high-quality, high-speed laser printer is needed in order to print large volumes of information. The print server controls the location where documents are printed and controls the work queue or order in which a document prints. The fastest way to print is to use a print file server to control and facilitate the printing process. There must be an electronic or computerized print tracking log, similar to an audit log, that indicates who requested or submitted the print order, where the printing occurred (which printer was used and in what area of the healthcare facility), date and time of printing, what forms or reports were printed, and any other pertinent information the healthcare facility deems appropriate.

Annotation

One of the functions of a DMS is the ability to annotate the images. Annotation is the ability to add to the image in some way. Because the image may be a legal document, the image itself cannot be altered; however, an overlay to the document will show the annotation. These annotations are useful to call attention to some data on the form and to enhance viewing. There are several ways to annotate a document:

- Note—The note tool will allow the physician or other user to add a note to the image. This may be useful if additional data have become available and the physician wants to call it to the reader's attention.
- Highlighting—The highlighting tool emphasizes important sections of text, much like a highlighter pen on paper. The purpose is to call the reader's attention to specific test results or other documentation.
- Drawing—The drawing tool can be used to draw circles, arrows, or other markings. This is another way to bring the reader's attention to specific data or, in the case of radiology imaging, the anomaly.
- Zoom and reduction—The zoom and reduction tool enlarge or reduces the size of the image to enhance viewing. This is helpful if the writing is small or there is a lot of writing on the page that is difficult to read. It is very helpful in the interpretation of radiology reports because the radiologist can enlarge portions of the image to better see any anomalies.
- Rotate—The rotate tool allows the user to flip an image. This is useful if a document has been scanned upside down or sideways.

Advantages and Disadvantages

There are many advantages and disadvantages to the DMS. Some healthcare facilities choose to focus on the advantages and implement the DMS in their progression toward the EHR; others choose to skip this step and go directly to the EHR. Some advantages are space savings, productivity gains, and immediate access to patient information. Disadvantages include lack of manipulation and reporting capabilities and fear of change to work processes.

Space Savings

Space savings is a definite advantage of the DMS because paper health records take up a lot of space. Space in a healthcare facility is a valuable commodity, and healthcare facilities are always looking for ways to improve space utilization. To realize the space savings, many healthcare facilities destroy the paper health records after a predetermined period of time. This practice ultimately eliminates the need for the long-term file area, opening the space for other needs, such as expansion of the HIM department or reallocation to other departments. The elimination of the file room may take several years as health records are destroyed, scanned, or microfilmed.

Retrieval of Large Number of Records

The HIM department is constantly pulling large numbers of health records for audits, research, and other purposes. HIM staff must pull the health records for review and later refile them once the review is complete. This process takes up a lot of time and space because the health records have to be stored during the review process and space has to be allocated for the reviewers to work. With a DMS, health records are stored electronically. If a researcher or auditor needs to access large numbers of health records, these records can be placed in a work queue. The reviewer can view the health record from any location as long as proper authorization is provided, thus eliminating the need to pull, manage, and refile the health records.

Productivity Gains

Through the use of DMS and workflow technology, employee productivity is improved because they no longer have to look for health records or move them from one location to another. A DMS eliminates health record retrieval and assembly and many other routine paper-based traditional health record functions. Other functions, such as coding, analysis, and qualitative and quantitative analysis, can be done electronically. With the DMS, patient care providers have 24-hour access to patient information without the need for around-the-clock staff. Another productivity gain comes from the elimination of lost or misplaced health records. Hours spent looking for health records could be better spent on other tasks such as eliminating duplicate health record numbers, documentation improvement, compliance audits, and privacy audits.

Online Availability of Information

When it comes to emergency patient care, minutes count. The availability of the patient's past medical history can be the difference between life and death. For example, if the patient has an allergy and the physician does not know, an inappropriate medication could be prescribed to the patient, thus resulting in harm to the patient and possibly death. The ability to access critical information in seconds—not minutes or hours—improves the quality of the care to patients and can prevent unnecessary or duplicate testing. Another benefit to the online availability of information is that multiple users view the same health record simultaneously, even the same document at the same time. This accessibility improves user satisfaction and ultimately improves patient care through improved communication and accessibility.

System Security and Control

With access controls, audit trails, and other security measures, the security of the health record is improved over that of the traditional paper health record. With the paper health record, there is only one point of access, but there is no way to know who viewed the health record and what they looked at. With proper security measures, only authorized individuals will be able to view what they have a need to know and there will be a record of not only the health record viewed but also the specific documents.

Database Retrieval

The DMS allows for searches based on indexed data. For example, a search could retrieve all patients who were discharged from the healthcare facility on December 1, 2013, or all of Dr. Smith's patients, or John Brown's health record. This function is great for research and saves time from having to identify patients and then retrieve their data individually. The searching is limited to the data elements captured during indexing.

Lack of Manipulation or Reporting

Because the images are pictures of the health record document and not entries into the EHR, the user is unable to manipulate the data to show trends or other views. Likewise, the user cannot generate reports related to the images rather than entered data.

Fear of Change

People are inherently afraid of change. Research on DMS implementations has shown that, at least initially, the number of employees needed increases because the HIM department is still managing the paper health record in addition to the EHR. Because of this, management must let the employees know the status of their positions. Usually, staff members will maintain their current jobs, but some jobs may change or even be eliminated. Instead of filing reports in the health record, they may be scanning documents. Keeping employees informed of the changes will keep their fear manageable and may prevent the department from losing good employees. Fear can develop not only in staff but also within management. Fears such as the risk of not being able to access information because of technology failure, power outages, bad media, or other reasons add to the responsibility and accountability expected of management.

Implementation

Healthcare facilities must manage the existing paper health records when a DMS is implemented. The healthcare facility has to decide if these existing records will be scanned into the information system and, if so, how many. Healthcare facilities' decisions on this matter vary widely. Some scan only health records with a discharge date on or after the DMS implementation date. Other healthcare facilities choose to backscan some or all existing health records to provide users electronic access to the old health records. **Backscanning** is the process of scanning past health records into the DMS so there is an existing database of patient information, making the DMS valuable to the user from the first day of implementation. Although this methodology provides an immediate database of health records in the DMS on the first day of the go-live, it also gives the healthcare facility a long backlog of information to be scanned, preferably before implementation. Many patients may never come back to the healthcare facility, so it will not realize any benefit from many records scanned into the DMS. The healthcare facility should choose how far back to go with the scanning, such as six months or two years. Healthcare facilities that choose to backscan documents typically participate in medical research and have high readmission rates to the healthcare facility. An example of this research could be a pediatric longitudinal study that looks at patient care or treatment protocols over a number of years or decades, such as in the case of babies born with certain birth defects. Other healthcare facilities choose to backscan on a patient-by-patient basis upon future admittance. The decision should be based on the needs of the healthcare facility, cost, filing space, and other resources. The decision should balance the needs of the user and the resources available. Many healthcare facilities only provide the HIM department access to the DMS initially if they decided not to backscan. The logic behind this decision is to prevent users from going to the DMS and not locating health records on a patient, which can lead to assumptions that records do not exist or frustration with the DMS. Once there is a strong repository of data, access should be rolled out throughout the healthcare facility. Record scanning can be performed by the healthcare facility HIM or other designated staff or it can be outsourced to a vendor. If the facility decides to scan the health records themselves, additional staff would be needed to manage the current workload and to add backscanning to their tasks. Many facilities overcome this need by hiring temporary employees to cover the difference in workload. Healthcare facilities that choose vendors to scan (because of their high productivity and experienced staff) enable the scanning to be completed more quickly. The vendor usually charges by the number of images scanned and the actual tasks performed. These tasks may include preparation of the health record for scanning, indexing, and quality control.

Many hospitals begin implementation of the DMS by scanning the current emergency department patient records and gradually working up to inpatient records. Emergency department records are smaller, more controllable, and easier to manage than the inpatient records. An inpatient health record can have 75 to 100 pages or more for a three- to four-day stay on a regular nursing unit, whereas an emergency department record may be 5 to 15 pages.

Scanning may be performed in either a centralized or a decentralized approach. In the centralized approach, all scanning is performed in one location, generally the HIM department. In the decentralized approach, scanning is performed throughout the healthcare facility—wherever the documentation is created. These locations include admissions, nursing units, emergency department, and many more.

Justification of Cost

Healthcare facilities justify the cost of DMS with the savings that occur from decreasing the operating costs of the HIM department and the healthcare facility as a whole. The savings come from reductions in clerical staff, improvement in accounts receivable as health records are no longer misplaced and are therefore able to be coded, and increased revenue due to decreased expenses. Although staffing may increase at first while both the existing paper health record and the DMS are managed, over time staffing can be reduced below original levels. Additionally, operating cost reductions of the HIM department can be achieved, including elimination of file folders and other supplies related to processing the paper health record.

Because costs may actually go up in the short term, the return on investment may be calculated over a 5- to 10-year period. When the file area is eliminated, the healthcare facility can reallocate that space to a revenue-generating department. Productivity is also increased, thus offsetting the cost of staffing. For example, the release of information coordinator no longer has to stand in front of a copy machine and the coder does not have to wait for health records to be assembled and analyzed in order to code them.

Forms

Forms management is a key implementation issue that must be addressed. At least six months prior to implementation of the DMS, forms should be evaluated and redesigned to facilitate the scanning process. The weight of the paper used should be appropriate for use in a scanner. Paper that is too heavy or too light may jam the automatic feeder. White paper is recommended for all forms because the color of the document is scanned along with the content of the form. This significantly increases the size of the computer file and the quality of the printed document. The forms should be standardized to 8.5 by 11 inch dimensions where possible. The redesign should include the addition of barcodes to each form. The barcode makes indexing more efficient because the barcode can enter metadata automatically. Standards for the use of barcodes must be established to facilitate scanning. These standards should include the size of the barcode, the standardized location of the barcode, and the amount of white space between the barcode and any text. The new forms with the barcode should be in use at the time of implementation. The recommended barcode symbiology, or format, is Code 39, also known as Code 3 of 9. These barcodes should be placed on the form in a standardized location.

Staffing Changes

With the transition of employees from filing paper to scanning, indexing, and quality control, new job titles and job descriptions will be required, and staffing needs may be reduced. For example, the file clerk role could be replaced by a clerk who performs both scanning and quality control for the scanning process. These tasks require additional technology skills, which may elevate the clerk's pay grade. However, since the workload is electronic, fewer pages would need to be filed within a paper health record, reducing the time and, thus, the personnel required to complete the task. Test results and other documents would be entered into the EHR automatically, without the need of human assistance. Over time, fewer paper documents would need to be scanned and incorporated, further decreasing the workload. However, there would still be a need for quality control measures, including both electronic precautions and physical monitoring procedures performed by the staff, to ensure that the information incorporated would go to the appropriate health record.

Changes in job titles and job descriptions must be in place at the time of the DMS implementation and would be decided after discussions with administration and the human resources department. The HIM department and other affected staff must be trained on the DMS prior to implementation to prevent backlogs from occurring, which would impact user satisfaction.

Process Redesign

The implementation of a DMS will have a tremendous impact on the workflow of an HIM department. As a result, the HIM department will have to reengineer workflows to adapt to an electronic environment and review and update policies and procedures, among many other tasks, to aid in the transition. The HIM department will no longer have to assemble the health record; they will prepare the health record for scanning instead. The way the traditional discharge processing, such as coding and chart analysis, is done will also drastically change. For instance:

- Analysis is done online.
- Physician completion of records can be completed from any location.
- Electronic signatures are used.

When to Scan the Health Record

Ideally, scanning should be performed as documents are created to allow immediate online access to orders, progress notes, and other written documentation. In practice, however, the health record is not usually scanned until after discharge. Some healthcare facilities scan the health record immediately following discharge and use workflow technology to facilitate the record discharge processing. Other healthcare facilities complete the health record, obtaining all necessary documents and signatures, and then scan it.

Immediately Following Discharge

Many healthcare facilities scan the health record immediately following the patient's discharge from the hospital. There are a number of advantages to scanning the health record at this point. This timing allows coding and analysis to be performed remotely if the healthcare facility so chooses. It also allows immediate access to the health record for patient care, coding, analysis, and other healthcare operations. In the traditional paper environment, the discharge processing of the health record is a linear process. One step has to be completed before the next because only one employee can access the health record at a time. With DMS and workflow technology, coders, analysts, and other users no longer must wait for other steps in the discharge process to be complete before accessing the health record because imaging allows concurrent access. This speeds up the discharge processing function. Many patients are readmitted to the healthcare facility immediately after discharge, so having the recent discharged health record scanned and available to the emergency department or other patient care areas improves the quality of care provided.

There are also disadvantages to scanning immediately after discharge. Not only do staff members have to be trained to use the DMS as part of their discharge processing, but physicians must also be trained on how to complete health records online. In addition to retrieval of images, the physician would need to know how to use the annotation tools discussed earlier in this chapter and how to sign the documents electronically. The physician would also need to know how to complete forms electronically and to dictate discharge summaries and other documents.

The healthcare facility must have sufficient staff and equipment in place to ensure that the scanning is performed quickly so that the records are available to HIM staff, physicians, and other users in a timely manner. If scanning is not done promptly, health record users quickly become disillusioned with the DMS and not want to use it. It is especially important to have records available in the appropriate time period in the early days of the DMS, when everyone is getting used to it and learning about its benefits.

Scanning Upon Completion

Some healthcare facilities choose to scan the health record after the completion of the health record discharge processing. This method does not impact physician chart completion, and it does not allow coding and analysis to be performed remotely. Those who need access to the health record in the immediate discharge period still must wait for it to be processed in the traditional linear method—that is, the process in which the health record goes from the first step in discharge processing (usually putting all pages in the correct sequence) to each subsequent step and is completed when the final deficiency analysis is complete. The health record is scanned once all final paperwork (such as lab results) is received, all forms signed by the appropriate medical/nursing personnel, and transcribed reports are incorporated.

There are expenses related to the management of the paper record during the discharge process, such as the cost of folders and space for health record completion.

Retrieval of Images

To retrieve and view document images stored in the DMS, one must be an authorized user with the proper permissions. A user enters one or more of the indexed fields, such as a patient's health record number, to retrieve the appropriate health record and its associated document images for review.

Future of Document Management System

It is unlikely that imaging itself will be outdated anytime soon because there continue to be paper documents brought by the patient or from an outside source that will need to be scanned into the appropriate health record in the EHR.

CHECK YOUR UNDERSTANDING 8.1

1. What method encodes text from analog paper into bitmapped images so that the computer can read it?

    a. CPOE
    b. PACS
    c. OCR
    d. DMS

2. Pages that tell the scanner information about the page(s) that follow are called _____.

    a. Target sheets
    b. Automatic forms processing
    c. Barcodes
    d. Indexing

(Continued)

3. What term is used for the process of getting and listing specific information about a document so that it can be retrieved easily from a DMS?

   a. Scanning
   b. Target sheets
   c. Indexing
   d. Routing

4. A print tracking log is similar to what other function in an EHR or clinical information system?

   a. Provider authentication
   b. Password protection
   c. Audit log
   d. Biometric authentication

5. In a DMS, altering an image in some way, such as highlighting or enlarging, is referred to as _____.

   a. Annotation
   b. Abstracting
   c. Analytics
   d. Auditing

Radiology Information System

A radiology information system (RIS) is used to collect, store, and provide information on radiological tests such as x-rays, ultrasound, magnetic resonance imaging (MRI), computed tomography (CT), and positron emission tomography (PET). The RIS also supports other radiological procedures performed in radiology such as ultrasound-guided biopsies and upper and lower gastrointestinal series. A RIS is designed to assist the technician by identifying the steps required to prepare for each test or procedure. The RIS can also assist the technician with taking x-rays and other radiological examinations by controlling radiation exposure, positioning of the patient, and image quality. Ultimately, the RIS provides patients with follow-up instructions to take home after the procedure.

The RIS can be used to assist in the management of the radiology department as well as document patient care. A RIS can perform many administrative tasks:

- Schedule patient examinations and procedures
- Report charges to the financial information system
- Generate management reports
- Generate radiology reports
- Track nuclear materials
- Transcribe documents
- Retrieve test results
- Fax radiology reports to the ordering physician
- Monitor supply inventory

Some of the management reports generated by the RIS include number of tests performed, types of tests or procedures performed, productivity by technicians, utilization of the various radiology machines, and productivity levels for each radiologist.

A RIS frequently has a picture archival communication system (PACS). A PACS is an integrated information system that obtains, stores, retrieves, and displays digital images. In a PACS, x-ray films,

MRIs, mammograms, and other radiological examinations (such as cardiac catheterization films and ultrasounds) are stored digitally, thus eliminating the need to store and manage the physical film. The digital image is immediately available for patient care, which is especially important in emergency department and intensive care situations. The filmless radiology saves the healthcare facility money and physical space by eliminating steps such as making copies for patients or purchasing folders for storage. As a result, radiology departments are able to provide improved (more efficient) customer service because there is no waiting for films to be pulled and copied. In addition, the PACS eliminates lost files.

The ability to view radiology images from any location by the radiologist and other users is called teleradiology. The images can even be viewed at multiple locations at the same time. A radiologist can read images from home in the middle of the night, from another city, or even from other countries. Teleradiology is also used frequently for consultations between radiologists who are in distant locations.

Because radiology images must have high resolution to be of diagnostic quality, the image must be compressed as it is transported across the network or Internet and then decompressed in a lossless manner to maintain its original form. PACS provides this capability.

A PACS affords the radiologist many conveniences. He or she can easily compare previous films to current ones, zoom in on suspicious areas, enhance an image, relocate or reposition an image, and apply pointers to identify problem areas. Once the images are pulled up in the PACS, the radiologist is able to magnify, rotate, measure, and use many other tools to view the images. When an image is read, the radiologist is able to dictate the report for transcription or use voice recognition software to create the report from within the information system.

Laboratory Information System

The laboratory information system (LIS) collects, stores, and manages laboratory tests and their respective results. The LIS can speed up access to test results through improved efficiency from various locations, including anywhere in the hospital, the physician's office, or even the clinician's home. The LIS has the necessary functionality to be used in all areas of the laboratory, including blood chemistry, blood banks, microbiology, virology, and pathology. Currently, LISs involve many interfaces because they are still typically standalone information systems, separate from the EHR. It is important for these interfaces to work seamlessly with the specified EHR system to ensure integration with the clinical and communications needs of the healthcare facility (Biedermann and Dolezel 2017, 84). The healthcare facility must get assurances from the EHR vendor that the interfaces between the new EHR and the existing information systems are complete and sustainable to avoid issues with transmission of the data.

The physician order for a laboratory test is generally received from a CPOE or other order entry system. The CPOE identifies what tests need to be run, schedules them, and creates a list that indicates where the patient is located and if the test is routine or urgent. Test results can be entered into the LIS manually or collected automatically from the instruments running the test. The LIS can also print out various laboratory reports needed, such as all of the tests performed on a single day or during a patient's entire hospitalization. Other functions include:

- Identifying normal ranges for each laboratory test
- Generating laboratory reports
- Marking laboratory values as high, low, or panic
- Notifying laboratory staff and physicians of panic (very high or low) values via alerts (such as an audible ping or alarm, results highlighted in a different color, or a note sent to the "to-do list")
- Printing barcode labels to track specimens
- Recording quality control activities
- Generating management reports
- Submitting charges to the financial information system

The LIS can assist management in running the laboratory department through the management reporting capabilities. It should be able to generate reports such as the number of tests run per month, the tests ran, turnaround time, and productivity reports on individual laboratory technicians.

CHECK YOUR UNDERSTANDING 8.2

1. A PACS system allows the x-ray department to be totally digital, so there is no need for the use of physical _____.

   a. Coding
   b. Certification
   c. Invoices
   d. Film

2. An RIS system may perform all of the following radiological tests except _____.

   a. PET
   b. MRI
   c. CT
   d. Complete blood count

3. The term used to describe viewing images from a remote location is _____.

   a. PACS
   b. Teleradiology
   c. RIS
   d. Symbiology

4. A computer program that allows two different information systems to communicate with each other is referred to as an _____.

   a. Interface
   b. Interchange
   c. Integration
   d. Annotation

5. Which of the following data or documents would not be used in a PACS?

   a. CT scan
   b. Ultrasound
   c. Discharge summary
   d. X-ray

Nursing Information System

A nursing information system (NIS) assists in the planning and monitoring of overall patient care. A NIS will document the nursing care provided to a patient. Clinical documentation is any manual or electronic notation or recording made by a physician or other healthcare clinician related to a patient's medical condition or treatment. There may be different NISs available for the emergency department, intensive care areas, and other nursing areas because of the differing needs of each specialization. The capabilities of a strong nursing information system are flexible to accommodate the needs of the nurse. Conveniences such as efficient and quality documentation practices as well as easy access to quick reference guides are important. Advantages to NIS include:

- Reduction in costs of providing nursing care
- Improved patient care
- Immediate access to information on services rendered by the nursing staff
- Immediate notification of results from laboratory, radiology, or other ancillary departments
- Reduction in lost charges

- Reduced average length of stay
- Submitting charges to the financial information system

Many of these advantages result from the documentation of information at the time of care.

An NIS must be designed to support and promote quality documentation and practices through the use of protocols and vocabularies. Based on information entered into the NIS, such as the patient's diagnosis or procedure, the appropriate nursing protocol is selected.

The nurse plans the patient's nursing care needs based on this protocol. Nursing documentation traditionally includes:

- Admission assessment
- Nursing activities
- Intake and output
- Graphic information
- Activities of daily living
- Nursing care plans
- Nurses' notes
- Medication administration record

The NIS can also assist in the administrative management and daily operations of the nursing department by:

- Monitoring staffing allocation
- Scheduling nursing staff
- Generating performance improvement reports

Pharmacy Information System

A pharmacy information system (PIS) assists providers in ordering, allocating, and administering medication. With a focus on patient safety issues, especially medication errors, the PIS is a key tool in providing optimal patient care. The PIS stores the patient's demographic information, allergies, medication history, diagnoses, laboratory results, and other key information.

Data contained within the hospital information system and the functions of the PIS help providers reduce medication errors by using the hospital information system, the EHR, and the PIS, combined with information from medical databases and drug formularies. For example, a patient may have indicated an allergy in her history and physical exam, which may have been performed many days or weeks ago. If the physician attempts to prescribe a medication that is contraindicated by the documented allergy, the PIS would alert the physician to this contraindication and suggest another medication.

The PIS can stand alone or be integrated with other systems in the healthcare facility such as CPOE. The greatest benefits come from the integration of data. For example, CPOE can record the medication order in the pharmacy system, which, in turn, can automatically update inventory levels—thus, automatically charging the patient.

PISs are used in hospitals, drugstores, and other healthcare settings. Functions vary according to the needs of the setting and facility. For example, a drugstore might need to track the number of refills remaining on a prescription, whereas this function would not be as important to a hospital.

PISs check for drug interactions, food and drug interactions, and other contraindications. When problems are identified, the PIS alerts the pharmacist or end user. It should also determine whether or not the dosage and administration method is appropriate for the size and age of the patient. The PIS can also manage the inventory of drugs in the pharmacy. This includes:

- Ordering drugs
- Inventory control
- Managing the formulary
- Tracking the costs of drugs
- Reporting on the usage of controlled medications

The pharmacy can analyze data stored within the information system, such as looking for patterns of drug usage and signs of abuse. These patterns may identify potential abuse by patients or physicians.

PISs can assist in the dispensing of medications in the pharmacy, which can help the nursing units in a number of ways:

- Creating individual dosages
- Use of secure storage systems
- Robotics
- Secure access to medications
- Documentation of medications administered, including when and by whom
- Barcodes

Interdisciplinary Charting System

An **interdisciplinary charting system** can be used by any healthcare professional to collect and store patient assessments, progress notes, and care plans. Examples of these healthcare professionals include physicians, nurses, physical therapists, respiratory therapists, pharmacists, dietitians, and the like. The information system can also collect data, such as vital signs and input and output, automatically. Handheld devices such as tablets are frequently used to allow for documentation at the bedside.

Emergency Department System

The **emergency department system (EDS)** is designed to meet the unique needs of the emergency department, including tracking patients from triage to discharge. The EIS is also able to record test results and other clinical information. Demographic information is obtained from the hospital information system. The emergency department system can also assist in the department's workflow and generate management reports such as turnaround times, patient wait times, and more. This information system has become increasingly important in population health reporting.

There is a need to notify state health authorities regarding diagnoses of newly emerging diseases, such as Zika virus infection or multidrug-resistant tuberculosis; injuries due to mass casualty events, such as terrorist bombings or train derailments; and injuries due to natural disasters, such as tornadoes and hurricanes.

Anesthesia Information System

An **anesthesia information system** collects information on preoperative, operative, and postoperative anesthesia-related clinical information. This system follows the patient through the surgical process. The information system collects information on risk factors, vital signs, type of anesthesia, anesthetic agents used, dosage of anesthetic agents, and much more. The information system uses the information that is captured to create charges for billing purposes. As with other clinical information systems, the demographic information comes from the hospital information system. The data captured can also be used for quality improvement. Management reports can be created to provide statistics on a number of operations, frequency of anesthetic agents, and such.

Patient Monitoring System

The **patient monitoring system** automatically collects and stores patient data from various information systems used in healthcare. Data collected include fetal monitoring, vital signs, and oxygen saturation rates. Patient monitoring systems are typically utilized in the intensive care units and other specialty areas such as the operating and recovery rooms.

A patient monitoring system must be able to capture the desired data automatically. The nurse or other user should be able to monitor a patient's condition from the nursing unit, physician office, or other remote location if necessary. This may require the use of the Internet to access the information system. A nurse or other user must be able to create notes if needed to document and report variations in results, such as if the fetal monitor slipped out of position.

Vital signs and other data collected must be also reviewed and approved by the user regularly to ensure proper system functioning.

Telehealth

Telehealth has two aspects:

- Professional services given to a patient through an interactive telecommunications system by a practitioner at a distant site
- A telecommunications system that links healthcare facilities and patients from diverse geographic locations and transmits text and images for (medical) consultation and treatment

These locations can be across town, in rural areas, or in another country. Most specialists are located in urban areas, leaving patients in rural areas without easy access to them. Telehealth allows a physician to examine and treat a patient remotely. Telehealth can utilize video telephone, computers, smart phones, and other medical devices with wireless capabilities, such as cardiac pacemakers, glucose monitors and insulin pumps, or neuromonitors that can be checked remotely. Access to the patient or the device through the healthcare facility's EHR is also feasible. A nurse may be required to interact directly with the patient in order to support the physician's evaluation and treatment.

Benefits of telehealth include:

- Improved access to healthcare, such as specialty consultations, biomedical monitoring, and second opinions
- Improved continuity of care, patient education, and timely treatment—follow-up visits for chronically ill patients, reduced travel time for all involved, increased care to underserved areas
- Cost efficiency—managing chronically ill patients more efficiently decreases admissions and shortens length of stay
- Improved access to health records and patient information with online health information available for learning, peer support groups, research information
- Improved training and education for medical/clinical personnel as well as patients, clinical trial research, improved interactions with medical personnel for disease management (Johnson and Warner 2013)

Physicians find clinical telehealth a benefit in giving patients medical consultations and monitoring those living in rural areas or those who are homebound. Telemonitoring is used at the patient's home to monitor cardiac rhythms, blood sugar, blood pressure, and other values to be submitted to the care provider. This type of monitoring can be performed through the use of the telephone or the computer. The data collected at the patient's home are digitally submitted into a CIS and thus made a part of the EHR.

Telehealth is a very sophisticated technology. Technology used includes virtual reality and robotics, which may be used to assist with the examination or treatment of a patient. The use of robotics to perform surgery is called **telesurgery**. This allows surgery to be performed on a patient in a different location.

Issues that healthcare facilities need to consider when developing or using **telemedicine**—a subset of telehealth that focuses on the provision of care whereas telehealth includes administrative uses and education—programs:

- Privacy, confidentiality, and security must be ensured during the telemedicine event.
  - Safeguard patients' privacy
  - Network security among hospitals, clinics, practitioners
  - Contract specialties, such as radiology and mental health, with private networks with point-to-point connections
- Liability is usually shared between referring provider and consulting provider, but for telemedicine vendors and technical staff there is no legal precedent yet.
- Licensure and accreditation rules differ by states for both licensure and accreditation; there is no federal legislation for telemedicine at this time.
- Fraud—vendor services, billing for healthcare services provided, and contracts need clear legal analysis.
- Policies and procedures must be developed and agreed to by all parties.
- Documentation requirement for patient information and services is provided. (Johnson and Warner 2013)

Telehealth provides many advantages, such as improved access to care, treatment provided via communication tools, and home monitoring. The problem is that the infrastructure is expensive, and because physicians are licensed to practice medicine by state, the geographic range in which the physician can consult is limited.

Telehealth records must be managed as with any other patient care encounter. There are no differences in the documentation requirements between patient care provided remotely or at bedside, so the current documentation practices and forms are adequate. The American Health Information Management Association (AHIMA) recommends the following minimum information:

- Patient name
- Identification number
- Date of service
- Referring physician
- Consulting physician
- Provider facility
- Type of evaluation performed
- Informed consent
- Evaluation results
- Diagnosis and impression
- Recommendations for further treatment (Johnson and Warner 2013)

The HIM professional must take the necessary steps to ensure that the privacy and security of patient's health information is protected according to HIPAA requirements and any applicable state laws. For example, procedures in the administrative, technical, or physical safeguards domains may require revision to remain HIPAA-compliant while accommodating telehealth. This may involve providing a secure area where physicians can consult with the patient, ensuring additional security and encryption capabilities on the HIS, and established procedures and training for conducting telehealth sessions. The HIM professional may also be involved in the medical staff credentialing process to ensure physicians are indeed licensed and qualified to practice within the state. Finally, specific attention must be paid to the varying state laws and regulations to ensure compliance with them.

Smart Card

A smart card is a plastic card, similar in appearance to a credit card, with a computer chip embedded in it. Smart cards have been widely adopted for use in banking, retail, government, and other applications. Three uses of smart cards in healthcare are emergency treatment, reducing fraud and abuse, and reducing administrative costs (Secure Technology Alliance 2017a).

Smart cards enable portable storage of health and insurance information. They are relatively inexpensive and are able to protect the information stored within them from unauthorized access. In an emergency situation, smart cards can provide a physician with the critical information needed for proper care and treatment of a patient such as allergies, significant conditions like diabetes mellitus, and more. There are two categories of smart cards: contact and contactless. The contact smart cards require a scanner through which the card is scanned in order to read it. The contactless card only has to be close to the scanner (Secure Technology Alliance 2017b).

Although smart cards are useful tools, the patient must manage and maintain the accuracy of information on the card. Some smart cards require a password or a personal identification number that the patient must remember for access. Another concern is privacy of the information on the card in the event that it is stolen.

Impact of Clinical Information Systems on HIM

The HIM professional is typically not a direct user of the various CISs discussed throughout this chapter, although the HIM professional accesses the information through either the CIS or the EHR. However, the HIM professional is the expert on the management of health records, and input from this individual is important to ensure that accreditation, regulatory, and other requirements are met. The same is true for privacy and security issues. HIM professionals are highly recommended to be a part of the information system implementation team to ensure that all HIM-related concerns such as quality documentation, confidentiality practices, and retention schedules are addressed up front. As each CIS submits charges to the financial information system, the HIM professional may be involved in developing the charges, similar to the involvement in the facility's chargemaster. Lastly, remember that every clinical information system can populate the EHR with information that is ultimately managed and maintained by HIM professionals.

CHECK YOUR UNDERSTANDING 8.3

1. Data such as graphic information and activities of daily living would be typically found within which of these clinical information systems?

   a. Telehealth
   b. Pharmacy information system
   c. Nursing information system
   d. Telemedicine

2. Which of the following clinical information systems easily operates with the CPOE?

   a. Telehealth
   b. Pharmacy information system
   c. Nursing information system
   d. Telemedicine

3. A portable method of storage of health data is known as _____.

   a. E-medicine
   b. Smart card
   c. E-health
   d. E-care

4. Another term used interchangeably with telehealth is _____.

   a. Teleconference
   b. E-health
   c. Teleradiology
   d. Telemedicine

5. Which of the following personnel typically does not use the clinical information systems directly in their daily tasks?

   a. Radiology
   b. Nursing
   c. Pharmacy
   d. HIM

Real-World Case

Due to the tropical nature of most of the state of Florida and the large influx of travelers from the southern Atlantic islands, and Central and South America, the spread of the Zika virus is a very real concern. The Florida Department of Health (FDOH) can receive real-time electronic notification of any suspected or confirmed diagnoses of Zika exposure from any hospital or laboratory in the state.

Using the patient demographic information received from the EHR's public health reporting systems, FDOH uses a geographic information system (GIS) to map and track the spread of the Zika virus anywhere in the state. Based on the tracking information, mosquito eradication efforts can be coordinated and focused on the most at-risk locations. The respective county health departments can then provide additional and more aggressive screenings on the identified at-risk populations.

REVIEW QUESTIONS

1. Which function is not under CIS?

   a. Quality improvement
   b. surgery
   c. nursing
   d. pharmacy

2. All of the following are advantages of a DMS except _____.

   a. Space saving
   b. Retrieval of a large number of records
   c. Lack of ability to manipulate data
   d. Multiple users can access data at one time

3. What is the term used for the processing of scanning past health records into the information system so there is an existing database of patient information, making the information system valuable to the user from the first day of implementation?

   a. CPOE
   b. OCR
   c. Backscanning
   d. Barcoding

4. Which health record should be scanned first when implementing a DMS?

   a. Inpatient
   b. Outpatient surgery
   c. Newborns
   d. Emergency department

5. The return on investment for a DMS is usually calculated using what time period?

   a. 5–10 years
   b. 6–12 months
   c. 1–3 years
   d. 1–3 months

6. What makes the indexing of scanned health record more efficient because it can enter metadata automatically?

   a. Barcodes
   b. Backscanning
   c. OCR
   d. CPOE

7. Which of the following is not a component of a DMS?

   a. Scanner
   b. LIS
   c. File server
   d. Workstations

8. Which of the following is not a diagnostic test completed in a RIS?

   a. MRI
   b. PET
   c. CPOE
   d. CT

9. Which of the following systems obtains, stores, retrieves, and displays digital images?
   a. CPOE
   b. OCR
   c. PIS
   d. PACS

10. In which area would you find robotics performing specific and complex tasks?
   a. Telehealth
   b. Telesurgery
   c. EDS
   d. Telemedicine

References

Biedermann, S. and D. Dolezel. 2017. *Introduction to Healthcare Informatics,* 2nd ed. Chicago: AHIMA.

Johnson, M. L. and D. Warner. 2013. Practice Brief: Telemedicine services and the health record (2013 update). http://bok.ahima.org/doc?oid=300269#.Wduo3GhSxRa.

Miliard, M. 2012. Healthcare IT News. Bringing the ED to the C-suite. http://www.healthcareitnews.com/news/bringing-ed-c-suite.

Secure Technology Alliance. 2017a. Smart Card Applications in the U.S. Healthcare Industry. http://www.smartcardalliance.org/smart-cards-applications-healthcare/.

Secure Technology Alliance. 2017b. Smart Card Primer. http://www.smartcardalliance.org/smart-cards-intro-primer/.

Electronic Health Record

Learning Objectives

- Create a development and implementation plan for an electronic health record (EHR).
- Explain the role of clinical vocabularies in the EHR.
- Support the need for and address issues related to the EHR.
- Educate the provider on benefits of the EHR.
- Identify the need for the multiple information systems required to support the EHR.
- Support the need for the personal health record.

Key Terms

Audit log
Barcode medication administration record (BC-MAR)
Certified EHR technology
Clinical decision support (CDS) system
Clinical messaging
Computerized provider order entry (CPOE)
Continuity of care record (CCR)
Core data set
Digital signature
Digitized signature
Document management system (DMS)
Electronic medical record (EMR)

Electronic medication administration record (EMAR)
Electronic signature
Health information blocking
Health information technology (HIT)
Health Level Seven International (HL7)
Hybrid record
Interoperability
Longitudinal health record
National Voluntary Laboratory Accreditation Program (NVLAP)
Office of the National Coordinator for Health Information Technology (ONC)

ONC–Approved Accreditor (ONC-AA)
ONC–Authorized Certification Bodies (ONC-ACBs)
Order entry and results reporting
Patient-provider portal
Personal health record (PHR)
Population health
Radiofrequency identification devices (RFIDs)
Reminders
Source systems
Structured data
Template-based entry
Unstructured data

As defined in chapter 1, an EHR is an electronic record of health-related information on an individual that conforms to nationally recognized interoperability standards and that authorized clinicians and staff across more than one healthcare organization can create, manage, and consult. With its seminal publication, *To Err Is Human: Building a Safer Health System*, the Institute of Medicine, now the National Academy of Medicine

(NAM), advocated for the use of **health information technology (HIT)** to help prevent many of the mistakes that regularly occur in the delivery of healthcare and that lead to the injuries and deaths of tens of thousands of patients (NAM 2000, 1). HIT includes the hardware, software, integrated technologies or related licenses, intellectual property, upgrades, or packaged solutions sold as services that are designed for or support the use by healthcare entities or patients for the electronic creation, maintenance, access, or exchange of health information. Included under the umbrella of HIT is the EHR. Among its many recommendations, the NAM promotes the EHR to include the following:

> (1) longitudinal collection of electronic health information for and about persons, where health information is defined as information pertaining to the health of an individual or health care provided to an individual; (2) immediate electronic access to person- and population-level information by authorized, and only authorized, users; (3) provision of knowledge and decision-support that enhance the quality, safety, and efficiency of patient care; and (4) support of efficient processes for health care delivery (IOM 2003, 1).

A **longitudinal health record** is a permanent record of significant information listed in chronological order and maintained across time, ideally from birth to death. Access to the EHR should not be limited to the healthcare facility, but rather be accessible remotely for providers as well as the consumer.

The EHR should not be confused with an **electronic medical record (EMR)**. An EMR is an electronic collection of all of the patient's health information and clinical care that is stored, managed, and referred to by authorized members of one healthcare entity, much like the actual paper health record only in digital or electronic form. An EHR includes everything in an EMR, but is much more comprehensive in terms of the patient's overall health, the care and services provided to the patient, and all healthcare providers participating in the patient care. The EHR must meet national standards for interoperability set by the Office of the National Coordinator for Health Information Technology (ONC). **Interoperability** is the ability of different information technology systems and software applications to communicate; to exchange data accurately, effectively, and consistently; and to use the information that has been exchanged. (Standards for the EHR and interoperability are addressed in detail in chapter 12.) Additionally, an EHR is a system in which the clinical information is utilized for the following purposes:

- Reimbursement, diagnostic and procedural coding, claims processing
- Computerized provider order entry (CPOE) and results reporting for laboratory, radiology, and other diagnostic tests
- E-prescriptions sent to the patient's pharmacy
- Medication management
- Population health reporting
- Quality improvement activities
- Clinical decision support
- Healthcare facility administrative reports and analytics
- Other additional authorized activities (Sandefer 2016, 370)

The EHR is designed to not only be used by the originating healthcare entity but be able to be referred to and transmitted to authorized and authenticated users at other healthcare entities (Amatayakul 2017, 9).

Purpose and Components of the Electronic Health Record

The EHR is not like a software program that can be bought, loaded on a server, and used immediately. It can take years to properly implement an EHR because of the number and complexity of the system components. The EHR is a collection of multiple technologies and systems that work together. **Source systems** are information systems that capture and feed data into the EHR. Source systems include the electronic medication administration record (EMAR), laboratory information system, radiology information system, hospital information system, nursing information systems, and more. Source systems are not just clinical systems, but also include administrative and financial systems (Sandefer 2016, 367). To realize the full benefits of the EHR, data should be captured at the point of care or data origination. Data can be captured in a multitude of ways, which can include personal computers, handheld devices, voice recognition, handwriting recognition, and other methods of data entry.

The healthcare facility must have the necessary infrastructure, the underlying framework and features of an information system, to integrate data. Much of the infrastructure for the EHR is the same as that for any information system—computers, monitors, network, printers, operating system, and application software.

The EHR infrastructure may also include a clinical data repository to centralize the data from the source systems. Another component of the EHR infrastructure is clinical decision support that controls alerts, reminders, order sets, and protocols (Amatayakul 2017, 14). The EHR should have access to knowledge-based resources such as MEDLINE, electronic drug references, and research databases.

EHRs include a **continuity of care record (CCR)** and a personal health record. The CCR is a **core data set**, which is the most relevant administrative, demographic, and clinical information about a patient's healthcare, covering one or more healthcare encounters. The CCR is *not* the minimum dataset for the EHR; it is information that is deemed most important for the continued care of the patient who is transferred to or seen by another healthcare practitioner (Amatayakul 2017, 302). It provides a means for one healthcare practitioner, system, or setting to aggregate all of the pertinent data about a patient and forward it to another practitioner, system, or setting to support the continuity of care. ASTM International, a standards development organization, has established a core data set defining the minimum requirements for the CCR. In addition to these minimum requirements, the CCR core data set has some optional data elements. Data contained in the CCR (shown in figure 9.1) can be provided to care providers in electronic format using extensible mark-up language (XML) or Health Level 7 International formats as well as traditional paper format. **Health Level Seven International (HL7)** is a not-for-profit, American National Standards Institute–accredited standards-developing organization dedicated to providing a comprehensive framework and related standards for the exchange, integration, sharing, and retrieval of electronic health information that supports clinical practice

Figure 9.1.   Core data set for CCR

1. CCR identifying information
   a. Referring ("from") practitioner
   b. Referral ("to") practitioner
   c. Date
   d. Purpose or reason for CCR
2. Patient identifying information—required information to uniquely identify the subject patient; not a centralized system or national patient identifier but a federated or distributed system identifier
3. Patient insurance or financial information—basic information from which eligibility for insurance benefits may be determined for the patient
4. Advance directives—indicators that resuscitation efforts are to be either unrestricted or limited in some way; includes what is commonly known as the Do Not Resuscitate status of the patient as addressed in such documents as living wills, healthcare proxies, and powers of attorney
5. Patient health status
   a. Conditions, diagnoses, problems
   b. Family history
   c. Adverse reactions, allergies, clinical warnings, and alerts
   d. Social history and health risk factors
   e. Medications
   f. Immunizations
   g. Vital signs and physiologic measurements
   h. Laboratory results and observations
   i. Procedures and imaging (this section may be expanded in extensions for clinical specialty-specific information regarding the patient.)
6. Care documentation—details of the patient—practitioner encounter history, such as:
   a. Dates and purposes of recent pertinent visits
   b. Names of practitioners seen (this section may be significantly expanded in future extensions)
7. Care plan recommendation—includes planned or scheduled tests, procedures, or regimens of care for the patient
8. Practitioners—information about those healthcare practitioners who are participants in the patient's care; links as appropriate to 5a (conditions, diagnoses, problems) and 6 (care documentation) encounters

Source: ONC 2013, 38.

and the management, delivery, and evaluation of health services (HL7 2018). HL7 is an important standards development organization most focused on data exchange standards across health information systems (Amatayakul 2017, 401).

The **personal health record (PHR)** is an electronic or paper health record maintained and updated by individuals that can be used to collect, track, and share past and current information about their health or the health of someone in their care. PHR information includes a wide range of data including allergies, diagnoses, medications, health status tracking (such as diet, nutrition, and fitness activities; blood pressure or glucose monitoring), healthcare provider contact information, and social and family history.

There are many benefits in having an EHR. Healthcare is facing many changes with reductions in reimbursement, the focus on reducing medical errors, increased use of technology, escalating healthcare costs, and a need to coordinate care of the patient. The traditional paper health record is not meeting the needs of patients or healthcare professionals because of the fragmentation of the health record, difficulty in analyzing data in a paper environment, and frequent accessibility issues because of missing information or lost health records. EHRs can help to improve efficiency and quality of care throughout a healthcare facility. For example, alerts built into the EHR can prevent a medication error before the prescription is executed and the EHR can eliminate issues encountered with handwriting and illegibility. Also, health record accessibility will not be lost or delayed, thus preventing treatment errors such as removing the wrong kidney. **Reminders** can notify physicians of screenings that should be performed based on the patient's age and gender. For example, the physician would be reminded that the patient needs an annual mammogram or a colonoscopy.

Healthcare today can be complicated depending on care and treatment needed. It may require patients to go to multiple physicians and possibly multiple hospitals. The fragmentation of the health record that results from these patient visits results in a lack of consistency and completeness of the health information, which impacts the quality of care provided to the patient. For example, a patient may be placed on medications that his or her primary care physician is not aware of. The primary care physician may also be unaware of past serious medical or surgical conditions, restricting the thoroughness and accurateness of the patient care rendered. The EHR allows for patient information to be complete and accurate because the system can be programmed to require that key data elements be entered before a user can proceed to the next screen, ultimately improving the quality of the documentation captured. Patients can also receive individually designed and detailed patient instructions (Hamilton 2009).

In 2016, the United States spent 3.3 trillion dollars on healthcare expenditures, which makes up about 17.9 percent of the Gross Domestic Product (CMS 2018). This percentage continues to escalate. A large percentage of these expenses are a result of performing administrative tasks, and the EHR is designed to help reduce these tasks to save time and money (ONC 2018a). For example, e-prescribing decreases turnaround time for patient prescriptions; laboratory and diagnostic tests are received faster; coding, billing, and claims management are more efficient; improved documentation provides for higher-compensating codes; and streamlined communication improves care coordination (ONC 2018).

CHECK YOUR UNDERSTANDING 9.1

1. A reason to implement an EHR is to _____.
   a. Determine the cost of care
   b. Improve patient care
   c. Eliminate medical errors
   d. Meet Joint Commission mandate for the EHR

2. Which of the following is an example of a reminder?
   a. Use of anticoagulant is contraindicated.
   b. Patient is due for MMR immunization.
   c. Patient is allergic to sulfa drugs.
   d. Drug does not come in this format.

3. The system that includes patient information from both the patient and the healthcare provider is called the _____.

    a. CCR
    b. PHR
    c. Core data set
    d. Mini-EHR

4. A health record that contains all health information on a patient from birth to death is referred to as _____.

    a. CCR
    b. PHR
    c. EHR
    d. Longitudinal

5. Which of the following activities and applications is not within the scope of an EHR system?

    a. It is maintained by the patient.
    b. It can be used in clinical decision support processes.
    c. Orders for lab tests and x-rays can be entered and results are reported back.
    d. Medication prescriptions can be sent electronically to the patient's pharmacy.

Status of EHR Adoption

Prior to the 2004 Presidential Directive for the development and implementation of HIT and EHRs, many healthcare facilities had been slow to implement the EHR for reasons such as financial constraints, concerns about the technology, privacy and security, a lack of standards, lack of resources, and conflicting standards. Many of these issues have been addressed by Congress, federal agencies, and independent organizations. The Office of the National Coordinator for Health Information Technology (ONC) is the lead federal agency spearheading this national effort to improve patient safety and health outcomes. ONC is responsible for advising the secretary of the Department of Health and Human Services (HHS) and for establishing guidelines and requirements for the adoption of HIT and to coordinate all efforts to develop and implement the nationwide health information exchange and its infrastructure to help improve healthcare in the United States. The ONC created the Meaningful Use (MU) program as a way to spur the acceptance and adoption of HIT and EHR usage in healthcare so that certified EHR technology is used to improve quality, safety, and efficiency; reduce health disparities; engage patients and family; improve care coordination and population and public health; and maintain privacy and security of patient health information. MU sets specific objectives that eligible professionals (EPs) and hospitals must achieve to qualify for CMS Incentive Programs. It is a monetary incentive plan for healthcare providers to implement certified EHR technology and to make healthcare more patient-centered, improve health outcomes, and increase the productivity of healthcare services in any setting. In addition to providing incentives, MU also incorporated quality of care indicators and reporting requirements to evaluate the impact of EHR adoption on healthcare quality, patient safety measures, and provider efficiency (Leventhal 2017).

As of 2015, approximately 97 percent of hospitals had certified EHR technology (ONC 2016a). However, only 77 percent of office-based physicians were using a certified EHR system (CDC 2017). Certified EHR technology (CEHRT) is a complete EHR that meets the requirements included in the definition of a qualified EHR and has been tested and certified in accordance with the certification program established by the ONC. While the actual EHRs are being used, the health information exchange among providers still lags behind. Almost 75 percent of hospitals have exchanged health information electronically with other providers, but physician practices lag behind at only 26 percent. It is encouraging that health information exchange has improved public health reporting. Almost 90 percent of healthcare providers participating in the MU program had reported immunization information to local or state public health departments. Patients are also showing interest in using the EHR. Approximately 40 percent were offered online access to their health information through an EHR, and 55 percent of those individuals electronically viewed their health information within a 12-month period (ONC 2016a).

Of course, there are still obstacles to be overcome. Many healthcare providers are not eligible, for a variety of reasons, for the MU program, and their adoption of EHRs still trails behind those who participated in the MU program significantly. Interoperability is still a sticking point. Standards for EHR systems and implementation lack specificity, resulting in variability as to how HIT stakeholders interpret and apply federal policies and regulations. More information about HIT standards can be found in chapter 12. Although HIT has improved patient safety in many areas, best practices have yet to be refined, publicized, and consistently implemented. HIT vendors and developers are hesitant to collaborate with competitors regarding data use agreements, hindering the exchange of health information. In addition to the lack of collaboration, health information blocking is also an issue. Health information blocking occurs when "persons or entities knowingly and unreasonably interfere with the exchange or use of electronic health information" (ONC 2016a). Blocking stems from healthcare providers or HIT vendors protecting their own proprietary and business interests above the interests of the patient and healthcare improvement. These efforts actively impede the progress sought by the concept of EHRs and health information exchange. The ONC has established a complaint process whereby health information blocking efforts can be reported and investigated.

Certified EHR Technology

Certified EHR technology has been evaluated by a member of the Office of the National Coordinator–Authorized Certification Bodies (ONC-ACBs) and verified that it meets the criteria set by the MU incentive programs. There are two programs, one for Medicare providers and the other for Medicaid providers. Providers must choose one or the other, as participating in both programs is prohibited. The MU incentive EHR program created first a temporary certification organization, which was then replaced with permanent certification organizations. The testing of the EHR product is performed by Accredited Testing Laboratories (ATLs). Once the testing confirms that all standards have been met, the ONC-ACB awards the certification status. "A single organization can serve as both an ONC-ACB and an ATL, as long as a firewall is established between testing and certification activities" (ONC 2017a).

It is the responsibility of these organizations to evaluate EHR technologies to ensure that they perform specific functions and developed standards for structured data. The EHR certification program has evolved to encompass other HIT initiatives, interoperability, care quality improvement plans. HIT that is certified is subject to surveillance activities as a condition of certification. Surveillance of certified EHR products and vendors ensures the continued maintenance of the functionalities required by certification (ONC 2016b). The National Voluntary Laboratory Accreditation Program (NVLAP) maintains the Healthcare Information Technology Testing Laboratory Accreditation Program and accredits organizations that contract to perform HIT conformance testing in the ONC Health IT Certification Program (ONC 2017a).

As shown in figure 9.2, the ONC oversees the Health IT Certification Program while delegating the specific function areas (testing, accreditation, and surveillance) and program operations to the designated and vetted agencies and entities. These vetted groups then accredit the testing organizations and certification bodies that evaluate specific products from HIT vendors. The ONC–Approved Accreditor (ONC-AA) is an entity designated by the ONC to accredit and oversee the certification bodies (ONC-ACBs). The ONC approves only one ONC-AA at a time, and approval status lasts for three years (ONC 2017a).

Organizations that wish to become accredited certification bodies must seek authorization from ONC-AA to participate in the ONC Health IT Certification Program. Once authorized, the responsibility for certifying EHR products is delegated to them, and they are called ONC-ACBs.

As shown in figure 9.3, when developers and vendors seek ONC certification, they must contact an ATL to have their product tested. Only after the HIT product meets administrative requirements and passes all analyses and evaluations can the vendor apply to have its product certified. The vendors can then apply to an ONC-ACB to have their product certified (ONC 2017a).

An ONC-ACB certifies a vendor's HIT product has been successfully tested against the certification criteria by an ATL. The ONC-ACB submits the certifications of the HIT product for posting on the Certified Health IT Product List (CHPL) on the ONC's website. The CHPL provides the authoritative, comprehensive listing of Health IT Modules that have been tested and certified through the ONC Health IT Certification Program. The CHPL is updated, at minimum, once per week (ONC 2017a).

The ONC Certified Health IT Mark Certification and Design (Mark) is available to represent products that have been certified by an ONC-ACB under the ONC Health IT Certification Program and meet the 2014 Edition

Figure 9.2.   ONC Health IT Certification Program schematic

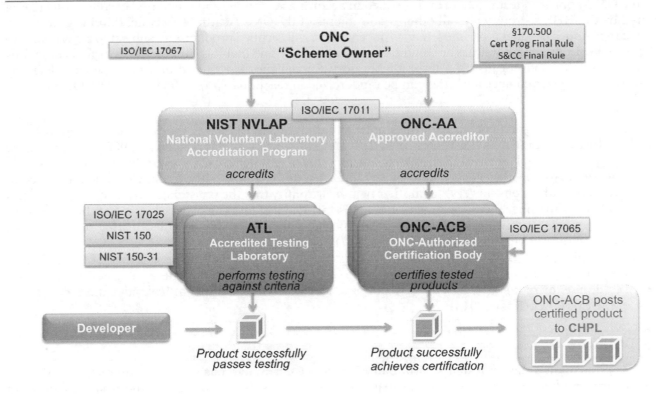

Source: ONC 2017a.

Figure 9.3.   ONC certification process

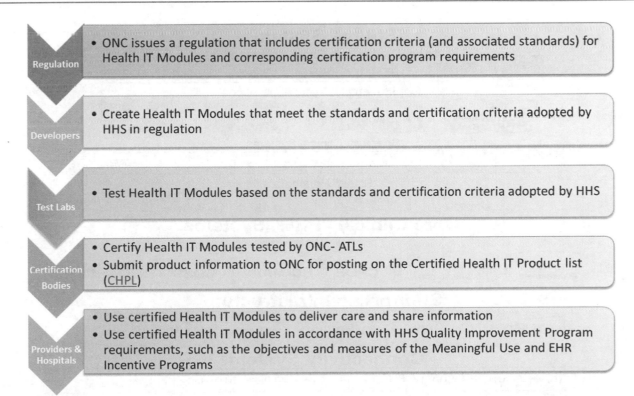

Source: ONC 2018b.

or 2015 Edition Standards and Certification Criteria. This means that a product was tested in accordance with the ONC-approved test method, and certified in accordance with the standards and certification criteria adopted by the HHS secretary and all other requirements of the ONC Health IT Certification Program.

Once a vendor's product is certified, it does not end there. All certified products are subject to surveillance to make sure the product's capabilities are maintained by the vendor and that it is capable to perform its functions "in the real world" and not just in a testing laboratory. Surveillance is required and must be completed by ONC-ACBs. These surveillance activities can be randomized in reaction to a specific issue (ONC 2017a).

Stark Law Exception

Another way that Congress encouraged the implementation of the EHR was the Stark law exception. The Stark law (formally known as the Ethics in Patient Referrals Act) was established in 1989 to decrease the amount of physician self-referral. Self-referral means that a physician refers or sends a patient (who is covered by Medicare or other government payer) to have a designated healthcare service (such as an x-ray, physical therapy, outpatient surgery) to another healthcare entity that the physician or one of the physician's immediate family member owns, operates, or benefits from financially. The original intent of the law was to remove any financial motivation for the physician to send patients for unwarranted testing or procedures that could raise overall healthcare costs (Ellison 2017).

Since hospitals and physicians are so intricately tied to one another in the delivery of many health services, many of these providers share or coordinate EHR products. Under the exception, hospitals are allowed to donate or monetarily assist physician practices without fear of penalties under the Safe Harbor clause of the Stark Act (Rosin 2014).

Components of EHR

There are four main areas or systems within an EHR, and each system has specific components. Although there is variation between inpatient and outpatient EHR systems, figure 9.4 shows the basic systems and components of an EHR.

Figure 9.4. Conceptual model of EHR

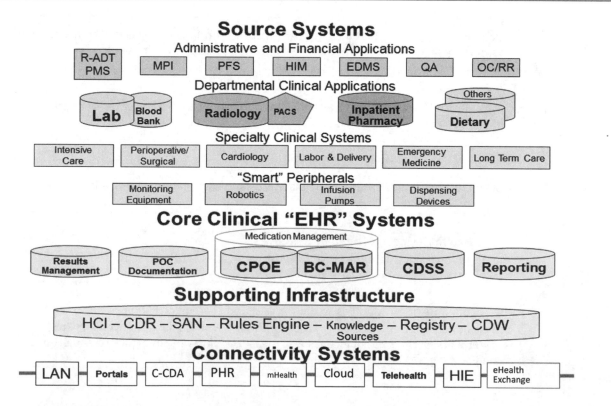

Source: Amatayakul 2017, 14.

The consolidation of these functions and systems allows health information to be used in ways that were impossible with the paper health record. The time and staff required to go through a paper health record to analyze data are much more costly compared to the readily available information contained within the EHR. For this reason, EHRs can be a significant source of information for identifying trends and ensuring that protocols are followed. For example, a healthcare facility can analyze data to determine that compliance practices are being followed, such as whether or not physicians performed a routine foot examination for patients with diabetes. A brief overview of each of these components follows.

Registration—Admission, Discharge, Transfer

The registration—admission, discharge, transfer (R-ADT) system collects patient demographic information such as name, address, and phone number. It also collects insurance information that will be used in billing and includes the master patient index. Refer to chapter 7 for details on the R-ADT system.

Patient Financial Services

The patient financial services (PFS) department receives the information collected by the R-ADT system. It then adds further information including charges for services provided and then creates the bill. It also has the capability to verify insurance coverage and copayments, determine the status of a claim, and manage prior authorizations (Amatayakul 2017, 17).

Order Communication and Results Retrieval

The order communication system notifies clinical departments, such as the laboratory, radiology, physical therapy, and dietary departments, of orders made by the physician. These orders are not typically entered by the physician, but rather by the nurse, unit secretary, or other authorized user (Amatayakul 2017, 18). When the orders are generally written down on paper and then transcribed into the order communication system, the facility does not receive the benefits of a computerized provider order entry (CPOE) system. The CPOE contains preprogrammed clinical decision support designed to assist the user through making an entry appropriately (Amatayakul 2017, 21). Once tests are performed, results of the diagnostic studies are compiled from their respective clinical information systems (that is, laboratory information system or radiology information system) and transferred into the EHR. The results are then available for viewing, which in turn speeds access to the information because the report does not have to be printed, filed in the health record, and transported to the provider before it is available for use.

Ancillary, Clinical, and Department Applications

Various clinical systems are used throughout the hospital and include the laboratory information system and the radiology information system. Clinical systems both manage the department as well as document the findings of the tests performed. Specialty clinical applications collect and manage information in specialty areas, such as the intensive care units, anesthesia, and labor and delivery. The information collected can include nursing notes, anesthesia records, delivery records, and more. Refer to chapter 8 for more information.

Patient Monitoring Systems

Patient monitoring systems are biomedical monitoring systems that capture data such as vital signs and fetal monitoring. Vital signs include the patient's heart rate, respirations, and blood pressure. Other smart systems collect electrocardiograms, electroencephalograms, and more advanced tests. The data captured by the smart peripherals are accessible through the EHR.

Document Management System

The document management system (DMS) may utilize scanning to capture patient information from the paper health record. DMS also uses electronic document and content management systems that collect data from forms. Data may also be captured from an electronic source in another system or through voice recognition, e-mail, and e-fax systems. The DMS may utilize workflow technology to direct specific documents or patient health records to coders, risk management, analysts, and other users. Most DMS systems have the capability for indexing of forms. These systems are referred to as electronic document/content management (ED/CM) systems and have methods to manage and retrieve some of the data on these forms (Amatayakul 2017, 17). For more information on DMS, refer to chapter 8.

Clinical Messaging and Provider-Patient Portals

Clinical messaging connects the medical staff and hospital by providing access to information systems such as order entry and results reporting and DMS. Order entry and results reporting is a software application in which healthcare professionals can enter patient care orders and then see the test results. Web-based technology often is utilized to access information in an internal system such as an intranet, or it can use the Internet. Clinical messaging is the function of electronically delivering data and automating the workflow around the management of clinical data. Clinical messages can use e-mail, portals, virtual private networks, and other means to provide the secure means of communication needed for patient information. These messages are shared in such a way as to protect the privacy of the patient (Amatayakul 2017, 19). Standards have been established to control clinical messaging. These standards are discussed later in this chapter.

The patient–provider portal is a secure method of communication between the healthcare provider and the patient, just the providers, or the provider and the payer. The patient–provider portal may include secure e-mail or remote access to test results and provide patient monitoring. Monitoring may include tracking pacemaker activity, blood sugar, and breathing sounds. Patients could also have access to patient education materials to help them manage their own care. This would be especially valuable for chronic conditions such as diabetes mellitus and chronic obstructive pulmonary disease (Amatayakul 2017, 15).

Results Management

Results management systems receive data from diagnostic tests and procedures. Laboratory test results, x-ray studies, and other scans are electronically reported to the originating provider. This data can be incorporated with other data such as medication administration and vital signs to get an accurate and timely view of how the patient is progressing with treatment (Amatayakul 2017, 14). The data can then be used to evaluate effectiveness in treating a patient. This ability makes the results management systems more sophisticated than results reporting systems (Amatayakul 2017, 14).

Point-of-Care Charting

Point-of-care (POC) charting, also called clinical documentation systems, may utilize many different systems to accommodate all of the different healthcare professionals who document in the health record (Amatayakul 2017, 20). There may be separate systems for physicians, nurses, physical therapists, respiratory therapists, and others. These POC systems may use bedside terminals, personal digital assistants (PDAs), and other wireless devices to enable the care provider to document in the health record as the information is obtained from the patient. These systems generally allow entry of both structured and unstructured data. Structured data are generally found in checkboxes, drop-down boxes, and other data entry means whereby the user chooses from options already built into the system. Unstructured data, also called narrative data, can be entered in a free text format by the user, usually by typing (Amatayakul 2017, 20). To ease the workload, these clinical documentation systems use handheld wireless devices, such as tablets or smartphones, so that nursing personnel can document at the patient's bedside. In some cases, laptops on movable carts are used, and are referred to as workstation on wheels or wireless on wheels (WOW) (Amatayakul 2017, 20).

Computerized Physician or Provider Order Entry System

As previously discussed, the computerized physician or provider order entry system (CPOE) is designed for orders to be entered by the healthcare providers. The use of a CPOE can lead to significant improvements in patient safety because of the reminders and alerts built into the system, improved legibility, reduced risk of data entry errors, and integrated clinical decisions support capabilities (Amatayakul 2017, 21). These alerts and reminders are provided to the physician or other healthcare provider as data are entered, thus identifying problems and key information at the point of capture rather than after review by nurses, pharmacists, or others. These alerts and reminders are controlled by clinical decision support built into the system, which is able to help prevent medication errors and improve the quality of care through its validation mechanisms (Amatayakul 2017, 21). Alerts may notify the physician of medication contraindications or that a prescription is about to expire. Reminders usually notify the physician of laboratory test results and preventive measures such scheduling for a mammogram.

Figure 9.5.   Sample clinical decision support screen

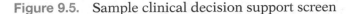

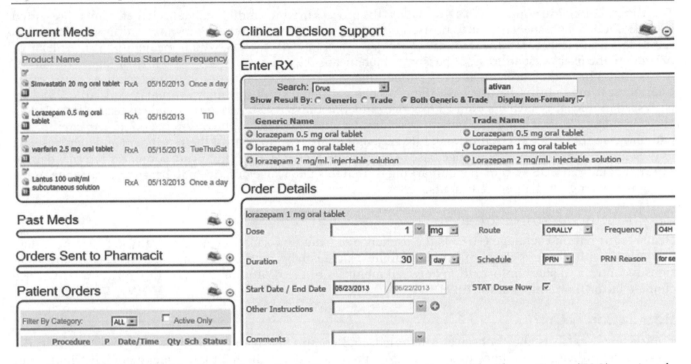

Source: CPOE developed by The Shams Group (n.d.). Reprinted with permission. The Shams Group (TSG), a privately held healthcare software and service provider, has served over 400 hospitals and healthcare systems worldwide.

Although alerts and reminders are useful, too many can become frustrating to the physician who is constantly interrupted during data entry to address the alerts and reminders (Amatayakul 2017, 21). CPOE can be used to avoid duplicate testing and ordering of medications not covered by the patient's insurance by reminding the physician a recent test or by telling the physician that the test is not covered or requires preapproval from the insurer.

Using CPOE can be time consuming for physicians; many are reluctant to adopt the systems or try to pass the responsibility of entering the orders to the nurses or other support staff. The benefits of CPOE are realized when the physicians are the users of the system. Because of the importance of physician users and the decision support such as recommending alternative medications, catching inappropriate dosages, and other edits, the providers must be involved in developing it.

Electronic Medication Administration Record

The **electronic medication administration record (EMAR)**, also referred to a **barcode medication administration record (BC-MAR)** automates many of the medication administration processes in a healthcare facility. The level of sophistication varies by system and can be as simple as printing out a list of medications to be administered to the patient and documenting the medications given to the patient. It can be much more sophisticated by using barcodes or **radiofrequency identification devices (RFIDs)** to properly identify the patient. RFID is a microchip implanted in an item to allow tracking of that item (Sandefer 2016, 372). The EMAR can also provide alerts to assist in medication timing and provide the nurse with reference material on the medication itself (Amatayakul 2017, 22). Some EMARs can automate the entire medication administration process. This process includes identifying the drug to administer, identifying the patient, and documenting the administration of the medication or the exception. An example of an exception would be to record that medication was administered late. Some EMAR systems are designed to store commonly used medications in the nursing unit for dispensing through the use of kiosks. This capability is particularly important when addressing the eight rights of medication administration: the right patient, right medication, right time, right dose, right route, right position, right documentation, and the right of the patient to refuse medication.

Clinical Decision Support System

The **clinical decision support (CDS) system** is the process in which individual data elements are represented in the computer by a special code to be used in making comparisons, trending results, and supplying clinical reminders and alerts (AHIMA 2017, 45). The CDS system may be active, which means that it has alerts or reminders the user must address, or passive, which means the user may choose to utilize or ignore the alerts. Alerts may notify the care provider of patient allergies or contraindications for the medication or other treatment. It may notify the user that the drug being ordered is off-formulary (Amatayakul 2017, 23). The CDS system may also have the clinical practice guidelines advice installed and provide access to knowledge-based systems. Clinical guidelines advice provides recommendations to the physician on how to care for the patient given the patient's circumstances. Rules engines are used to control the reminders and alerts as well as the clinical practice and knowledge base (Amatayakul 2017, 23). Benchmarking compares internal data to external data. In a CDS system, benchmarking is used to standardize practice patterns and reduce the usage of high-cost drugs and other treatments.

Health Information Exchange

Health information exchange (HIE) is the exchange of health information electronically between providers and others with the same level of interoperability, such as laboratories and pharmacies. The organization signs a contract to share information between members of the health information organization (HIO). See chapter 11 for more information on HIE.

Population Health

Population health is the "cohesive, integrated, and comprehensive approach to health considering the distribution of health outcomes in a population, the health determinants that influence the distribution of care, and the policies and interventions that impact and are impacted by the determinants" (Jacobson and Teutsch 2012). The population health component in an EHR is designed to capture and report healthcare data that are used for public health purposes. It allows the healthcare provider to report infectious diseases, immunizations, cancer, and other reportable conditions to public health officials. This reporting is required at the local, state, and national levels and includes infectious diseases. A population health system also can connect with public health officials to receive alerts regarding health issues (Amatayakul 2017, 635). The traditional methods are cumbersome because of the manual processes and disparate information systems. The use of technology can speed up the reporting process, thus speeding up the management of disease outbreaks.

HIT has a significant role in improving the health of not only a medical practice's population, but the population on the community level. The Affordable Care Act (ACA) and the Healthy People 2020 campaign set forth the following as goals to be achieved through the monitoring of population health:

- Attain high-quality, longer lives free of preventable diseases, injury, and disability and premature death
- Achieve health equity, eliminate health disparities, and improve health for all groups
- Create social and physical environments that promote good health for all
- Promote quality of life, healthy development, and healthy behaviors across all life stages (NCHS 2015)

CHECK YOUR UNDERSTANDING 9.2

1. The component of the EHR that allows patients to manage their own data is _____.
   a. Population health
   b. PHR
   c. Patient-provider portal
   d. Clinical decision support system

2. Which component of the EHR allows physicians to direct the patient's care by sending orders for prescriptions, lab tests, or x-rays?

   a. Order communication and results reporting
   b. PHR
   c. CPOE
   d. Patient-provider portal

3. What is the trend of adoption of the EHR in the United States?

   a. All healthcare providers use an EHR throughout the United States.
   b. The United States adoption rate is rapidly decreasing.
   c. The United States is rapidly increasing the rate of adoption of EHRs.
   d. The United States adoption rate is gradually decreasing.

4. Which of the following is not a goal for the health of the general population?

   a. Health equity
   b. Prevent injuries
   c. Decrease physical environments that promote healthy behavior
   d. Promote healthy behaviors across all life stages

5. Which of the following technologies support the eight rights of medication administration for patients?

   a. CPOE
   b. EMAR
   c. DMS
   d. PHR

Benefits of the EHR

The many benefits to the EHR, some of which are listed below, are economic, clinical, and administrative:

- The EHR offers easier access to clinical information. The EHR provides immediate access, which in turn speeds diagnosis and treatment to improve the quality of care provided.
- The EHR provides current information on tests, medications, allergies, and past diagnoses and treatments (among many more) required for decision making and disease management.
- As previously discussed, the use of tools such as reminders and alerts can remind a physician to schedule mammograms and colonoscopies and to avoid adverse drug events and allergies.
- The EHR can also enhance the documentation captured because the traditional paper health record is frequently illegible, incomplete, inaccurate, and redundant. These problems can be avoided with the use of required fields, uniform data entry practices, and trained personnel. Patient education is important for the continued improvement of a patient's condition. The EHR supports patient education materials such as discharge instructions and medication information can be personalized for the individual patient.
- The EHR allows healthcare providers to spend more time with patients because of the benefits in workflow and administrative tasks; for example, most documentation can occur at the bedside (Amatayakul 2017, 9).
- Test results can also be available immediately upon completion.
- The EHR supports various data analytics functions such as predictive modeling and application and contribution of evidence-based medicine to improve health outcomes (Sandefer 2016, 363).
- It provides accurate, up-to-date, and complete information about patients at the point of care.
- It enables quick access to patient records for more coordinated, efficient care.
- It securely shares electronic information with patients and other clinicians.
- It helps providers more effectively diagnose patients, reduce medical errors, and provide safer care.

- It improves patient and provider interaction and communication, as well as health care convenience.
- It enables safer, more reliable prescribing.
- It helps promote legible, complete documentation and accurate, streamlined coding and billing.
- It enhances privacy and security of patient data.
- It helps providers improve productivity and work-life balance.
- It enables providers to improve efficiency and meet their business goals.
- It reduces costs through decreased paperwork, improved safety, reduced duplication of testing, and improved health. (ONC 2014)

Barriers to EHR Use

The EHR is a powerful tool that can revolutionize healthcare. The EHR provides a multitude of benefits, but there are many issues and barriers that must be addressed in order to encourage adoption and interoperability.

One of the primary barriers to EHR implementation is cost. Implementing an EHR is expensive, and many are hesitant to invest in one without a guarantee of a return on their investment. Accurate and flexible budget planning must be completed for a successful implementation. The facility must be sure to account for every cost in planning the budget. Costs will include items such as hardware, software, construction or reconstruction of space, training, and maintenance, to name a few. Additional technical staff may be required to address technical issues that arise, such as the system crashing or virus infection.

Other barriers include:

- Prohibitive cost of many EHR systems/limited access to capital and infrastructure
- Limited access to EHR vendor information and technical assistance
- Suitability of EHR products for practice and rural health care settings
- Difficulty connecting to or obtaining broadband service
- Limited health information technology (IT) workforce and training programs
- Difficulty in obtaining community buy-in
- Limited opportunities for collaboration with other health stakeholders
- Limited buy-in from practice/hospital/health center staff with multiple roles and busy schedules (ONC 2013a)

CHECK YOUR UNDERSTANDING 9.3

1. Money is an example of a(n) _____ to the EHR.

   a. Barrier
   b. Benefit
   c. Component
   d. Asset

2. Which of the following is a benefit of the EHR?

   a. Improved efficiency
   b. Costs
   c. Fear of technology
   d. Security concerns

3. Which statement is true about the EHR?

   a. The EHR is the same regardless of the setting in which it operates.
   b. The EHR does not utilize reminders.
   c. The EHR is different based on the setting in which it operates.
   d. The EHR does not allow for the use of CPOE.

4. What is one of the techniques that can be performed to lessen the barriers to implementing an EHR?

   a. Thorough and repetitive training and communication
   b. Buying the biggest EHR system the healthcare facility can afford
   c. Give all employees new job titles
   d. Implement one component at a time

5. When an EHR reminds a physician to schedule preventive medicine techniques such as mammograms and colonoscopies for all her patients that may have an impact within the surrounding community, the EHR is impacting which of the following?

   a. Population health
   b. Results reporting
   c. BC-MAR
   d. CPOE

Signatures

Signatures are an important part of the EHR because the authentication of health record entries is a requirement of state licensing, accreditation, and other standards. The purpose of signatures, in both the paper and electronic environment, is to record the identity of the individual who performed the entry.

With electronic systems, digital signature management technology is a key authentication mechanism. To be in compliance with Joint Commission, Health Insurance Portability and Accountability Act (HIPAA), and the Affordable Care Act requirements, authentication means the corroboration that a person is who he claims to be. Digital signatures are the most secure way for a healthcare provider to acknowledge the order, progress note, discharge summary, or any other patient care–related document (McTosh 2014). The security capability of an EHR system to identify the individual who digitally signed the document is called signer authentication. Another security aspect of the digital signature management technology is to ensure that the document and the signature cannot be changed or altered, which is referred to as document authentication (Sandefer 2016, 350).

One of the benefits of the electronic signature is that it automatically stamps medical record entries with the date and time of the entry. It also records user identification so that the identity of the individual who created the entry into the system is automatically recorded. There are three levels of signatures found in the EHR. The digitized signature is a scanned image of an individual's actual signature. This method is unsecure because anyone who has access to the image can use the signature. The next level is the electronic signature, which requires at least a password but can use a two-factor authentication method (discussed in chapter 13). The digital signature is similar to the electronic signature except that it uses encryption to provide nonrepudiation to prove the authenticator's identity, which makes it most secure (Downing 2013).

Copy and Paste Concerns

Copying is the process of moving information from an existing health record. Pasting is the process of entering the copied data into the current record. Using the copy and paste functions to enter data into the EHR saves time because the information does not have to be retyped, but the process is not without problems. The EHR is the legal health record for the healthcare facility and therefore must be managed in a way that protects the hospital from risk. The health record must contain quality information that can be used for patient care and other purposes.

Using the copy and paste functions without checks and balances can cause legal issues, quality of care issues, and other problems. For example, a user could copy information from one patient's health record and accidently paste it into another patient's record. This should not be condoned as it can easily enter data into a patient's health record that does not apply. Health record problems, such as those that follow, can result from improper use of the copy and paste functions:

- An entry can be nullified.
- An entire record can be suspect.
- Healthcare practitioners may not notice additional information.

- Healthcare practitioners may not notice missing information.
- The entry may misrepresent the case.
- Fraudulent claims for reimbursement may be made.
- The patient is harmed.
- There might be a sentinel event that must be reported. (Amatayakul 2017, 352)

There should be policies and procedures in place to specify when copy and paste functions can be used and when they cannot. Productivity is important, but the accuracy of the information is more important because of the impact that erroneous information can have on patient care and in the courtroom. Audit logs must be checked on a frequent and regular basis to determine the usage of the copy and paste function. An audit log, or audit trail, is an electronic footprint of the actions that occurred in a particular file in an information system or that were performed by a specific individual. It maps when a file was accessed, who accessed it, how long they were in the file, what was done to the file (including printing and saving), which terminal or device was used to access the file, and so forth. As a key security feature, it is permanently maintained within the information system. See chapter 13 for additional information regarding this security feature.

EHR Tools

The EHR utilizes a multitude of tools to assist in the usability of the EHR. The software controls screen layout, data entry, and data retrieval. The flexibility of the presentation layer is what allows the various healthcare providers to manipulate it. This flexibility allows users to control the screens to meet their needs. The EHR also makes it possible for users to graph information to identify trends over time. Other tools in the EHR are used to facilitate data retrieval, alerts, and data entry.

Data Retrieval

When developing the EHR, the healthcare facility should understand how the data are to be used to ensure that all data will be present and in the desired format for retrieval. Data retrieval should also take into account printing format. Because of privacy issues, the EHR should also allow for identifying information to be removed automatically. This process is called deidentification.

Graphical User Interface

Graphical user interface (GUI) technology is used to navigate through an information system. Tools such as icons, colors, buttons, menus, and other tools are used to help make the system user-friendly by being visually appealing and intuitive. For example, an icon containing an image of a printer would notify the user that clicking it will trigger printing the document.

Color and Icons

Color and icons can be used to assist in retrieval, ease of use, and functionality in the EHR. Icons are graphic indicators that can be used to alert the user to important information. The user can click on the icon to access data, such as text, audio, pictures, or video. The icon picture would indicate the data type. For example, a picture of an ear might be used to indicate audio. The picture should be self-explanatory so that the user understands what lies behind the icon. Color can be a useful tool but must be used judiciously as some people are color blind. The colors used and the amount used must be carefully chosen; otherwise, they can put a strain on the user's eyes.

Data Entry

Data entry is important to the EHR. Data entry can take a lot of time, and errors can cause mistakes that could be detrimental to the patient. Because of this, a lot of care should be taken to improve data quality and speed data entry. A full discussion of data quality is presented in chapter 2. Typing, voice recognition, transcription, and other means of data entry can be used to get data into the system. When entering data, unstructured and structured data—or a combination of these—may be used.

Unstructured Data

Unstructured data, also called narrative or free text data, are usually entered using a keyboard, but other methods such as dictation may also be used. Unstructured data allow the data entered to be more specific and detailed for each patient than structured data. In these fields, the provider could enter a patient's history of present illness, level of compliance with medical regimen, or anything else not captured in the structured data. The user can use his or her own words to enter the data. A disadvantage of unstructured data is that reporting is not as strong as with structured data entry for reporting purposes. Because unstructured data do not have a data model, it will be difficult for the system to identify and gather desired information provided in a report.

Structured Data

Drop-down lists, checkboxes, radio buttons, and other forms of controlled data entry are used in structured data entry. The choices must be clearly defined, comprehensive, applicable, and mutually exclusive. "Structured data enable standardized values to be supplied for specific variables, so the data can be used in clinical decision support systems and provide standardized meaning for reporting purposes" (Amatayakul 2017, 20). Once the user learns the structure, data entry is quick and easy. There is a learning curve in the beginning while users get familiar with the choices and the graphical user interface (a style of computer interface in which typed commands are replaced by icons that represent tasks). For example, when entering a patient's gender, the options are male, female, and unknown; or if the data being entered were the number of dilation centimeters for an obstetrical patient, the choices would range from 0 to 10.

Structured data entry is frequently used for physician EHRs, with the menus developed specifically for the physician's medical or surgical specialty. Because it is easy for the user to overlook entry, defaults should not populate an entry but rather should be left blank, forcing the user to address the field. The EHR should be able to convert structured data into a narrative format. An example would be structured data of "no tobacco use" and "no alcohol use" converts to "Patient denies the use of tobacco and alcohol." One of the advantages of structured data is that it can be used for reporting purposes. Data can also be graphed, allowing for trending. An example of the use of graphing is the ability to trend blood sugar or blood pressure levels over time.

Template-Based Entry

Template-based entry is a blending of both free text and structured data entry. The user is able to pick and choose data that are entered frequently, thus requiring the entry of data that change from patient to patient. Templates can be customized to meet the needs of the organization as data needs change by physician specialty, patient type (surgical, medical, newborn), disease, and other classifications of patients.

Natural Language Processing

Natural language processing (NLP) is the conversion of unstructured data into structured data through the use of computer algorithms or statistical methods (Sayles 2016, 69). This requires sophisticated computer software to separate the narrative into little packets. These packets can be used for storage, analysis, and retrieval (Amatayakul 2017, 354). NLP has the ability to mine and obtain dictated and transcribed structures or unstructured words or phrases and convert this data into CPT Current Procedural Terminology (CPT) or *International Classification of Diseases, 10th Revision* (ICD-10) codes for health record coding or patient bills (Sandefer 2016, 348). Uses of NLP include dictation and computer-assisted coding. NLP is sophisticated enough to consider the different meanings of terms in order to correctly identify the word; one use of NLP is automated coding of diagnoses and procedures. NLP can analyze data entered and apply algorithms or statistical methods to the data to determine the correct code from either the *International Classification of Diseases, 10th Revision, Clinical Modification* (ICD-10-CM) or other coding systems. To be successful, automated coding must be able to understand the relationships between the terms. For example, the ICD-10-CM code for hypertensive heart disease is different from hypertension and heart disease; thus, algorithms must be able to understand these differences. NLP may also be utilized in clinical information systems and the EHR to convert narrative text into data that can be easily analyzed.

Legal Issues

There are a number of legal issues facing the EHR. Some of these issues are being addressed as laws and regulations catch up with technology. The EHR must be designed so that it is admissible in court. State laws vary as to what is and is not acceptable in a court of law regarding EHRs. Healthcare providers frequently receive subpoenas requesting the production of the health record. Data in the EHR will be used to meet the requirements contained in the subpoena. The documentation provided to the court must be in a usable and readable format, not just screen prints or other unformatted data. The subpoena may require the production of audit trails, decision support rules, clinical guidelines, and other information that was never an issue with the paper health record. A number of other legal issues that must be addressed are retention, storage, security, privacy, signatures, and data quality.

Unanticipated Issues in EHR Use

Several unanticipated consequences have arisen with the use of the EHR:

- Increased work for clinicians
- Unfavorable workflow changes
- Ongoing demands for system changes
- Conflicts between electronic and paper-based systems
- Unfavorable changes in communications
- Negative user emotions
- Generation of new kinds of errors
- Unexpected and unintended changes in institutional power structure
- Overdependence on technology (ONC 2017b)

Healthcare facilities must anticipate a variety of issues that will arise. Adequate planning, efficient decision-making, and early responses to problems can mitigate the negative effects of these unintended consequences. There must be acknowledgment of the trade-offs of implementing this new technology; indeed, this new way of thinking and performing medical care will be worthwhile in the end when increased patient safety and improved outcomes justify all of the angst that accompanied this massive undertaking (ONC 2017b).

Interoperability

Interoperability is divided into three levels: basic, functional, and semantic. With basic interoperability, a computer can send data to another computer but the receiving computer is unable to interpret the data. Functional interoperability defines the structure of messages so that the receiving computer can interpret the data. The most advanced level—semantic interoperability—allows the information to be used in a meaningful way. Interoperability will require uniform standards for data capture, storage, and transmission (Palkie 2016, 153). See chapter 11 for additional information on interoperability.

Transition Period—Hybrid Record

The conversion to an EHR does not happen overnight. Throughout the information system and implementation life cycle, the healthcare facility will have to manage paper health records, microfilms, scanned images, and the EHR. Because the health information is fragmented, there may be some risk to the quality of patient care. The fragmentation comes from the information being on several different sources such as paper, microfilm, and the EHR. The healthcare facility must have a means of pulling all information together when it is needed.

In order to make paper health records available, facilities have provided many different options. Some facilities backscan paper health records into the EHR, while others manually enter in basic information so that it is quickly available for patient care. Some even keep the paper health records as they are and maintain the same system and processes until the EHR is fully functional. The **hybrid record** is a combination of paper and electronic health records. Hospitals need policies and procedures to define the sources of the components of the patient's health information and to ensure easy and accurate access, use, and disclosure.

Some facilities print out documents from the electronic sources to compile the contents of the legal health record. This practice prevents the healthcare facility from realizing the benefits of the electronic system. Unnecessary printing is not only costly but also complicates operational issues in managing the hybrid health records; healthcare facilities frequently establish policies that discourage superfluous printing of documents.

Impact on Health Information Management

The EHR does not eliminate the health information management (HIM) department; however, the functions performed by the HIM department undergo significant changes and evolve to meet the current and future challenges that new technology brings. Issues facing the HIM department in a hybrid environment include authoring and printing issues, and access and disclosure issues.

As the EHR is implemented, some of the traditional HIM functions, such as assembly, are eliminated. Other functions, such as analysis, are significantly reduced as the information systems require authentication at the time of entry. Many functions such as coding are significantly changed. For example, computer-assisted coding technologies can be used to assign codes but coders are still needed to audit and monitor the codes assigned.

Transcription is a very labor-intensive process. The EHR decreases the dependence on transcription as providers more often perform data entry, including voice recognition, into the EHR, and the system can create discharge summaries and other documents automatically from data entered into the system.

Release of information traditionally has been a slow process because the paper health record had to be retrieved, copied or faxed, and then refiled. With the EHR, a few keystrokes will print or fax the document(s) needed to fulfill requests.

Health record processing varies widely by facility but generally includes assembly, analysis, and health record completion. The assembly process is eliminated completely with the implementation of the EHR because there is no need to organize paper documents. Dependent on healthcare facility's policy and quality levels, the analyst may or may not have to verify that all pages belong to the same patient, which will reduce the time needed for analysis. Finally, the information system will not allow an entry to be made without a signature, thus reducing the number of deficient health records.

In a hybrid health record environment, paper health records do not cease to exist immediately with the advent of the EHR but rather the paper health records disappear over time. The file room will ultimately be eliminated as the existing paper health records are destroyed according to the retention schedule or the health records are scanned into the EHR. For a discussion of disposal of electronic data, see chapter 13.

These changes do not signal the end of the HIM department or the HIM profession; rather, this is only the beginning. The knowledge and skill set of the HIM professional are needed to maintain and manage data quality, evaluate the system, evaluate standards, perform project management, and more. The HIM profession as we know it will change with some tasks being eliminated, others changed, and still others created. AHIMA has developed a plan to address these issues and move the profession forward. It is referred to as Health Information Management Reimagined (HIMR). See chapter 15 for additional information regarding HIMR.

CHECK YOUR UNDERSTANDING 9.4

1. Checkboxes are a method of data entry used in _____.

   a. Structured data entry
   b. Unstructured data entry
   c. Narrative data entry
   d. All types of data entry

2. The ability of different information systems and software applications to communicate and exchange data is referred to as _____.

   a. Interoperability
   b. Certification
   c. NLP
   d. Meaningful Use

(Continued)

CHECK YOUR UNDERSTANDING 9.4 (*Continued*)

3. As healthcare facilities transition to EHRs, what is the term that is used to describe the combination of the paper and electronic medical record?

   a. Mash-up
   b. Hybrid
   c. Cross mix
   d. Fusion

4. Which of the following is not an unanticipated effect of the implementation of EHRs?

   a. Increased work and effort for physicians
   b. Increased and ongoing demands for system changes and upgrades
   c. Improved workflow changes
   d. Unfavorable changes in communications between patients, staff, and providers

5. What is the software that converts unstructured data into structured data to help assist in automated coding functions and other processes in the EHR?

   a. SQL
   b. C++
   c. HTML
   d. NLP

Real-World Case

Many new assisted living and memory care complexes are being constructed in north Florida due to a significant increase in the population of individuals over age 50. Local medical societies and HCO administrators are actively working with these companies to establish relationships for continuing care services. As director of HIM at a local hospital, Larry Green has been asked to develop a slide presentation on the EHR and patient portals to members of these assisted living complexes and active senior citizens' educational centers.

Since the audience has somewhat limited medical terminology and technology knowledge, he is tailoring the presentation to meet their needs. Within the presentation, Larry stresses the importance of the EHR and the benefits it provides to patients, such as increased communication between providers, enhanced continuity of care, and improved patient safety.

He gives a brief overview and examples of the basic functions such as e-prescribing, CPOE, results management, and public health reporting. Larry also gives a demonstration of the patient portal for his hospital. He shows the audience how they can access their patient information, follow-up on lab test results, monitor their blood pressure or glucose levels, ask questions about prescriptions, request or change appointments, schedule educational or health-monitoring sessions, and address their insurance and account issues.

Larry is aware that confidentiality is a topic of concern. Therefore, he addresses interoperability and secure transmission of data between HCOs and providers in his presentation. He also incorporates the HIPAA confidentiality and security information audience members receive when visiting their physicians. Larry concludes his presentation with a discussion of frequently asked questions, and then he allows a significant amount of time to address any other questions the audience may have.

REVIEW QUESTIONS

1. The ability of the EHR system to identify the person who signed the document electronically is called
   _____.

   a. Signer authentication
   b. Document authentication
   c. Password authentication
   d. Biometric authentication

2. What publication highlighted the large number of medical mistakes that kill thousands of patients every year?

   a. The *Federal Register*
   b. *To Err is Human*
   c. The Affordable Care Act
   d. *Crossing the Quality Chasm*

3. What term is used to describe the hardware, software, and other integrated technologies used in the creation of electronic patient health information?

   a. HIPAA
   b. HIM
   c. HIT
   d. ACA

4. Identify the example that can be used to justify a policy against using the copy and paste function.

   a. Improves the quality of care
   b. Decreases the chances of fraudulent claims
   c. Provides more detailed documentation
   d. Documentation cannot be used for quality improvement purposes

5. Identify the concept that is considered an electronic footprint of what has occurred within a file.

   a. Audit log
   b. Digital signature
   c. Template-based entry
   d. Unstructured data

6. What term is used to describe health information technologies that have been tested and certified to perform up to national standards?

   a. CEHRT
   b. CERT
   c. CPOE
   d. ONC

7. What is the term used to describe foundation systems that collect administrative and clinical data that make up the EHR?

   a. Source systems
   b. Connectivity systems
   c. Specialty clinical systems
   d. Smart peripherals

(Continued)

REVIEW QUESTIONS (*Continued*)

8. What term is used to describe activities and charting that happen at the patient's bedside or while the patient is actively receiving care?

   a. POC
   b. CPOE
   c. CDS
   d. BC-MAR

9. Which of the following is not a barrier to EHR adoption?

   a. Cost
   b. Limited HIT workforce
   c. Suitability of products to meet practice needs
   d. Enabling safer more reliable prescribing

10. The combination of paper and electronic health records is called _____.

   a. Hybrid
   b. Half and half
   c. Mixed
   d. Interoperable

References

Amatayakul, M. K. 2017. *Health IT and EHRs: Principles and Practice*, 6th ed. Chicago: AHIMA.

Centers for Medicare and Medicaid Services (CMS). 2018. Historical National Health Expenditure Data. https://www.cms.gov/Research-Statistics-Data-and-Systems/Statistics-Trends-and-Reports/National HealthExpendData/NationalHealthAccountsHistorical.html.

Centers for Disease Control and Prevention (CDC). 2017. Electronic Medical Records/Electronic Health Records (EMRs/EHRs). https://www.cdc.gov/nchs/fastats/electronic-medical-records.htm.

Downing, K. 2013. Practice Brief: Electronic Signature, Attestation, and Authorship (2013 update). http://bok.ahima.org/doc?oid=107151#.WlFawN-nFRY.

Ellison, A. 2017. Becker's Hospital Review—15 Things to Know About the Stark Law. https://www.beckershospitalreview.com/legal-regulatory-issues/15-things-to-know-about-stark-law-021717.html.

Hamilton, B. 2009. *Electronic Health Records*. Boston, MA: McGraw-Hill Higher Education.

Health Level 7 (HL7). 2018. About HL7. Accessed 1/22/2018. http://www.hl7.org/about/index.cfm?ref=common.

Institute of Medicine (IOM). 2003. Key Capabilities of an Electronic Health Record System. https://www.nap.edu/catalog/10781/key-capabilities-of-an-electronic-health-record-system-letter-report.

Jacobson, D. M. and S. Teutsch. 2012. An environmental scan of integrated approaches for defining and measuring total population health by the clinical care system, the government public health system, and stakeholder organizations. Public Health Institute and County of Los Angeles Public Health Department. http://www.improvingpopulationhealth.org/PopHealthPhaseIICommissionedPaper.pdf.

Leventhal, R. 2017. CMS Finalizes 90-Day MU Reporting Period, Pushes Back Stage 3 Mandate. https://www.healthcare-informatics.com/article/payment/breaking-cms-finalizes-90-day-mu-reporting-period-2018.

Markle. n.d. Overview and principles. Accessed 7/11/2017. http://www.markle.org/health/markle-common-framework/connecting-professionals/overview.

McTosh, P. 2014. Implementing Electronic Signatures. https://www.hitechanswers.net/implement-e-signatures-ehrs/.

National Academy of Medicine (NAM). 2000. *To Err Is Human: Building a Safer Health System*. The National Academies Press. https://www.nap.edu/download/9728#.

National Center for Health Statistics (NCHS). 2015. Healthy People 2020. https://www.cdc.gov/nchs/healthy people/hp2020.htm.

National Library of Medicine. 2011. About the UMLS. http://www.nlm.nih.gov/research/umls/about_umls.html#Metathesaurus.

Office of the National Coordinator for Health Information Technology (ONC). 2018a. https://www.healthit.gov/providers-professionals/medical-practice-efficiencies-cost-savings.

Office of the National Coordinator for Health Information Technology (ONC). 2018b. https://www.healthit.gov/policy-researchers-implementers/about-onc-health-it-certification-program

Office of the National Coordinator for Health Information Technology (ONC). 2017a. About the ONC Health IT Certification Program. https://www.healthit.gov/policy-researchers-implementers/permanent-certification-program-faqs#a1.

Office of the National Coordinator for Health Information Technology (ONC). 2017b. Introduction to Unintended Consequences. https://www.healthit.gov/unintended-consequences/content/module-i-introduction-unintended-consequences.html.

Office of the National Coordinator for Health Information Technology (ONC). 2016a. 2015 Report to Congress on Health IT Adoption, Use, and Exchange. http://bok.ahima.org/PdfView?oid=301962.

Office of the National Coordinator for Health Information Technology (ONC). 2016b. Health IT Certification Program Overview. https://www.healthit.gov/sites/default/files/PUBLICHealthITCertificationProgram Overview _v1.1.pdf.

Office of the National Coordinator for Health Information Technology (ONC). 2014. Advantages of Electronic Health Records. https://www.healthit.gov/providers-professionals/faqs/what-are-advantages-electronic-health-records.

Office of the National Coordinator for Health Information Technology (ONC). 2013. Implementing Consolidated-Clinical Document Architecture (C-CDA) for Meaningful Use Stage 2. https://www.healthit.gov/sites/default/files/c-cda_and_meaningfulusecertification.pdf.

Palkie, B. 2016. Clinical Classifications, Vocabularies, Terminologies, and Standards. Chapter 5 in *Health Information Management: Concepts, Principles, and Practice*, 5th ed. Edited by P. Oachs and A. Watters. Chicago: AHIMA.

Rosin, T. 2014. Becker's Hospital Review—The Stark Act: 30 Things to Know. https://www.beckershospitalreview.com/legal-regulatory-issues/the-stark-act-30-things-to-know.html.

Sandefer, R. 2016. Consumer Health Informatics. Chapter 12 in *Health Information Management: Concepts, Principles, and Practice*. Edited by P. Oachs and L. Watters. Chicago: AHIMA.

Sayles, N. B. 2016. Health Information Functions, Purpose, and Users. Chapter 3 in *Health Information Management Technology: An Applied Approach, 5th ed*. Edited by N. B. Sayles and L. L. Gordon. Chicago: AHIMA Press.

The Shams Group. n.d. CPOE Portal. Accessed February 12, 2018. http://shamsgroup.com/healthcare-solutions/clinical-innovation/cpoe-portal/.

Consumer Informatics

- Explain consumer informatics.
- Differentiate between the patient portal and a personal health record.
- Explain impact of health literacy on patients.

Blue Button	Consumer informatics	Patient portal
Consumer	E-patients	Population health
Consumer engagement	Health literacy	Shared data record
Consumer health applications	Jargon	Social media

A consumer is a patient, client, resident, or other recipient of healthcare services. Therefore, consumer informatics, also known as consumer health informatics, is "the field devoted to informatics from multiple consumer or patient views" (AMIA 2017). More and more consumers are using technology to keep in touch with their healthcare providers and to access health information. Consumer informatics includes health literacy, consumer health applications, patient portals, personal health record (PHR), health information literature, and other consumer applications.

Health Literacy

Health literacy is "the degree to which individuals have the capacity to obtain, process, and understand basic health information and services needed to make appropriate health decisions" (Selden et al. 2000, vi). According to the Institute of Medicine (n.d.a), 90 million adult Americans have limited health literacy. Even patients with advanced education frequently do not understand their health information and the healthcare delivery system, which are complex even for healthcare professionals. The Department of Health and Human Services is working to solve this problem. The National Action Plan to Improve Health Literacy has established seven goals to improve health literacy:

- Provide access to health and safety information.
- Create change in the healthcare system that would improve health information and communication of that information.

- Implement health information into schools and universities.
- Support local adult education efforts.
- Conduct research on health literacy.
- Use evidence-based health literacy practice. (HHS 2010, 1–2)

Health literacy is not necessarily about a patient's reading ability or education level, but about understanding the terms and concepts related to their healthcare (Health and Human Services, Office of Disease Prevention and Health Promotion 2010, 4). "Health literacy includes the ability to understand prescription medications, discharge instructions, consent forms, appointment scheduling, requests for information, and the ability to negotiate complex healthcare organizations that offer a variety of services in multiple locations" (myPHR 2017a). Anything that affects the patient's ability to make decisions related to his healthcare, including understanding insurance coverage and billing or his rights as a patient, is related to health literacy.

A number of factors contribute to an individual's health literacy:

- Communication skills of the patient and the healthcare professional providing the information
- Level of educational knowledge of healthcare
- Culture-based experiences with or knowledge of healthcare
- Demands on the healthcare facility (HHS 2010, 5)

Other health literacy factors include:

- Age greater than 65
- Nonwhite ethnicity
- Recent immigrant
- Poverty level or below
- English is second language (HHS 2010, 8)

Patients for whom English is a second language may struggle with everyday communications, much less the complex language of medicine. However, communication goes far beyond the words or language used by the patient and the physician, extending to the ability of the patient to understand implications beyond the fundamental meaning. This can be connected to culture, which is what members of the group have in common including their ideas and values (Nielsen-Bohlman et al. 2004). Culture can be based on "ethnic heritage, nationality of family origin, age, religion, sexual orientation, disability, or socioeconomic status" (ACOG 2013). These factors influence patients' beliefs and the way that they communicate, as well as how they understand and react to health information (National Library of Medicine n.d.b).

Health literacy is important for a number of reasons, including the patient's:

- Ability to find the way through the healthcare delivery system
- Knowing what information to share with the healthcare provider
- Ability to care for himself
- Ability to understand risk (HHS 2010, 3)

The patient's struggle to find the way through the healthcare delivery system is shown in many ways including having trouble completing forms, understanding the healthcare claim, knowing who to call, and knowing what questions to ask. The inability to understand health information and remember instructions is even more difficult when the patient is not feeling well (HHS 2010, 5).

At one time, medical reference books and journals were the only sources of information, other than physicians, on diseases and medicine. Today, the patient has access to what can be an overwhelming amount of information. Patients get their medical knowledge from many different sources including:

- Magazines and other news sources
- Commercials and other marketing campaigns
- Family and friends
- Websites (Nielsen-Bohlman et al. 2004)

Some websites provide quality information on diseases, procedures, and other healthcare issues. Others provide erroneous, outdated information. Consumers do not always know how to determine the difference.

Basing healthcare decisions on erroneous or outdated health information can have a negative impact on the patient. For example, a patient may decide not to take the physician's advice based on the outdated information.

Medical terminology is sometimes called the language of medicine. People who do not understand it often feel like the healthcare provider is speaking a foreign language. Patients may be too embarrassed to tell the physician or other healthcare provider that they do not understand. This results in them leaving the healthcare facility without really understanding what was said or what to do. This can then harm their health if they take medications on the wrong schedule or do something else incorrect. Healthcare providers should encourage patients to ask questions (Graham and Brookey 2008).

The healthcare provider may believe that he is explaining the patient's condition in simple terms when, in fact, jargon is being used. **Jargon** is specialized terminology used by a specific group; in this case healthcare professionals. For example, in health information management (HIM) terms such as MS-DRGs, health information exchange, and notice of privacy practices are familiar to providers and HIM professionals, but patients do not necessarily understand them if they have heard of them at all. Problems with understanding healthcare jargon makes it difficult for patients to make informed decisions about their healthcare or for them to understand the decisions that they make. This can lead to negative outcomes. For example, a patient may agree to have her "tubes tied" and not realize that it means she cannot have any more babies. Medicaid requires patients undergoing surgical sterilization to sign a document stating that the patient realizes he or she cannot have a baby. This form came about because patients did not realize the significance of the procedure.

A number of ways can help improve compliance and understanding instructions:

- Bringing family member or friend to appointments
- Using terms that are easy to understand
- Avoiding jargon
- Not overwhelming patients with information
- Providing a comfortable environment to discuss their health (Graham and Brookey, 2008)

When confused, patients may take an overdose or underdose of a medication because they do not understand the instructions on the bottle or what the physician said. One research study showed that patients frequently misunderstand even simple instructions such as take a medication every 6 hours or twice a day (Wolf et al. 2011).

There are tools, such as pictures, and strategies, such as Teach Back and Ask Me 3, available to healthcare providers in order to help improve patient's understanding of their health.

There is an old adage that says a picture is worth a thousand words. Pictures, graphs, and other visual aids can present health information in a way that is easy to understand. These pictures should not be the only method of communication but rather reinforce the verbal communications (CDC 2014).

The Teach Back communication strategy involves using simple language to explain the patient's condition and then asking the patient to repeat the information in their own words. This enables to the healthcare provider to ensure that the patient understands her condition, her plan of care, and the provider's directions (Always Use Teach-Back n.d).

The Ask Me 3 initiative is a method promoted to patients to help them get the information that they need. It consists of three questions:

- What is my problem?
- What should I do?
- Why do I need to do this?

These three questions are designed to bring patients into their own care process, alongside providers, to achieve improved communication (IHI 2018).

Consumer Health Applications

Consumer health applications are healthcare-based applications designed for use by the patient or provider on smart phones, tablets, and other computers. Patients use consumer health applications to:

- Access health information
- Promote a healthy lifestyle

- Track calories and other information
- Manage their conditions
- Access the PHR (FDA 2015)

The healthcare provider uses it to:

- Access patient information
- Communicate with patients and other healthcare professionals
- Monitor patients
- Provide telemedicine (Athenahealth 2017)

Telehealth

Telehealth is defined as "the use of electronic information and telecommunication technologies to support and promote long-distance clinical health care, patient and professional health-related education, public health and health administration. It is used in dentistry, counseling, both physical and occupational therapy, disease management, patient information, and more (Center for Connected Health Policy 2018). Telehealth technologies include video conferencing, the internet, store-and-forward imaging, streaming media, and terrestrial and wireless communications" (HRSA 2015). Telemedicine is a subset of telehealth that focuses on the provision of care whereas telehealth includes administrative uses and education.

Telehealth technology can be used for electronic visits (e-visits), which can take the form of real-time videos, or use a patient portal whereby the patient logs in to an information system and asks the physician questions. When using live video for an e-visit, the patient and provider communicate synchronously (both online at the same time). Synchronous communication requires an appointment, but an appointment is not necessary to communicate with a provider through asynchronous (not online at the same time) methods, such as store-and-forward. The store-and-forward method includes videos that have been prerecorded, pictures, e-mail, and more. To qualify as an e-visit, the interaction must include obtaining the patient's history, assigning a diagnosis, assigning a diagnosis code, submitting a healthcare claim, and performing some type of treatment (Adamson and Bachman 2010). E-visits provide a number of benefits to patients and physicians as well as the healthcare delivery system, including improved access to care, flexibility in care provided, quality of care, improved efficiency, and a decrease in costs (Hicks et al. 2015). It is important to note that e-visits should be used with only minor conditions such as sinus problems, urinary problems, diarrhea, and so forth. It is not appropriate for all situations such as when the patient is pregnant or breastfeeding (Premier Health 2015).

In addition to live video and store-and-forward, telehealth also includes remote patient monitoring (collecting and reviewing health data patients submit remotely) and mobile health, which is using cell phones, tablets, and other mobile devices to share information to improve lifestyle, notify patients of disease outbreaks, and more (Center for Connected Health Policy 2018).

Telehealth offers a number of benefits to the patient:

- Patients who live in rural areas can reduce or eliminate trips to the city to see specialists.
- Patients are able to be monitored while going about their day-to-day business.
- Hospitalizations may be reduced as health issues may be identified early.
- Amount of time out of work is less as travel time is reduced and monitoring is performed remotely.
- Patients can submit blood sugar, blood pressure, and pulse results to the healthcare professional.

In addition to being more convenient for patients, telehealth has led to better outcomes, reduced cost of care, and higher patient satisfaction. As a result, the number of patients using telehealth is rapidly increasing. Estimates show that approximately 250,000 patients used telehealth in 2013 (AHA 2015). This figure is expected to increase to 3.2 million patients by 2018. One study shows that 64 percent of patients are willing to consult their physician via video (American Well 2015).

Several factors are contributing to this increase:

- Patients are more engaged in their healthcare.
- Affordable Care Act provided incentives to healthcare facilities to implement various telehealth models.

- Some states are mandating that insurers pay for telehealth services.
- Employers are offering telehealth to employees as part of their benefit program. (AHA 2015)

Despite its many benefits, telehealth has its disadvantages:

- Lack of funds to start telehealth program
- No face-to-face interaction
- Issues with patient's technology
- Reimbursement for e-visits (AHA 2015)

The costs of creating a telehealth program include more than the hardware. It also includes planning, training, new technologies, and staff to manage the technologies. Because the patient and healthcare provider are not actually face to face, efforts must be taken to create a personalized, interactive environment in which the patient is engaged so that the experience does not feel impersonal. Although many Americans have computers or other technology and access to the Internet, their computers often do not have the security measures and speed required for the best experience. This can result in issues such as low-quality video. In spite of the fact that telehealth is a significant trend, many insurers do not cover it (Anderson et al. 2017, 13–14).

Patients are also using telehealth to take daily ownership of their healthcare by using wearable devices, such as fitness trackers, to monitor a number of aspects of their health including exercise, blood sugar, and vital signs. These wearable devices can notify the patient when there is a problem. For example, the technology could notify the patient of a spike or drop in blood sugar. This notification could be through a text or a message on the device. When a problem is identified, the patient or the technology can contact the physician (Grebner and Mikaelian 2015). One prediction is that there will be 213 billion wearable devices, including watches, wristbands, clothing, and eyewear, sold by 2020 (Marbury 2017). For additional information on technical aspects of telehealth, refer to chapter 8.

Consumer Informatics Applications

One of the benefits of consumer informatics is that these technologies encourage consumer engagement. Consumer engagement is "a diverse set of activities that can include interacting with healthcare providers, seeking health information, maintaining a PHR, and playing an active role in making decisions in regard to personal healthcare" (Aschettino et al. 2016a, 7). Research shows that for consumer informatics to have a positive impact on patient's health, three factors are key: individual tailoring of the interaction based on the characteristics of the patient; personalization, which is customizing the program specifically for the patient; and behavior feedback, which provides messages to the patient about how well he is doing and where he is in the program (AHRQ 2009, 97).

In order to encourage patient engagement, the Blue Button campaign was established by The Office of the National Coordinator for Health IT (ONC). It is a consumer-motivated method to improve healthcare by having the patient or caretaker actively involved in decisions and planning by having direct access to personal health information. Many healthcare providers, health plans, pharmacies, laboratories, and other healthcare businesses are now offering this service. The Blue Button logo signifies that consumers can electronically access their health information in a secure and easy manner. Many studies have shown that the more actively involved patients are in their healthcare, the healthier they are likely to be (ONC 2016). "Individuals who are equipped, enabled, empowered and engaged in their health and health care decisions" are called e-patients (Society for Participatory Medicine 2017).

The benefits of consumer engagement include reduced costs, increased communication between physicians and patients through the use of technology, improved patient satisfaction, and population health. Population health is the capture and reporting of healthcare data that are used for public health purposes. If each individual patient's health is improved then the health of the population is improved (Rangaswamy 2015). Population health allows the healthcare provider to report infectious diseases, immunizations, cancer, and other reportable conditions to public health officials. Population health benefits through the information collected by healthcare providers and health departments that can be used to identify trends and improve the quality of care (Foisey 2015). For more on population health, refer to chapter 11.

Three key consumer informatics applications are patient portals, PHR, and social media.

Patients using these consumer informatics applications, described in the following sections, provide additional information about their health habits, care, and outcomes.

Patient Portals

A patient portal is an information system established and maintained by the healthcare facility that allows patients to log in to obtain their health information, register for appointments, and perform other functions such as using secure e-mail, downloading forms, updating demographics, scheduling appointments, and requesting a prescription refill. The information contained in the patient portal is a subset of the patient's electronic health record (EHR). Patients can access their health information through the patient portal at all times. Information available in the portal varies but can include lab results, summary of hospitalization, medications, radiographic reports, and much more. Patients must log in, typically with a username and password to protect the patient's privacy. The benefits of using patient portals include:

- Strengthening communication between the healthcare provider and the patient
- Providing patients with healthcare information
- Providing resources to the patient between patient visits
- Promoting patient engagement (Aschettino et al. 2016b)
- Reducing the amount of time that healthcare staff spend answering the phone, processing requests for information, and related activities (Kadlec et al. 2015)

Unfortunately, little if any training in the portal is provided to patients, and many patients are unable to understand the information available to them because of health literacy issues (Grebner and Mikaelian 2015). The healthcare provider can supply training for patients that addresses how to log in and navigate the site, privacy concerns, and health literacy.

There are two types of patient portals: standalone and system integrated. Standalone portals do not have all of the features of a system integrated portal and are typically used by smaller healthcare providers. System integrated portals are typically a function of the EHR and are, therefore, a fully functioning system (Aschettino et al. 2016b). The portal itself is owned by the healthcare provider or some other agent, such as a vendor or insurance company, who controls the portal, but the information is owned by the patient.

Some of the trends in patient portals include personalization, mobile devices, wearable technology, and communication. Personalization allows the healthcare provider to dispense educational material and other resources specific to the patient's condition. Mobile devices are used by the patient to enter data, such as blood sugar levels, into the portal for review by the physician. Data captured by wearable technology, such as fitness trackers and other monitoring devices, can be uploaded and reviewed by the physician. The patient portal supports two-way communication, which allows the patient to work with physicians between patient visits, request appointments, and receive reminders (Aschettino et al. 2016b). These reminders can be for appointments, need for follow-up, and more.

Personal Health Record

The personal health record (PHR) is an electronic or paper health record maintained and updated by an individual for himself or herself; it is a tool that individuals can use to collect, track, and share past and current information about their health or the health of someone in their care. The PHR contains health information that comes from both the physician and the patient, but the PHR is controlled by the patient. It is estimated that 75 percent of adults will be using PHRs by 2020 (Landi 2016).

The PHR is important because it links health information from all of the patient's care providers into one central location, which will help to improve the overall quality of the care provided. The PHR has no uniform format and is independent of any specific provider's EHR or patient portal and therefore not constrained by those requirements. The patient's health information from a provider can be downloaded to the PHR. A shared data record is a popular and effective model for a PHR. The shared data record is maintained by the patient and provider, health plan, or employer. The PHR may be managed by a healthcare provider, vendor, employer, or other (Amatayakul, 2016, 305).

Several items should be included in the PHR:

- Personal identification, including name and birth date
- People to contact in case of emergency
- Names, addresses, and phone numbers of your physician, dentist, and specialists

- Health insurance information
- Living wills, advance directives, or medical power of attorney
- Organ donor authorization
- A list and dates of significant illnesses and surgical procedures
- Current medications and dosages
- Immunizations and their dates
- Allergies or sensitivities to drugs or materials, such as latex
- Important events, dates, and hereditary conditions in your family history
- Results from a recent physical examination
- Opinions of specialists
- Important tests results; eye and dental records
- Correspondence between you and your provider(s)
- Current educational materials (or appropriate web links) relating to your health
- Any information you want to include about your health, such as your exercise regimen, any herbal medications you take and any counseling you may receive
- Dietary practices, such as whether you are vegetarian, or on a temporary diet; especially if changes in your diet have produced changes in your health in the past (MyPHR 2017b)

Much of the information in the PHR is the same as in the patient portal. The distinction between the two is that PHR is created and controlled by the patient whereas the patient portal is created and controlled by the healthcare facility (Aschettino et al. 2016b). There are currently four common formats of PHRs: paper, personal computer, Internet, and portable devices such as smart phones and tablets. Obtaining copies of health records and organizing them into a folder or a three-ring binder is one way to start a PHR. However, because there is only one source, accessibility is limited. The health information can also be scanned documents on a USB drive or other portable device. Although much more portable than a folder or three-ring binder, the physical nature of the USB format still limits accessibility. A personal computer-based product uses the patient's computer for storage of information that can be printed or copied to a portable device to take to the care provider. The Internet PHR provides access at any time from anywhere. Internet PHRs can be obtained by the patient in several ways. One way is for the patient to purchase a PHR service from a vendor who stores the data and provides basic services to the user. In this case, the patient must collect health records from his or her physicians and other providers and enter the information into the PHR. The patient's healthcare provider or insurer may provide the service automatically, populating it with clinical information and claims data.

Internet-based PHRs may be tethered or untethered. Tethered PHRs are connected to the EHR and allow patients to access information contained within the EHR. Untethered PHRs are not connected to the EHR. One of the benefits to tethered PHRs is that patients can identify any errors and therefore request a correction to the EHR (Lester et al. 2016). The PHR allows the patient to share information from other healthcare providers, exercise regimen, medications, dietary supplements, and other information that the patient wants the healthcare provider to know. The patient controls who has access to this information and what information it contains.

The PHR is not without its challenges. Figure 10.1 addresses some issues related to the PHR.

The use of the PHR has created roles for health information management professionals. For a discussion of these roles, refer to figure 10.2.

Social Media

Social media are online tools that allow people to communicate. Healthcare facilities use social media to advertise services, promote wellness, provide health education, provide support forums, and provide other communications to their patients and the general public (Backman et al. 2011). The benefits of using social media in healthcare include:

- Building a sense of community for patients with chronic diseases
- Patients are better informed and can track their health
- Patients can search for clinical trials that they might quality for
- Building awareness of conditions (Glaser 2016)

Figure 10.1. Challenges the PHR presents

1. **Who owns the data?** The consumer, employer, insurance carrier, or provider? Can you take the data with you when you switch doctors or stop paying the subscription fee?

2. **Who can access that data?** Will the information be sold to or shared with a third party? If personal health information is stored on an employer's database, will employers have access to it?

3. **How does the PHR get populated** with the patient's health information? Data must be accurate and traceable so that physicians know information is the right information about the right patient.

4. **Is there adequate technology** in place to keep personal health information secure in an Internet-based PHR?

5. **Are there adequate laws and regulations** that protect privacy and security of health information in a PHR or EHR format? For example, independent, third-party PHR websites are not subject to HIPAA regulations. Some states are filling the gap, but others do not.

6. **How can information from an EHR populate the PHR** securely and conveniently—and at the same time meet privacy and security guidelines?

Source: AHIMA 2008, 3–4.

Figure 10.2. Roles of health information management in PHR

Design and testing of PHRs. HIM professionals can be active advocates in designing PHR tools that are sensitive to underserved populations. Well-designed forms can overcome health literacy deficits. They should be designed to capture accurate information and be understandable to both the patients and providers. Testing of resources in development should include minority populations so their concerns are identified.

Distribution of PHRs to consumers. Cultural differences can be a barrier to PHR adoption. HIM professionals can address various groups using lay terminology to tout the benefits of PHRs and train consumers to become effective users.

Training providers and consumers. Having active, informed patients is often a paradigm shift for both providers and consumers. HIM professionals can facilitate information exchange between providers and patients, who often use differing language to describe medical conditions. They can also assist consumers, especially the elderly, in overcoming the digital divide.

Protecting confidentiality. HIM professionals can communicate safeguards to protect privacy for various PHR formats. Many consumers do not trust electronic systems to protect their privacy. HIM professionals are experts on privacy regulations and procedures for both the paper and the electronic world.

Source: Garvin et al. 2009.

Other uses of social media include online communities, exchange of information between healthcare providers, and communication between patients and healthcare providers via mobile devices (Kohn 2012). Patient information cannot be exchanged via social media due to privacy laws, but healthcare facilities may use social media to share emergency room wait times, list new services, gain information about patient satisfaction, and more (Glaser 2016). However, healthcare facilities must be careful when using social media because patient privacy can be compromised, statements can be misinterpreted, and unhappy patients can use it as a sounding board (Backman et al. 2011). The healthcare facility's policies and procedures should address:

- Who can access social media websites from within the healthcare facility
- Improper usage of social media
- Penalties for improper use of social media
- Responsibility of employees to report improper use
- Ensuring that employees know that statements on their personal social media accounts can impact the healthcare facility (Backman et al. 2011)

Patients can use social media to text, blog, and post status updates to share information about their condition with their family and friends, access support groups for their particular disease, and raise money for medical research.

CHECK YOUR UNDERSTANDING 10.1

1. Identify the accurate statement about health literacy.

   a. Health literacy is all about the patient's reading level.
   b. Health literacy is not impacted by the patient's culture.
   c. Health literacy includes understanding discharge instructions.
   d. Health literacy applies to healthcare professionals only.

2. The term used for specialized terminology for a specific group is _____.

   a. Jargon
   b. Culture
   c. Telehealth
   d. Portal

3. The patient wants to schedule an appointment. What should he use?

   a. Health record
   b. PHR
   c. Telehealth
   d. Patient portal

4. The patient wants to ensure the physician knows about the dietary supplements he is taking. Where should he record this?

   a. Health record
   b. PHR
   c. Telehealth
   d. Patient portal

5. Social media is best used to _____.

   a. Share test result with patients
   b. Communicate between nursing shifts
   c. Share healthcare experiences with family and friends
   d. Share healthcare status with physician and other healthcare professionals

Real-World Case

Louise is an 89-year-old woman who was discharged from the hospital after having a cardiac valve replacement for mitral valve stenosis. After going home, she had home health services for a few weeks. Louise had both Medicare and a secondary insurance. She received a bill requesting payment for the home health services provided. She was prepared to write a check for the total amount. Fortunately, her granddaughter, Marie, a HIM professional, was visiting and reviewed the bill. Marie immediately saw that neither Medicare nor the secondary insurance had been billed. Marie assisted her grandmother by calling the home health agency to discuss the bill. She was told that the home health agency did not have the insurance policy numbers. Marie provided the policy numbers. When she was about to hang-up, the billing office representative told Marie that when Louise received a Medicare Summary Notice from Medicare to call them back to let them know so that they could bill the secondary insurance. Marie explained to them that it was their responsibility to identify this. If Marie had not gotten involved, then Louise would have paid the bill and her insurance companies would never have been billed. Also, Louise would have called the home health agency to ask them to bill the secondary insurer.

CHAPTER REVIEW

1. Consumer informatics includes which of the following?

   a. Health information literature
   b. EHR
   c. Telehealth
   d. Health record

2. Health literacy is important because patients need to be able to

   a. Understand risk
   b. Use patient portal
   c. Utilize telehealth technologies
   d. Use social media

3. An e-patient is one who _____.

   a. Is engaged in her healthcare
   b. Is using telehealth technologies
   c. Has not signed up to use patient portal
   d. Uses social media

4. Social media includes _____.

   a. Support groups
   b. Sharing clinical information with physician
   c. Obtaining clinical information from physician
   d. Wearable technology

5. The healthcare facility's social media policies should address _____.

   a. Improper usage of social media
   b. How patients can use social media
   c. How employees can use social media at home
   d. Use of wearable technology

6. PHRs allow patients to _____.

   a. Add information
   b. Experience e-visits
   c. Request prescription refill
   d. Schedule appointments

7. Benefits of patient engagement include _____.

   a. Focus on the individual
   b. Improved patient satisfaction
   c. Telehealth
   d. Social media

8. The information system that is controlled by the healthcare facility that allows patients to register is known as _____.

   a. PHR
   b. Wearable device
   c. Social media
   d. Patient portal

9. Benefits to telehealth include _____.

   a. Access to patient information
   b. Reducing hospitalization
   c. Providing information to healthcare providers
   d. Population health

10. Critique this statement: Consumer health applications are used solely by patients.

   a. This is a true statement.
   b. This is a false statement as it is also used by insurers and healthcare providers.
   c. This is a false statement as it is also used by healthcare providers.
   d. This is a false statement as it is only used by physicians.

References

Adamson, S. C. and J. W. Bachman. 2010. Pilot Study of Providing Online Care in a Primary Care Setting. Mayo Clinic Proceedings. https://www.ncbi.nlm.nih.gov/pmc/articles/PMC2912730/.

Agency for Healthcare Research and Quality (AHRQ). 2009. Impact of Consumer Health Informatics Applications. https://www.ahrq.gov/downloads/pub/evidence/pdf/chiapp/impactchia.pdf.

Always Use Teach-Back. n.d. Welcome to the Always Use Teach-back Training Toolkit. Accessed February 11, 2018. http://www.teachbacktraining.org/.

Amatayakul, M. 2016. Health Information Technologies. Chapter 11 in *Health Information Management Technology: An Applied Approach*, 5th ed. Edited by N. B. Sayles and L. L. Gordon.

American Health Information Management Association. 2008. The Power of the PHR. *AHIMA Advantage* 12(3). http://bok.ahima.org/PdfView?oid=79608.

American Congress of Obstetricians and Gynecology (ACOG). 2013. Cultural Sensitivity and Awareness in the Delivery of Health Care. https://www.acog.org/Resources-And-Publications/Committee-Opinions /Committee-on-Health-Care-for-Underserved-Women/Cultural-Sensitivity-and-Awareness-in-the Delivery of Health Care.

American Hospital Association (AHA). 2015. The Promise of Telehealth for Hospitals, Health Systems and Their Communities. http://www.aha.org/research/reports/tw/15jan-tw-telehealth.pdf.

American Medical Informatics Association (AMIA). 2017. Consumer Health Informatics. https://www .amia.org/applications-informatics/consumer-health-informatics.

American Well. 2015. American Well 2015 Telehealth Survey: 64% of Consumers Would See a Doctor Via Video. https://www.americanwell.com/press-release/american-well-2015-telehealth-survey-64-of -consumers-would-see-a-doctor-via-video/.

Anderson, R., B. Beckett, K. Fahy, E. Gordon, A. Gray, S. Kropp, S. LePage, E. Liette, F. McNicholas, B. Phillips, K. Pulda, and L. Renn. 2017. Telemedicine Toolkit. http://www.bok.ahima.org/doc?oid=302358.

Aschettino, L., K. M. Baldwin, L. Bouma, B. Burton, D. Collier, M. Davis, M. Dolan, K. Fahy, C. Gardner, E. Gorton, L. Grebner, M. Hennings, L. Kadlec, A. Kirby, N. LaFianzo, M. Nelson., P. Reinger, and A. R. Smith. 2016a. Consumer Engagement Toolkit. http://bok.ahima.org/PdfView?oid=301404.

Aschettino, L., L. Bouma, B. Burton, M. Davis, C. Gardner, E. Gorton, L. Grebner, M. Hennings, N. LaFianza, K. Baldwin, M. Nelson, P. Reisinger, A. Rose, and A. Smith. 2016b. Patient Portal Tool Kit. http://bok.ahima.org/PdfView?oid=301419.

Athenahealth. 2017. What is mobile health technology? https://www.athenahealth.com/knowledge-hub /mobile-health-technology/what-is-mobile-health-technology.

Backman, C., S. Dolack, D. Dunyak, L. J., Lutz, A. Tegen, and D. Warner. 2011. Social Media + Healthcare. *Journal of AHIMA* 82(3), 20–25.

Center for Connected Health Policy. 2018. What is Telehealth? http://www.cchpca.org/what-is-telehealth.

Centers for Disease Control and Prevention (CDC). 2014. Health Literacy: Visual Communication Resources. https://www.cdc.gov/healthliteracy/developmaterials/visual-communication.html.

Department of Health and Human Services (HHS). 2010. Office of Disease Prevention and Health Promotion. https://health.gov/communication/HLActionPlan/pdf/Health_Literacy_Action_Plan.pdf.

Department of Health Resources and Services Administration (HRSA). 2015. Telehealth Programs. https://www.hrsa.gov/rural-health/telehealth/index.html.

Foisey, C. Q. 2015. Challenges and Upsides of Patient Engagement. http://www.medicalpracticeinsider .com/news/challenges-and-upsides-patient-engagement.

Food and Drug Administration (FDA). 2015. Mobile Medical Application. https://www.fda.gov /MedicalDevices/DigitalHealth/MobileMedicalApplications/ucm255978.htm.

Garvin, J. H., B. Odom-Wesley. W. J. Rudman, and R. S. Stewart. 2009. Healthcare Disparities and the Role of Personal Health Records. http://bok.ahima.org/doc?oid=91677#.WoCi9-Ry5jo.

Glaser, J. 2016. Five Reasons to "Like" Patients' Use of Social Media. *Hospitals & Health Networks*. http://www .hhnmag.com/articles/7090-five-reasons-to-like-patients-use-of-social-media.

Graham, S. and J. Brookey. 2008. Do Patient's Understand? *The Permanente Journal* 12(3). https://www .ncbi.nlm.nih.gov/pmc/articles/PMC3037129/.

Grebner, L. A. and R. Mikaelian. 2015. Best practices in mhealth for consumer engagement. *Journal of AHIMA* 86(9), 42–44.

Hicks, R., J. Talbert, W. W. Thombury, N. R. Perin, and A. J. Goodin. 2015. Online medical care: the current state of "eVisits" in acute primary care delivery. *Telemedicine and e-Health*. https://www.ncbi.nlm.nih .gov/pubmed/25474083.

Institute for Healthcare Improvement (IHI). 2018. Ask Me 3: Good Questions for Your Good Health. http://www.npsf.org/page/askme3.

Kadlec, L., A. D. Rose, and D. Warner. 2015. HIM engaging the patient portals. *Journal of AHIMA* 86(1).

Kohn, D. (2012). AHIMA Advance: The Impact of Social Media on the Integrity of Patient Record Information.   http://www.mobihealthnews.com/news/ahima-advance-impact-social-media-integrity -patient-record-information.

Landi, H. 2016. Study: 75% of Adults Will Use Personal Health Records by 2020, Exceeding MU Targets. https://www.healthcare-informatics.com/news-item/study-75-adults-will-use-personal-health-records -2020-even-without-mu-incentives.

Lester, M., S. Boateng, J. Studeny, and A. Coustasse. 2016. Personal health records: Beneficial or burdensome for patients and healthcare providers? *Perspectives in Health Information Management*. 13(Spring):1h.

Marbury, D. 2017. Top 10 Healthcare Wearables. http://managedhealthcareexecutive.modernmedicine. com/managed-healthcare-executive/news/top-10-healthcare-wearables-watch.

MyPHR. 2017a. What Is Health Literacy? http://www.myphr.com/HealthLiteracy/default.aspx.

MyPHR. 2017b. How to Create a Personal Health Record. http://www.myphr.com/StartaPHR/Create_a _PHR.aspx.

National Library of Medicine. n.d.a. Clear Communication. Accessed February 10. 2018. https://www.nih .gov/institutes-nih/nih-office-director/office-communications-public-liaison/clear-communication/.

National Library of Medicine. n.d.b. Health Literacy. Accessed February 7, 2018. https://nnlm.gov /professional-development/topics/health-literacy.

Nielsen-Bohlman, L., A.M. Panzer, and D. A. Kindig. 2004. *Health Literacy: A Prescription to End Confusion*. Washington, D.C: National Academies Press. https://www.ncbi.nlm.nih.gov/books/NBK216032/.

Office of the National Coordinator of Health Information Technology (ONC). 2016. About Blue Button. https://www.healthit.gov/patients-families/blue-button/about-blue-button.

Premiere Health. 2015. E-Visits Convenient, Efficient for Minor Health Problems. https://www .premierphysiciannet.com/Health-and-Wellness/Health-Topics/E-Visits/.

Rangaswamy, N. 2015. The Five Pillars of Population Health Management: Consumer Engagement. http://www.zeomega.com/2015/05/the-five-pillars-of-population-health-management-consumer -engagement/.

Selden, C. R., M. Zorn, S. Ratzan, and R. M. Parker. 2000. Health Literacy. https://www.researchgate .net/publication/230877250_National_Library_of_Medicine_Current_Bibliographies_in_Medicine _Health_Literacy.

Society for Participatory Medicine. 2017. About Us. https://participatorymedicine.org/epatients/about-e -patientsnet.

Wolf, M. S., L. M. Curtis, K. Waite, S. C. Bailey, L. A. Hedlund, T. C. Davis, W. H. Shrank, R. M. Parker, and A. J. J. Wood. 2011. Helping patients simplify and safely use complex prescription regimens. *Archives of Internal Medicine* 171(4): 300–305. https://jamanetwork.com/journals/jamainternalmedicine /fullarticle/226687.

Learning Objectives

- Illustrate why the health information exchange (HIE) is a positive step for healthcare.
- Describe the role and function of the health information organization (HIO) in the HIE efforts.
- Explain the concept of interoperability and its importance in healthcare.
- Juxtapose the benefits and barriers of HIE.
- Compare and contrast the models and methods of HIE.
- Explain the requirements of Meaningful Use.

Key Terms

American Recovery and
  Reinvestment Act (ARRA)
Bring your own device (BYOD)
Consent management
Consolidated (centralized) model
Consumer-mediated exchange
Directed exchange
eHealth Exchange Sequoia Project
Federated (decentralized) model
Health information exchange
  (HIE)

Health information
  organization (IIIO)
Health Information Technology
  for Economic and Clinical
  Health (HITECH) Act
Hybrid model
Identity management
Identity matching
Interoperability
Local health information
  organization (LHIO)

Meaningful Use (MU)
Opt-in or opt-out consent
Population health reporting
Query-based exchange
Record locator service (RLS)
Regional health information
  organization (RHIO)
Value-based healthcare
Vetting

Currently, the federal government is encouraging statewide health information exchange (HIE) to support the nationwide health information network (NHIN), referred to as eHealth Exchange. HIE is defined as the formal agreed-upon process for the seamless exchange of health information electronically between providers and others with the same level of interoperability, according to nationally recognized standards. According to the Office of the National Coordinator for Health Information Technology (ONC), "health information exchange (HIE) allows doctors, nurses, pharmacists, other health care providers and patients to appropriately access and securely share a patient's vital medical information electronically—improving the speed, quality, safety and cost of patient care" (ONC 2014a).

HIE is a revolutionary and evolutionary step in the delivery of healthcare services. It is no longer sufficient to gather information and store it in health records (paper or electronic) or in secondary databases such as tumor registries and consider it a static resource. This data and information must become dynamic to be transformed into knowledge and wisdom not only to make better decisions for individualized patient care but also to make an impact on the health of the population, both regionally and nationwide. HIE requires collaboration between healthcare providers, patients, government and public health agencies, health information technology (HIT) companies, professional associations, and payers. These parties must work jointly and cooperatively in order to achieve individual, organizational, and national goals of improving health status, efficient coordination of services, financial viability, and producing valid and reliable healthcare research.

HIE requires a shift in mindset for healthcare professionals, from treating individuals within a specific practice or facility to understand how healthcare organizations (HCOs) impact the health of the entire community in which they practice. HIE can improve patient outcomes by reducing medical errors and increasing the efficiency of care by decreasing unnecessary tests and services because the health information is readily available for all providers. These steps, in turn, support healthy, productive citizens. HIE encourages patients to become active participants in their healthcare and well-being by offering information and education about health conditions, managing chronic diseases, working with diet and exercise tracking apps, and decreasing completion of repetitive paperwork needed by providers. HIE works to bolster community health by coordinating with public health officials by identifying disease trends, implementation of immunization programs, and developing health education programs for at-risk populations (ONC 2013a). These new cultural norms must permeate through every personnel layer and work process in the HCO. The traditional silos of information or territories exclusive to one aspect of care must be broken down to allow free exchange of information and ideas and foster better coordination of healthcare services for the duration of a patient's life. **Value-based healthcare** is an evolving concept focused on three areas: better care for the individual, better health for the community, and lower cost of healthcare through improvement of services and delivery methods (CMS 2017). HIE is a way to bridge the gaps in the disjointed healthcare system of the United States. Figure 11.1 shows the connectivity that can be achieved by the use of HIE.

Figure 11.1.   Health information connectivity with the HIE

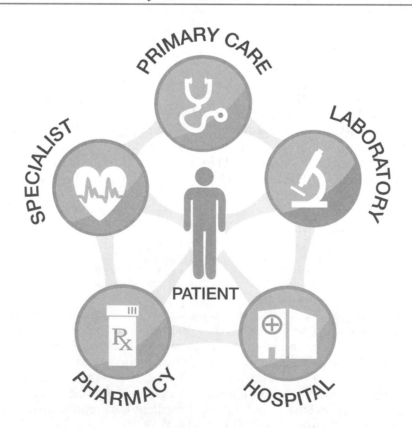

Source: ONC 2014a.

Interoperability and Health Information Exchange

The exchange of health information between entities is possible only if interoperability is in place. Interoperability is the capability of different information systems and software applications to communicate and exchange data. E-prescribing, in which pharmacies receive electronic prescriptions from hospitals, physician practices, and health departments, is an example of interoperability. It is likely that each of these HCOs has a different electronic health record (EHR) or information system. Nonetheless, the pharmacy must be able to securely receive a verified prescription from a licensed provider and accurately provide the correct medication and dosage for the specified patient. Another example is a primary care provider (PCP) referring one of her patients to a specialty provider, such as an oncologist or cardiologist. The PCP would electronically send, over a secure network, all pertinent medical and health information of the patient to the specialist for the specialist to have all the background health information to develop a tailored and comprehensive care plan. Again, each of these practitioners would have different EHRs, but these systems must be able to communicate effectively to benefit the patient.

Interoperability must be both an internal and external application and can be difficult to achieve. To achieve interoperability internally, software across an HCO's departments must communicate and exchange information with each other. Many HCOs have several information systems to coordinate internally, and some could be years older (and, therefore, potentially obsolete) compared to others. For example, coordinating and converting a radiology information system that is five years old with a newly implemented EHR will be a challenge for the HCO, the EHR vendor, and the old radiology software vendor, who must work together to make sure all old information on the original system can be accessed and used. Other challenges of coordinating with older systems include a change in workflow because the newer system may have automated functions that were manual in the older system, software programming most likely would be different, and reporting functions and formats would change. The HCO may be using the phased-in approach to implementing the EHR, and the new radiology administrative information system may be two years out. Converting or updating these older information systems can put a financial strain on even the most efficiently run facilities.

If the HCO is part of a large corporation of healthcare providers, each satellite facility must be able to exchange information with the others easily. Because most HCOs are independent, this is where external interoperability gets very problematic. As mentioned in chapter 9, health information blocking has created a challenge to interoperability by impeding the flow of data between HCOs or providers, which may be detrimental to the patient. HCOs that are owned by corporations typically have similar systems, but this is not necessarily the case with independent providers. Four types of interoperability can facilitate a successful exchange of health information:

- **Technical**: Based on the hardware and equipment connectivity used in the exchange, this type of interoperability allows any computer or device to exchange data with another computer or device without corrupting the data or creating errors.

- **Syntactic**: Message format standards identify how the data should be formatted or structured to allow the exchange. Interface software (programming where one application or entity is told how the other application or entity formats its data so that the receiving entity can appropriately convert the data it receives for processing) must be employed for compatibility to enable the exchange. These interoperability standards are not specific to healthcare, as they are applied to any electronic transmission between two entities.

- **Semantic**: This process involves the use of standardized terminologies (such as SNOMED-CT which is covered in chapter 12) to provide clarity, consistency, and appropriate meaning in HIE. This area of HIE is still undergoing development.

- **Process**: The most difficult of all the types of interoperability, process refers to the "degree to which the integrity of workflow can be maintained between systems and includes maintaining and conveying information such as user roles, data protection, and system service quality between systems" (Amatayakul 2017, 398). An example of this would be the patient authorization for release of information, which varies by state. HCOs requesting protected health information (PHI) (any individually identifiable health information of the patient) across state lines or with other HCOs that have less reputable security and access standards impede the exchange of data (Amatayakul, 2017, 398–399).

The Office of the National Coordinator for Health Information Technology (ONC) is the principal federal entity charged with the coordination of nationwide efforts to implement and use the most advanced HIT and the electronic exchange of health information and, in so doing, establishing interoperability among all health information systems (ONC 2017a). The ONC was established in 2004 as a result of an executive order by President George W. Bush and is a permanent agency within the Department of Health and Human Services (HHS). The ONC was the first federal agency empowered to coordinate and modernize the use of HIT and infrastructure to seamlessly and securely transmit electronic health data to improve patient care and administrative functions. It has grown to include branches that address standards and technology, ethics and compliance, care transformation, quality and safety, planning, evaluation, and analysis (ONC 2017a). This allows for improved strategic planning and communication to address concerns from healthcare providers and organizations, patients, HIT industry leaders, other stakeholders to effectively confront the challenges of this massive overhaul of the US healthcare system.

In 2007, the American Recovery and Reinvestment Act (ARRA) was enacted to stimulate the US economy during a recession. A significant portion of ARRA was dedicated to expanding the use of HIT to improve the business efficiency and effectiveness of HCOs while increasing patient safety and positive health outcomes. This part of the ARRA legislation is the Health Information Technology for Economic and Clinical Health (HITECH) Act which dedicated more than $19 billion to developing HIT, implementing workforce education and training, certifying EHR products, establishing standards and vocabularies, and driving electronic security and privacy regulations into the 21st century (Kellogg 2016, 28).

The HITECH Act was the foundational legislation for the development, adoption, promotion, and use of electronic and computerized applications to create an interoperable health information exchange system. The HITECH Act added new regulations and requirements toughening enforcement and increasing penalties for security breaches and privacy violations. Fortifying privacy and security standards in HIE helped foster more connectivity and communications and therefore interoperability between systems. It also mandated the establishment and strengthening of transmission standards and protocols to help establish interoperability among US health information systems. The HITECH Act emphasizes use of real-time health information on current and emerging technology at the time health services are administered to help providers make better decisions for the benefit of the patient and society (McCann 2016, 450).

In 2014, the ONC published *Connecting Health and Care for the Nation: A 10-Year Vision to Achieve an Interoperable Health IT Infrastructure,* which lays out the goals and objectives for the improvement of HIT interoperability. An infographic road map, shown in figure 11.2, was developed to visualize a path to achieving this goal.

Figure 11.2.   Shared nationwide interoperability roadmap

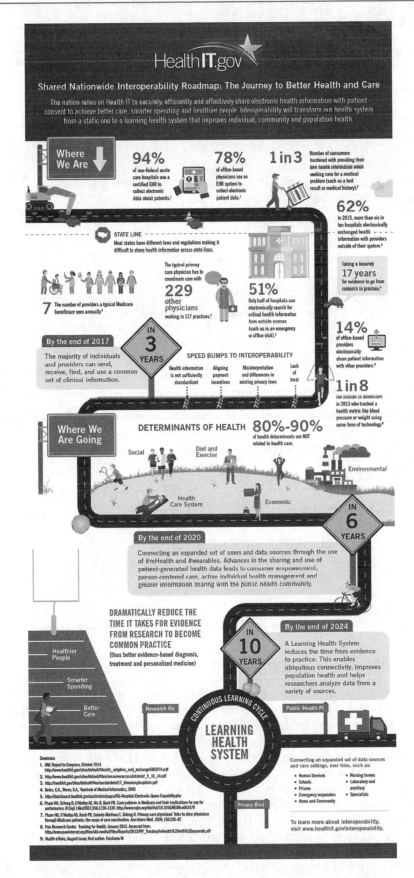

Source: ONC 2014b.

CHECK YOUR UNDERSTANDING 11.1

1. What term is used to describe the process of physician electronically ordering an antibiotic for a patient and for that patient to pick it up a specified drugstore?

   a. E-meds
   b. E-drugs
   c. Compu-drugs
   d. E-prescribe

2. What concept describes the ability for healthcare providers and their associates, regardless of location, to swap healthcare data seamlessly and meeting all interoperability and national standards to provide patient-centered care?

   a. RHIO
   b. HIE
   c. NHIN
   d. ONC

3. What principle describes the unified and smooth exchange of information among various healthcare providers and information systems and software applications?

   a. Privacy
   b. Confidentiality
   c. Infrastructure
   d. Interoperability

4. Which president is responsible for the establishment of the ONC and laying the foundation for HIE?

   a. Barack Obama
   b. Bill Clinton
   c. George W. Bush
   d. Donald Trump

5. What type of interoperability addresses the functions of actual computers and other hardware used during HIE?

   a. Process
   b. Technical
   c. Semantic
   d. Syntactic

History of Health Information Exchange

The HIE concept has evolved over the last several decades from a myriad of attempts at transmitting data from one HCO to another. However, without oversight and coordination from one designated governing body, previous attempts were piecemeal at best. Over these decades there have also been technological advances that could hardly have been imagined at the inception of the HIE.

HIE is typically conducted through an intermediary called an HIO. A **health information organization (HIO)** is typically a public–private partnership organization that oversees, governs, and facilitates the transmission of health data between different types of HCOs that have various EHR systems, according to nationally recognized standards. Many HIOs started as a **local health information organization (LHIO)** or **regional health information organization (RHIO)**. The Health Information Management Systems Society (HIMSS) defines RHIO as "a group of organizations with a business stake in improving the quality, safety and efficiency of healthcare delivery that comes together to exchange information for these purposes. The terms RHIO and Health Information Exchange, or 'HIE', are often used interchangeably" (HIMSS 2018). An LHIO is a small-scale version of an RHIO. LHIOs and RHIOs are groups of healthcare organizations in specific geographic areas that share electronic health information according to accepted standards. For a discussion on the organizations that set these standards, refer to chapter 12. HIOs help the HCOs and providers by delivering the services of patient identification functionality, identity management and security services, and data exchange management (Amatayakul 2017, 418). Inconsistent federal oversight and financial support, particularly prior to mid-2000s, has limited tracking of HIOs in the United States, making it difficult to determine exact numbers. Public–private partnerships with state governments have facilitated the stability of HIOs and contributed to the development of the eHealth Exchange, a network of HCOs and associated businesses that can exchange health information securely, privately, and efficiently through established transmission protocols (Amatayakul 2017, 422).

The Sequoia Project eHealth Exchange (originally known as Healtheway) is a group of "federal agencies and non-federal organizations that came together under a common mission and purpose to improve patient care, streamline disability benefit claims, and improve public health reporting through secure, trusted, and interoperable health information exchange" (McCann 2016, 468). The Sequoia Project is a private sector organization supplying and managing the data stewardship for the nationwide network. Currently, it provides exchange services in all 50 states for more than one million patients; 65 percent of US hospitals; 50,000 medical groups; 8,300 pharmacies; and the Department of Defense, Centers for Medicare and Medicaid, Veterans Administration, and the Social Security Administration (Sequoia Project 2017). Organizations taking part in the Sequoia Project "mutually to agree to support a common set of standards and specifications that enable the establishment of a secure, trusted, and interoperable connection among all participating Exchange organizations for the standardized flow of information" (Sequoia Project 2017). Although it initially found its footing with the guidance of the ONC under the title Nationwide Health Information Network (NHIN), eHealth Exchange is now an independent enterprise for secure health information transmission, but it does not store any data.

Benefits and Barriers to Health Information Exchange

In 2000, the Institute of Medicine (IOM), later renamed National Academy of Medicine, identified a conservative estimate of 98,000 people who die annually due to the lack of quality in healthcare, including incorrect medications; untimely or incomplete tests results; lack of timely access to health information that could influence healthcare decision making, and lack of continuity of care in all realms of medicine and healthcare (IOM 2000). In addition to the deaths, lack of quality in healthcare can also result in wrong-limb amputations, medication errors and poisonings, hospital-acquired infections, and faulty communication leading to delayed or incorrect treatment and follow-up. The IOM's data led to a call for action to reduce the number of quality-related deaths and improve health and safety of patients by implementing HIT and HIE. The authors of the IOM study hypothesized that better and more timely information and the use of technology for monitoring patient care and safety can contribute to the decrease in the number of medical mistakes.

Implementing and using current HIT and HIE has many benefits for healthcare entities, providers, patients, and society:

- Ability to improve quality of care by increasing the amount of patient-specific data available and decreasing the time it takes to make treatment decisions
- Reduction of healthcare costs by eliminating the repetition of diagnostic tests, unnecessary paperwork, and unnecessary diagnostic testing
- Use of clinical decision support software by healthcare providers to assist with more comprehensive and effective care
- Increased public health monitoring and reporting for immunizations, health screenings, communicable and infectious diseases such as influenza or Zika virus outbreaks, and other major health events
- Reporting and monitoring of population health trends such as a decrease in diabetic complications due to patient education and notification
- Increased use of mobile technology such as cell phones, tablets, laptops that can communicate anywhere and anytime; the new phrase is bring your own device (BYOD), which refers to healthcare practitioners using their personal smartphones or other devices rather than devices provided by the HCO. While acceptable, the personal device must meet specific encryption and other security protocols to protect PHI as required by the HCO.

- Increased and improved effectiveness and efficiency of healthcare treatments and business operations
- Improved connection between evidence-based health research and actual medical practice
- Provides basic level of interoperability among EHRs (Biedermann and Dolezel 2016, 112, 499; Giannangelo 2016, 337; ONC 2017b)

Because patients are the priority, their involvement, treatment, and successful outcomes must be evaluated to determine best practices to improve patient care. HIT and HIE benefits for the patients include:

- Patient safety—reduce unnecessary treatment and testing, decrease medication errors, more coordinated healthcare, longitudinal documentation of healthcare among all providers
- Automatic appointment and health reminders such as follow-up instructions, patient education information, and medication prescriptions sent directly to patient's pharmacy
- Saving patient's time throughout continuum of care by decreasing time spent on completing paperwork and briefing providers on health history allowing more time spent on interactive discussions regarding decisions about their health status and treatment with providers
- Equity of treatment and services with improved health outcomes leading to a reduction of health disparities
- Emergency and urgent care personnel can quickly determine the patient's medications, allergies, and other significant medical history to aid in diagnosing current episode of care
- More engaged patient education and patient involvement in the decisions that affect their health (Biedermann and Dolezel 2016, 506; Amatayakul 2016, 305; ONC 2017b)

Patient health affects more than just that individual, extending into his or her network of communities into society at large. Benefits to society include:

- Equity of treatment and services with improved health outcomes leading to a reduction of health disparities
- Decreased response time for disaster response—many population/public health issues have links to homeland security such as newly emerging diseases such as Ebola and bioterrorism attacks
- Public health surveillance of outbreaks or epidemics of large-scale food-borne illnesses, epidemics/pandemics of mutated influenza, and Zika virus spread
- Alerts can be sent to appropriate government and health officials to speed response and mitigation efforts. This is particularly helpful when outbreaks or epidemics cross state lines (Amatayakul 2017, 9; Biedermann and Dolezel 2016, 498)

However, along with the good comes the bad. Implementing computerization for a large portion of the healthcare industry creates many changes and problems. Barriers to implementing Health IT are numerous and include:

- Financial issues of supporting the HIOs and HIE and increased cost of hardware and software, trained professionals, and infrastructure
- Lack of complete operational and interoperability standards and vocabularies and inadequate computer interfaces across all vendors and organizations
- Healthcare information ownership between patients and providers
- Patient identification and matching capabilities and protocols along the entire continuum of care
- Competition and proprietary issues between HCOs
- Many rural hospitals lack financial stability and strength to provide new hardware, software, up-to-date IT personnel, and regional geographic infrastructure for reliable transmission of data (Biedermann and Dolezel 2016 268; ONC 2015a)

The ONC has developed an infographic (shown in figure 11.3) on how HIT can improve the state of healthcare in the United States.

Figure 11.3.   Infographic on HIT impact

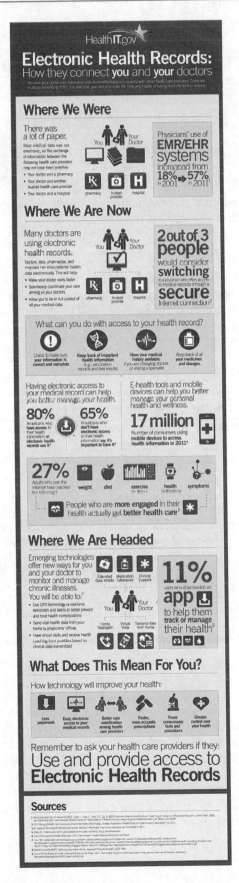

Source: ONC 2016.

CHECK YOUR UNDERSTANDING 11.2

1. The hospitals within a seven-county area in Montana have agreed to set up an information exchange for their area according to national standards to share electronic health data to meet the needs of their constituents. This describes which of the following?

   a. RHIO
   b. HCO
   c. HIO
   d. NHIN

2. Which of the following is a societal benefit of HIE?

   a. Ability to schedule appointments with healthcare provider
   b. Equality of treatments and decreasing health disparities
   c. Cost of implementation of HIT
   d. Reducing unnecessary tests and treatments

3. Recent research from Johns Hopkins University supports the original Institute of Medicine/National Academy of Medicine report identifying what leading cause of death could be decreased or prevented with the implementation of health information technology?

   a. Medical mistakes
   b. Physician shortage
   c. Nursing shortage
   d. Opioid overdoses

4. _____ is a nationwide project with federal and nonfederal agencies providing the data stewardship for 65% of hospitals in all 50 states initially starting as the NHIN.

   a. eHealth Exchange
   b. HIPAA
   c. BYOD
   d. NHIN

5. Healthcare providers using their personal smart phones and other devices and the increase in mobile technology can be summed up in which of the following abbreviations?

   a. eHealth Exchange
   b. HIPAA
   c. BYOD
   d. NHIN

Meaningful Use

Meaningful Use (MU) is a regulation that was issued by the Centers for Medicare and Medicaid (CMS) on July 28, 2010, outlining an incentive program for eligible professionals (EPs), eligible hospitals, and critical access hospitals (CAHs) participating in Medicare and Medicaid programs that adopt and successfully demonstrate meaningful use of certified EHR technology (CEHRT) (ONC 2013b). The EHR product in question must meet HIT and HIE criteria and standards for functionality and interoperability in order to be certified by the ONC or its designee. (See chapter 12 for more information on standards for the HIT and HIE.) HCOs using a CEHRT can then apply and qualify for the MU incentive program (Amatayakul 2017, 6).

ARRA and the HITECH Act specified three components for MU, all requiring the use of CEHRT:

- Must be used in a meaningful way such as e-prescribing (eRx) and computerized provider order entry (CPOE).

- The exchange of health information must be used to improve quality of health care.
- EHR must be used to submit clinical quality measures (CQMs) and other specified measures identified by the ONC and HHS (ONC 2013c).

Since 2004, when HIT became a major focus of healthcare delivery, most recent health legislation has addressed many of the negative issues that have been identified in the US healthcare system such as patient safety, healthcare outcomes, and health disparities. In order to tackle these negative issues, specific guidelines, standards, and levels of treatment and patient care must be followed. Using CQMs is one of the ways to evaluate the delivery of care and patient outcomes. CQMs are criteria and tools to measure or quantify healthcare processes, outcomes, patient perceptions, and organizational structure and systems that relate to one or more of the quality goals for healthcare: effective, safe, efficient, patient-centered, equitable, and timely. The CQMs were specifically designed to use HIT effectively to combat the negative issues (CMS 2015).

MU emphasizes population health reporting, the aggregate data on immunizations, communicable diseases, and other health events and CQMs that healthcare entities, providers, and public health agencies are required to report and is a standard function in EHRs. Population health, or public health, focuses on preventing, diagnosing, and treating an entire group of people rather than one person at a time. Figure 11.4 shows how the EHR and HIE used by acute care facilities is providing real-time reporting of diseases such as influenza to public health officials. Electronic reporting improves the timeliness and accuracy of health data to identify outbreaks and health trends (ONC 2017b). Using HIE, healthcare providers electronically submit reportable lab results, provide electronic syndromic surveillance data (health data which is used by community and public health officials to plan, respond, evaluate to a disease and its spread throughout the population), and submit electronic data to immunization registries to public health agencies.

Research on the state of health outcome disparities between genders, race, and socioeconomic status that exist within the United States has helped to identify priority populations where much of the work needs to be implemented to alleviate and eventually eliminate these inequities. Data collection of health outcomes and treatment patterns is used to identify specific disparities, and the subsequent epidemiological information is used to support evidence-based action plans for HIT and EHR adoption to improve healthcare delivery and help reduce health disparities. A health disparity occurs when there are unequal differences in health access, status, or outcome based upon factors such as gender, race, socioeconomic status, sexual identity/orientation, disability, and geography. After this phase, language barriers and health literacy can be addressed, and more effective and efficient communication can be employed to help educate specific populations about their health status. Refer to chapter 10 for additional information on health literacy. Healthcare coordination as well as planning and implementing identified services to best meet the needs of underserved populations can help to decrease the occurrence of health disparities. CMS has given priority to research and development of action plans that address health disparities in the following populations:

- Racial and ethnic minorities
- Immigrants (and those with limited English proficiencies)
- Individuals with low health literacy
- Socioeconomically disadvantaged
- Disabled and those with special needs
- Older adults
- Rural residents
- Children and adolescents
- Lesbian, gay, bisexual, and transgender (LGBT) people (CMS 2015)

Figure 11.4.   Public health syndromic surveillance

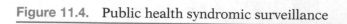

Models of Health Information Exchange Architecture

HIE architecture refers to the configuration, structure, and relationships of hardware (the machinery of the computers including input and output devices and storage devices) in an information system. There are three types of HIE architecture that are most commonly used in the United States.

Consolidated or Centralized Model

The consolidated (centralized) model of HIE was typical of the early years of HIEs. Many independent HCOs connected with the HIE and aggregate data was stored and shared within a central repository managed by the HIE (Amatayakul 2017, 417). This centralized data has a master patient index or a record locator service (RLS) (Biedermann and Dolezal 2016, 304). A RLS indicates where the patient's information is detected within the participating HCOs based on patient identity information and record data type. With robust access and security controls (see chapter 13 for more information), each HCO can access the appropriate information. However, because the US healthcare system is highly competitive and proprietary, HCOs were concerned about competitors having access to their data. Advantages to the consolidated model include consistency of the data availability and rapid response to requests. Duplication of data, data that is not completely up-to-date, and costs for supporting software are some of the disadvantages to this model (McCann 2016, 454).

Federated or Decentralized Model

The federated (decentralized) model of HIE occurs where there is no centralized database of patient information. The federated model is more common than the consolidated model because it works much like the Internet (McCann 2016, 454). Each HCO is responsible for maintaining its own patients' health records and is required to have the appropriate access and transmission safeguards operational. Each HCO is also responsible for vetting user access. Vetting is the process of critically appraising the abilities of an organization or person to determine if they meet the stated criteria. For example, an HCO establishes criteria for authorized access to the HCO's health information. The HCO uses the criteria to determine which external entities have authorized access the HCO's health information. The external entities are vetted for their authority and security mechanisms to access the health information.

The federated model has several key benefits, including the lack of data ownership. Because each HCO maintains its own data, the available data are always current, and this HIE has the capability to integrate with many EHR systems, providing redundancy, or the use of additional or back-up systems. This is particularly important in the case of disasters when an HCO could be damaged or completely shut down. Disadvantages include data availability problems due to technical issues of a specific HCO, and data may not always be available or complete because the patient may have data distributed across many of the HCOs involved (McCann 2016, 454).

Hybrid Model

The hybrid model combines the advantages of centralized and decentralized models. It has an RLS, and some data are stored in a central repository while the remainder stays with the other HCOs within the HIE. The hybrid model also has a patient portal to itself, and not to a specific HCO (McCann 2016, 455).

Methods of Health Information Exchange

There are three methods in which health information is exchanged between appropriate healthcare entities or providers: directed exchange, query-based exchange, and consumer-mediated exchange.

Directed Exchange

Directed exchange is frequently referred to as a "push exchange" because it pushes authorized and secure information from one HCO to another. For example, if a patient is being transferred from one hospital to another, the patient's health information would be "pushed" to the receiving hospital in order to provide the background health information to help the transition to continued care. As part of the stage 1 Meaningful MU requirements for EHRs, the Direct Project was initiated in 2010. The Direct Project is important for the secure messaging and transmission of laboratory results, summary care records, referrals, public health reporting, and conveying quality measures. Direct Project is a standards-based exchange platform to provide a secure, straightforward, scalable method to transmit encrypted information to collaborating providers. Direct messaging exchange acts like regular e-mail but with the added Health Insurance Portability and

Accountability Act (HIPAA) security mechanisms for protection of both senders and recipients with Direct addresses. Any messages sent from a Direct e-mail address are encrypted, and can only be opened when received by another Direct e-mail address. If a nurse at ABC Hospital used her employee e-mail address to send a patient's health information to an emergency department physician at XYZ Hospital, it would fail because it was not sent through a Direct address (ONC 2014c).

DirectTrust, which oversees the Direct Project, "is a federally recognized, non-profit policy and governance body that makes it possible for Direct exchange to operate smoothly and reliably, giving Direct users much needed confidence in their exchange partners' privacy and security practices" (DirectTrust 2017). It is a collaboration of 124 HIT companies and healthcare providers to further the interoperable HIE and is federally recognized by the ONC. DirectTrust currently has more than 94,000 HCOs, almost 1.5 million electronic addresses of DirectTrust participants, 300 EHR and personal health record (PHR) products, and 50 HIOs. For additional information on EHRs, refer to chapter 9. For additional information on PHRs, refer to chapter 10.

Query-Based Exchange

Query-based exchange is a find-and-seek request for information that is sent through the HIO to find any available health information on a specified individual. It is the opposite of the "push exchange," so it is thought of as a "pull exchange." This type of exchange is typically used in urgent and emergency care to seek information that would be relevant for the encounter at hand. In order to use a query-based exchange, an interface is required within the HIO. The HIO broadcasts the request for information through the eHealth Exchange. It uses the internal tools of its patient registry, identification matching, and other programs to locate the appropriate health information. This method requires higher security, audit logging, and additional protection protocols because of its wider scope of exchange (Amatayakul 2017, 425).

Consumer-Mediated Exchange

Consumer-mediated exchange is a type of HIE that is controlled by patients who want to control the use and access of their health information. According to the ONC, "consumer-mediated exchange provides patients with access to their health information, allowing them to manage their health care online in a similar fashion to how they might manage their finances through online banking. When in control of their own health information, patients can actively participate in their care coordination by:

- Providing other providers with their health information
- Identifying and correcting wrong or missing health information
- Identifying and correcting incorrect billing information
- Tracking and monitoring their own health" (ONC 2014a).

While some HIT professionals feel that consumer mediated exchanges would improve health information privacy and cooperation among HCOs, others feel that the complexity and volume of data would overwhelm consumers, who would not be able to effectively and efficiently manage and control their information (Pak 2017).

Patients may have the ability to incorporate their PHR because, as discussed in chapter 10, consumer engagement and getting patients more involved in their healthcare and well-being is a component of MU requirements. Although not administered by a federal entity, consumer-mediated exchange is encouraged through the Blue Button campaign and commercial EHR enterprises (Amatayakul 2017, 425).

CHECK YOUR UNDERSTANDING 11.3

1. What regulations require healthcare providers who participate in the incentive program to utilize computer-based patient health records effectively to improve patient outcomes?
   a. CEHRT
   b. MU
   c. HIPAA
   d. CQM

2. The requirement that vendors prove that their EHR products meet specific and optimal standards is termed _____.

   a. CEHRT
   b. MU
   c. HIPAA
   d. CQM

3. What is the name of the criteria that healthcare providers must meet to show that they are efficiently using the EHR to show a positive impact on patient care?

   a. CEHRT
   b. MU
   c. HIPAA
   d. CQM

4. MU is not just to improve the health of one patient but to have an impact on a large portion of patients in a particular geographic area or diagnosis classification. The way this is monitored is called _____.

   a. Population health reporting
   b. Vetting
   c. Record locator service
   d. Query-based exchange

5. What is the "find and seek" method of HIE performed through an HIO?

   a. Population health reporting
   b. Votting
   c. Record locator service
   d. Query-based exchange

Patient Identification

Making sure that the correct patient is identified within the HIE is one of the major issues. In large or densely populated geographic areas, there could be hundreds of individuals with common names, such as John Smith. Many methods have been used to address this issue, from smart cards with magnetic strips or chips with identifying information, to advanced computer algorithms, to biometrics using fingerprints, facial recognition, or retinal scans. No one method has been found to be completely correct in its matching capabilities. To make matters worse, all this additional technology is expensive, meaning that many HCOs cannot afford to implement these methods (Brinda and Watters 2016, 330).

Identity matching (also known as patient matching) is the process in which the HIO identifies the right person within the database to exchange information between HCOs. The process examines "different demographic elements from different health information technology (health IT) systems to determine if they refer to the same patient. From an interoperability perspective, the ability to complete patient matching efficiently, accurately, and at scale has long been identified as a key element of the nation's health IT infrastructure. Patient matching is almost universally needed to enable the interoperability of health data for all kinds of purposes. Patient matching also requires careful consideration with respect to its effect on patient safety and administrative costs" (ONC 2017c).

Owing to privacy concerns, Congress has banned the Department of Health and Human Services from trying to develop and implement a national unique patient identifier (Dimick 2016). However, because of the progression of EHR systems and the issues with patient identification and matching, Congress is now considering allowing HHS to lend technical assistance and to evaluate the current state of patient identification management (Monica 2017). In the meantime, HIOs must establish other methods for identity matching. The sophistication of the algorithms depends upon the type and amount of data needed to solve the query:

> Basic algorithms that compare selected data elements, such as name, date of birth, and gender, are the simplest technique for matching records. Intermediate algorithms use more advanced techniques

to compare and match records by assigning subjective weights to demographic elements for use in a scoring system to determine the probability of matching patient records. Advanced algorithms contain the most sophisticated set of tools for matching records and rely on mathematical theory and statistical models to determine the likelihood of a match (Lusk et al. 2018)

Identity management is different from identity matching. **Identity management** ensures "that [the] individual who has been identified is who they say they are, that they have the authority to do what they want to do, and that their actions are tracked" (Amatayakul 2017, 419). Traditionally, identity management was performed as a part of patient registration or in health information management when the paper health record or master patient index were reconciled (AHIMA Work Group 2014). Individual HCOs develop processes for identity management that are best suited to their needs. For example, at the time of registration, most HCO's require the patient to provide a driver's license or state-issued identity card, his insurance card, and employment identification card as proof of employment (if applicable). These methods enforce identity management procedures within the HCO and compel the patient prove that he is who he says he is.

Because of the HIPAA, patients have the right to refuse to participate in the HIE and to limit who can view their information. A component of identity management within HIE is **consent management**. Consent management has nothing to do with the consent for treatment but rather the patient consents or approves the HIO to transmit health information between two or more authorized entities. According to the ONC, electronic consent management is

> a system, process, or set of policies that enables patients to choose what health information they are willing to permit their healthcare providers to access and share. Consent management allows patients to affirm their participation in electronic health initiatives such as patient portals, personal health records (PHR), and health information exchange (HIE). (ONC 2014d)

Figure 11.5 shows key components for the implementation on an electronic consent management process.

Figure 11.5.   Implementing meaningful consent

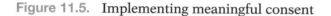

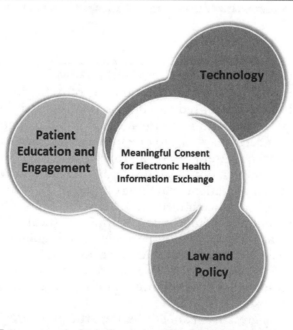

1. **Patient Education and Engagement**—including educating patients about their consent options, who may release their information and how, and the significance of the consent choice.
2. **Technology**—using technology to capture and maintain patient consent decisions, identify which sensitive portions of patient information are restricted from access, and communicate these restrictions electronically with others.
3. **Law and Policy**—ensuring alignment with federal and state law and other legal and policy requirements pertaining to consent, individual choice, and confidentiality.

Source: ONC 2014d.

The process of obtaining approval or consent to transmit health information has two components. The first is to obtain consent from an authorized HCO or provider to electronically request or transmit any patient's health information to or from other authorized healthcare entities. This part of the consent process is performed when healthcare providers enlist to be authorized users of an HIO. The second component involves the patient consenting to have the health information accessed and released. This is typically done the first time a patient is registered to receive healthcare services at the particular HCO and then confirmed during any subsequent encounters or admissions. This may be a complete consent allowing all information can be accessed by authorized users. There can also be constraints on the type of accessed data and by whom it may be released or accessed (Amatayakul 2017, 419).

Opt-in or opt-out consent sets the default for health information of patients to be included in the HIO automatically (opt-in), but the patient can choose not to be included (opt-out) completely. Opt-in consent means that the patient must specifically agree to have the personal health information accessible for the HIE (Biedermann and Dolezel 2016, 306). A variation of this consent is the opt-in with restrictions, in which the default is "no patient health information," which is automatically made available and the patient must define what information is to be sent, who it is sent to, and for what purpose the information may be used. "Each HIE must determine how patients and consumers will consent or not consent to have their data and information transmitted by or included in HIE operations" (Biedermann and Dolezel 2016, 306).

The opt-out consent means that the patient data can automatically be exchanged within the HIO by default (Amatayakul 2017, 419). A variation on this consent is the *opt-out with exceptions* model that sets the default for health information for patients to be included, but the patient can opt-out completely or allow only select data to be included (Biedermann and Dolezel 2016, 306).

The AHIMA Work Group has recommended specific data elements that help the HCOs and providers with patient identification issues. Some of the primary data elements include legal name (first, middle, last, maiden), date of birth (DOB), gender, race, mother's maiden name, and primary phone number. Examples of the secondary data elements are birth place, marital status, social security number, driver's license number, e-mail address, and some type of biometric. A biometric is a physical characteristic of the patient or users (such as fingerprints, voiceprints, retinal scans, iris traits) that systems store and use to authenticate identity of the patient or before allowing the user access to a system (AHIMA Work Group 2014). Patient identification integrity has always been a crucial principle of HIM. It is even more crucial now with HIE. Integrity refers to the ability of data to maintain its structure and attributes, including protection against modification or corruption during transmission, storage, or at rest. Maintenance of patient identification and data integrity are key aspects of data quality management and security.

Health Information Exchange Privacy Concerns

All health information is private, but mental health diagnoses, drug and alcohol treatment, and sexually transmitted disease identification are considered to be particularly sensitive. The HCO must determine what additional privacy and security protections are in place because some HIEs may not be able to adequately protect that sensitive information (Brinda and Watters 2016, 331).

Other best practices addressing privacy issues with the HIE include:

- Workforce education programs are robust and timely, including the right of the patient to request restrictions: All employees involved in any patient data or information transaction, access to ePHI, PHI, or HIE operations must receive regular and documented training regarding HIPAA and HCO rules, regulations, policies, and procedures.

- Up-to-date breach notifications policies and procedures for all HIPAA-covered entities: As recent news of data breaches and identity-theft events have shown, the public's trust has decreased regarding the ability of an organization to safeguard their information.

- All mobile devices have effective and strong encryption protection.

- Application of breach sanctions are as written in policy and procedures: Depending on the level of breach, sanctions must have commensurate severity of consequences and be established prior to the event following HIPAA guidelines.

- Business associate agreements are analyzed, evaluated, and updated on a regular basis: The rules are continually expanded and updated and the HCO must make certain it follows suit.

- Current risk analysis is implemented and revised on a regular basis: Follow-up with business associates, covered entities and any others must be verified by the HCO to be in compliance.

- Request for restrictions on release of information by patients is implemented and on the Notice of Privacy Practices: The enhanced privacy rule requires the HCO to have a method to note that the information has been restricted. (Downing 2014)

CHECK YOUR UNDERSTANDING 11.4

1. The process whereby the HIO has identified the correct person within a healthcare provider's database in order to send it to the requesting provider is termed _____.

    a. Identity matching
    b. Consolidated HIE
    c. Consent management
    d. Federated HIE

2. The protocols for approving that the HIO can exchange health information between two or more authorized healthcare providers is called _____.

    a. Identity matching
    b. CDA
    c. Consent management
    d. ePHI

3. What is the name of the method of patient identification that uses a physical characteristic of the patient, such as a fingerprint?

    a. CQM
    b. Biometric
    c. PHR
    d. RLS

4. If a patient does not want her ePHI exchanged with other HCOs, that is acceptable and allowable under HIPAA. What is this process called?

    a. Opt-in consent
    b. Opt-out consent
    c. Privacy
    d. Confidentiality

5. _____ refers to a patient giving consent for her personal information to accessible in the HIE.

    a. Opt-in consent
    b. Opt-out consent
    c. Privacy
    d. Confidentiality

Real-World Case

Florida's Agency for Health Care Administration (AHCA) oversees the health information exchange activities within the state. On a quarterly basis, it publishes a dashboard of metrics regarding HIE activities. It has been promoting the adoption of e-prescribing since 2007. Part of the dashboard includes e-prescribing adoption and use trending data. It also shows a comparison to the national adoption and trending status. Florida has seen a steady increase in the rate of e-prescriptions since 2007. In 2017, the rate reached almost 75 percent relative to all prescriptions that could have been e-prescribed.

Based on some modifications and clarification to existing federal and state regulations, Florida providers can e-prescribe controlled substances (EPCS) through EHR systems that are certified for that purpose, meaning they must not only have a certified EHR system, it must also be certified to EPCS. Pharmacies must also have certified systems to receive EPCS orders. AHCA has been collecting data on e-prescriptions of controlled substances since 2015. Since this is relatively new process, rates are low but expected to increase. As of 2017, 7.4 percent of active e-prescribers have been enabled to EPCS. The rate that pharmacies are enabled to receive EPCS is almost 87 percent.

REVIEW QUESTIONS

1. HIOs are managed by _____.

   a. ONC
   b. State agencies
   c. Private EHR vendors
   d. Public-private partnerships

2. Which of the following was a precursor to today's HIO?

   a. HIM
   b. RHIO
   c. HIE
   d. ePHI

3. What is the fourth stage in the following sequence of events: data, information, knowledge, and _____.

   a. Behavior change
   b. Wisdom
   c. Attitude
   d. Intelligence

4. Which of the following types of interoperability refers to how the data should be formatted and structured so that seamless exchange can take place?

   a. Technical
   b. Syntactic
   c. Semantic
   d. Process

5. What federal agency is responsible for the coordination and implementation of EHR technology for the exchange of ePHI?

   a. ONC
   b. NHIN
   c. Congress
   d. Department of Defense

6. What is the goal of the implementation of EHRs in healthcare?

   a. Improve patient safety issues
   b. Improve patient health outcomes
   c. Decrease health disparities
   d. Increase profitability of HCOs

7. What is the term used to describe the interconnected organizations that have the capability of sending and receiving confidential patient information anywhere in the country?

   a. eHealth Exchange
   b. LHIO
   c. ePHI
   d. EHR

(Continued)

REVIEW QUESTIONS (*Continued*)

8. Population health is also known as _____.

   a. Epidemiology
   b. Biostatistics
   c. Public health
   d. ePHI

9. Which HIE model does not have a centralized database of patient information, is more common, and works much like the Internet?

   a. Consolidated
   b. Federated
   c. Hybrid
   d. Direct exchange

10. What is the process that ensures that the person is who he says he is, has the authority to do what he needs to, and that his actions are tracked?

    a. Identity matching
    b. Identity management
    c. Consent management
    d. CDA

References

AHIMA Work Group. 2014. Managing the integrity of patient identity in health information exchange (2014 update). *Journal of AHIMA* 85(5): expanded web version. http://bok.ahima.org/doc?oid=300436# .WojcLainFRY.

Amatayakul, M. K. 2017. *Health IT and EHRs: Principles and Practice*, 6th ed. Chicago: AHIMA.

Amatayakul, M. K. 2016. Health Information Technologies. Chapter 11 in *Health Information Management Technology: An Applied Approach*, 5th ed. Edited by N. B. Sayles and L. L. Gordon. Chicago: AHIMA.

Biedermann, S. and D. Dolezel. 2016. *Introduction to Healthcare Informatics*, 2nd ed. Chicago: AHIMA.

Brinda, D. and A. Watters. 2016. Data Privacy, Confidentiality, and Security. Chapter 11 in *Health Information Management: Concepts, Principles, and Practice*, 5th ed. Edited by P. Oachs and A. Watters. Chicago: AHIMA.

Centers for Medicare and Medicaid (CMS). 2017. Value-based programs. https://www.cms.gov/Medicare /Quality-Initiatives-Patient-Assessment-Instruments/Value-Based-Programs/Value-Based-Programs .html.

Centers for Medicare and Medicaid (CMS). 2015. Clinical Quality Measures. https://www.cms.gov /Regulations-and-Guidance/Legislation/EHRIncentivePrograms/ClinicalQualityMeasures.html.

Cha, E. A. 2016. "Researchers: Medical Errors Now Third Leading Cause of Death in United States." *Washington Post*, May 3, 2016. https://www.washingtonpost.com/news/to-your-health/wp/2016/05/03/researchers -medical-errors-now-third-leading-cause-of-death-in-united-states/?utm_term=.64637f3a8bed.

Dimick, C. 2016. Petition calls for unique patient identifier solution. *Journal of AHIMA* 87(3) http: //journal.ahima.org/2016/03/21/petition-calls-for-unique-patient-identifier-solution/.

DirectTrust. 2017. What is DirectTrust?: DirectTrust overview. https://www.directtrust.org/about -directtrust/.

Downing, K. 2014. "Seven select questions to ask your privacy officer (or yourself)" *Journal of AHIMA* 85(4):42–44.

Giannangelo, K. 2016. Healthcare Information. Chapter 12 in *Health Information Management Technology: An Applied Approach*, 5th ed. Edited by N. B. Sayles and L. L. Gordon. Chicago: AHIMA.

HIMSS. 2018. Privacy & Security for RHIOs/HIEs. http://www.himss.org/privacy-security-rhioshies-0.

HL7. 2017. HL7/ASTM Implementation Guide for CDA® R2 Continuity of Care Document (CCD®) Release 1. https://www.hl7.org/implement/standards/product_brief.cfm?product_id=6.

Institute of Medicine (IOM). 2000. *To Err Is Human: Building a Safer Health System*. https://www.ncbi.nlm.nih.gov/books/NBK225179/.

Kellogg, D. W. 2016. Healthcare Delivery Systems. Chapter 2 in *Health Information Management Technology: An Applied Approach*, 5th ed. Edited by N. B. Sayles and L. L. Gordon. Chicago: AHIMA.

Lusk, K. N. Noreen, G. Okafor, K. Peterson, and E. Pupo. 2018 (Winter). Patient matching in health information exchanges. *Perspectives in Health Information Management*. http://perspectives.ahima.org/patient-matching-in-health-information-exchanges/.

McCann, P. 2016. Health Information Exchange. Chapter 15 in *Health Information Management: Concepts, Principles, and Practice* 5th ed. Edited by P. Oachs and A. Watters. Chicago: AHIMA.

Monica, K. 2017. National Patient Identifier Gains Congressional Support. https://ehrintelligence.com/news/national-patient-identifier-gains-congressional-support.

Office of the National Coordinator for Health Information Technology (ONC). 2017a. About ONC. https://www.healthit.gov/newsroom/about-onc.

Office of the National Coordinator for Health Information Technology (ONC). 2017b. Population/Public Health. https://www.healthit.gov/playbook/population-public-health/.

Office of the National Coordinator for Health Information Technology (ONC). 2017c. Demystifying Patient Matching Algorithms. https://www.healthit.gov/buzz-blog/interoperability/demystifying-patient-matching-algorithms/.

Office of the National Coordinator for Health Information Technology (ONC). 2016. Electronic Health Records Infographic.2016. https://www.healthit.gov/patients-families/electronic-health-records-infographic.

Office of the National Coordinator for Health Information Technology (ONC). 2015a. Key Barriers to Health IT Adoption. https://dashboard.healthit.gov/report-to-congress/2015-update-adoption-health-information-technology-full-text.php#key-barriers.

Office of the National Coordinator for Health Information Technology (ONC). 2015b. Public Health Surveillance. https://www.healthit.gov/sites/default/files/onc_public_health_surveillance_infographic-11042014.pdf.

Office of the National Coordinator for Health Information Technology (ONC). 2014a. Health Information Exchange (HIE). https://www.healthit.gov/providers-professionals/health-information-exchange/what-hie.

Office of the National Coordinator for Health Information Technology (ONC). 2014b. Connecting Health and Care for the Nation. A Shared Nationwide Interoperability Roadmap. https://www.healthit.gov/sites/default/files/hie-interoperability/nationwide-interoperability-roadmap-final-version-1.0.pdf.

Office of the National Coordinator for Health Information Technology (ONC). 2014c. Direct Basics: Q&A for Providers. https://www.healthit.gov/sites/default/files/directbasicsforprovidersqa_05092014.pdf.

Office of the National Coordinator for Health Information Technology (ONC). 2014d. Patient Consent for eHIE. https://www.healthit.gov/providers-professionals/meaningful-consent-overview.

Office of the National Coordinator for Health Information Technology (ONC). 2014e. Standards and Interoperability. https://www.healthit.gov/providers-professionals/standards-interoperability.

Office of the National Coordinator for Health Information Technology (ONC). 2013a. Why Is Health Information Exchange Important? https://www.healthit.gov/providers-professionals/faqs/why-health-information-exchange-important.

Office of the National Coordinator for Health Information Technology (ONC). 2013b. How to Attain Meaningful. https://www.healthit.gov/providers-professionals/how-attain-meaningful-use.

Office of the National Coordinator for Health Information Technology (ONC). 2013c. What Are Clinical Quality Measures? https://www.healthit.gov/providers-professionals/faqs/what-are-clinical-quality-measures.

Pak, H. 2017. Consumer Mediated Exchange. https://www.ehidc.org/sites/default/files/resources/files/Consumer%20Mediated%20Exchange-Pak.pdf.

Sequoia Project. 2017. About eHealth Exchange. http://sequoiaproject.org/ehealth-exchange/about/.

Chapter 12

Standards

Learning Objectives

- Explain the necessity for standards in health information technology (HIT).
- Explain how Health Level Seven International (HL7) influences healthcare data standards.
- Clarify the difference between the continuity of care record and the continuity of care document.
- Compare and contrast data content standards, vocabulary standards, and messaging standards.
- Describe how Systematized Nomenclature of Medicine Clinical Terms (SNOMED CT) works to achieve uniform terminology.
- Identify the need for mapping.
- Differentiate among national drug codes (NDC), RxNorm, and National Council for Prescription Drug Programs (NCPDP).

Key Terms

American National Standards Institute (ANSI)
ANSI Accredited Standards Committee X12N (ASC X12N)
Clinical document architecture (CDA)
Continuity of Care Document (CCD)
Continuity of Care Record (CCR)
Current Dental Terminology (CDT)
Data content standards
Diagnostic and Statistical Manual of Mental Disorders (DSM)

Digital Imaging and Communications in Medicine (DICOM)
Electronic data interchange (EDI)
General Equivalence Mappings (GEMs)
International Organization for Standardization (ISO)
Logical Observation Identifiers Names and Codes (LOINC)
Mapping
MEDCIN
Messaging standards
National Council for Prescription Drug Programs (NCPDP)

National drug codes (NDC)
Reference Information Model (RIM)
RxNorm
Semantics
Standard
Standards development organizations (SDOs)
Syntax
Systematized Nomenclature of Medicine Clinical Terms (SNOMED CT)
Unified Medical Language System (UMLS)
Vocabulary standards

A **standard** is a scientifically based statement of expected behavior against which structures, processes, and outcomes can be measured. Organizations of all kinds develop standards so that there is an uniformity in the products, tools, and technology that we use to perform almost all daily tasks, enhance performance of materials and products, and ensure consistency and quality of products. Standards are important to the electronic health record (EHR) because they streamline the communication method that allows information systems to speak to each other and for data to be stored using the same formats, language, and terms to describe and execute functions. Because technology changes so quickly, standards should be technology-neutral, meaning that they do not rely on any one type of technology in order to work. Standards must also be neutral to implementation processes, which vary widely, and not prefer one vendor over others (ONC 2017a).

Standards can be made by a number of entities. Government bodies can create them and require their use. Technology companies can incorporate their own standards into the software and hardware products they sell. These are referred to as de facto standards because of the influence of the technology company in the market (ONC 2017b). Groups of HIT vendors can also create standards. For example, Digital Imaging and Communication in Medicine (DICOM) is a set of imaging standards developed by imaging manufacturers.

The Office of the National Coordinator for Health Information Technology (ONC) is responsible for coordinating and guiding the development and establishment of standards for HIT. The HITECH Act allocated billions of dollars for the development of standards (ONC 2017b). The ONC works with standards development organizations to verify and corroborate standards that will benefit the EHR and electronic environment of healthcare at large. This chapter discusses the role of standards development organizations and categories of standards necessitated by the EHR, including data content, vocabulary, and messaging standards.

Standards Development Organizations

Standards development organizations (SDOs) are private or government organizations that create or approve standards at the national or international level. There are many SDOs for HIT and health information exchanges (HIEs). Some are specific to the United States, some are international, and some are both. Usually, an SDO develops standards for particular HIT software or hardware functions. For example, standards for interoperability allow health information from Mercy Hospital, who uses Vendor A's EHR, to pass through an authorized health information organization (HIO) and be read, used, and incorporated into Vendor B's EHR at Valley Medical Center.

Although each standard has value, some do not have an established best method or practice. Because of the many stakeholders involved in HIT, some standards overlap and can be interpreted differently by each stakeholder because they view the standard in a different context. For example, both HL7's clinical document architecture (CDA) and the American Society for Testing and Materials (ASTM) International's continuity of care record (CCR) address the need for electronic transmission of pertinent and timely health information. However, CDA has a required core data set and mandatory text and coded components while CCR has a flexible format "designed to permit easy creation by a physician using an electronic health record (EHR) system at the end of an encounter" (Conover n.d.). These two sets of standards conflicted until HL7 and ASTM worked together to create the continuity of care document (CCD) standard that addresses the competing and overlapping portions of their standards (Conover n.d.).

Unfortunately, although standards are meant to allow a smooth exchange to meld and incorporate data from all sites, vendors, and specialties across the healthcare continuum, conflicting standards sometimes leave HCOs struggling with interoperability issues. Interoperability, discussed in chapter 11, is required in order to share and reuse data based on the demands of the new models of healthcare, population health surveillance, and consumer/patient engagement (ONC 2017b). If there is an interoperability issue between EHRs, patient information might not be transmitted or could lose some of its integrity. As a result, one or both of the HCOs might need to send additional information possibly resorting to phone calls and faxes to resolve the transmission problem. To resolve the interoperability issue in this scenario, the affected HCOs would provide input on the impact of the EHR incompatibility. The HIT organization and HIE stakeholders for each EHR would be responsible for updating or modifying their EHR standards since their products are causing the interoperability issue. Together, these three groups could come to a secure and successful resolution.

Over time, SDOs have increasingly emphasized the consensus method, in which stakeholders determine the course of action based on the best interest of all for the current timeframe. Health Level Seven International (HL7) is an example of a consensus collaboration (ONC 2017b).

The **International Organization for Standardization (ISO)** is a large widely-recognized international SDO that has established many standards for EHR architecture and content (ONC 2017a). There are more than 22,000 standards for technology and manufacturing, and it takes approximately three years for the ISO to review and approve a standard. Some general areas of standards for HIT include the following:

- Vocabulary/terminology—a specific set of values for a specific data type; SNOMED CT and ICD-10 are examples.
- Transport messaging—how information is sent and exchanged between systems; TCP/IP and DIRECT are examples.
- Security—provides assurances that messages are protected; ASTM Committee E31 on Healthcare Informatics has E31.25 Healthcare Data Management, Security, Confidentiality, and Privacy standards is an example (ASTM 2018a).
- Content—identifies what data elements are included, where they are located, data type, field length, and so on; HL7, CDA, and ASC X12 are examples.
- Technical—usually a formal document that established uniform engineering or technical criteria, methods, processes, and practices (ISO 2018).

Many of the aforementioned examples will be discussed in further detail in this chapter.

The American National Standards Institute (ANSI) is the SDO for the United States and is a representative to the ISO. It is helpful to think of the ISO like the United Nations and its ambassadors from recognized countries (ANSI for the US, Standards Australia for Australia, and the Japanese Standards Association for Japan, for example) (Biedermann and Dolezel 2017, 151).

American National Standards Institute

ANSI does not develop standards but provides a neutral environment for organizations and entities to work together to settle on a common agreement for standards the format, content, requirements, and more. The types of standards that have been developed include clinical data exchange, standard vocabulary, and document architecture that facilitates sending, receiving and incorporating healthcare data into the EHR (ONC 2017c).

Before a standard can be approved, it must meet the rules of ANSI and the following requirements:

- Made from consensus—how agreements are determined
- Due process—procedures and specific committees that perform the critique, review the proposed standard, and eventually approve the proposed standard
- Openness—transparency of all procedures to all parties
- Balance—a platform for standards development that withstands scrutiny while protecting the rights and interests of all members (ANSI n.d.)

Through ANSI, diverse stakeholders, such as government agencies, private HIT companies, health insurance companies, and professional and trade organizations, work together to develop standards. The stakeholders must be willing to compromise to develop consensus-based standards. Due process comes from the fact that standards development must occur in an open manner that is responsive to the needs of the stakeholders, and the development should be equitable, thus balancing the needs of all of the stakeholders during the development process. The openness of standards development allows stakeholder representatives to participate in the development process (ANSI n.d.). The ISO has developed a six-step process for organizations that request approval for the specified standards:

1. Proposal: Stakeholders agree there is a need for a particular standard.
2. Preparatory: Draft of proposed standard is submitted.
3. Committee: Draft is analyzed and revised by committee until consensus is reached.
4. Enquiry: Proposed standard is available for review and comment by all stakeholders.
5. Approval: Final draft is voted upon for approval.
6. Publication: Standard is published (Biedermann and Dolezel 2017, 152).

ASTM International

ASTM is an international SDO, well known in other areas of industry, but its healthcare aspect is only in the United States (ONC 2017b). The US division, Committee E31, addresses standards for healthcare data management, privacy, confidentiality and security, as well as data analyses and information capture and documentation (Amatayakul 2017, 407). According to ASTM, its Committee E31 on Healthcare Informatics develops standards to help practitioners preserve and transfer accurate patient information using EHR technologies. Examples of the ASTM standards include the E2639 Continuity Care Record (more on that below) and the E1384 EHR content and structure, which allows clinical laboratory data to be integrated with other patient information in an EHR by providing a comprehensive structure for the data collected (ASTM 2015). HCOs and providers use products that have been built according to whichever set of standards the product falls under. Standards are typically voluntary, but in many cases government agencies cite them as requirements, codes, or laws (ASTM 2018b). HCOs can ensure the quality of an EHR and that it meets ASTM (and other pertinent SDO) standards by purchasing a EHR system that has been certified by the ONC (Certified EHR Technology [CEHRT]). In order to receive incentive payments from the Meaningful Use program, the HCOs must use a CEHRT (CMS 2015).

Data Content Standards

Data content standards are clear guidelines for the acceptable values for specified data fields. These standards make it possible to exchange health information using electronic networks, and they identify the structure and content of data elements to be collected by the EHR. Data content standards allow organizations to collect data once and use it many times in many ways. They also assist in data storage and mining as well as sharing data with external organizations for use in benchmarking and other purposes. The use of data content standards also assists in the HIE process (AHIMA Work Group 2013).

Health Level Seven International (HL7) was founded in 1987 as a not-for-profit ANSI-accredited SDO dedicated to providing a comprehensive framework and related standards for the exchange, integration, sharing, and retrieval of electronic health information that supports clinical practice and the management, delivery, and evaluation of health services. Its mission is to provide standards that empower global health data interoperability (HL7 2017). The National Committee on Health and Vital Statistics (NCVHS) has recommended that HL7's messaging and clinical encounters terminology be used in all healthcare information systems (ONC 2017c).

HL7 has developed standards for the electronic exchange of clinical documents, such as discharge summaries and progress notes, referred to as the clinical document architecture (CDA). CDA uses HL7 XML-based document markup standards for the electronic exchange model for the creation of clinical documents such as discharge summaries and progress notes. XML is a standardized computer language that allows the interchange of data as structured text. Implementation guides are included with each standard and define how to use the specific standard for specific purposes (ONC 2017e). The implementation guide removes optionality; it states what data elements are required and when, so that there is no room for interpretation (ONC 2017d). The implementation guide contains a library of CDA templates, incorporating and harmonizing previous efforts from HL7; the Integrating the Healthcare Enterprise (IHE); and the Health Information Technology Standards Panel (HITSP). It includes all required CDA templates for Stage I Meaningful Use, and HITECH final rule. It is commonly referred to as consolidated CDA or C-CDA. These documents are designed to be read by an individual on any standard web browser without special software.

ASTM International created the Continuity of Care Record (CCR), which identifies a core data set of patient information that must be passed on to the next healthcare provider in order to efficiently and effectively continue the patient's healthcare (Palkie 2016, 162). The CCR was designed for all patient referrals and transfers. At the end of the admission or care encounter, the originating healthcare provider generates an electronic summary document with a core data set of the most pertinent health information of the patient's care and status for the receiving healthcare provider to continue the care for the patient. The core data set for the CCR contains the following:

- Document identifying information
- Patient identifying information
- Insurance and financial information of the patient
- Patient's health status
- Care documentation and plan recommendations
- Advanced directives
- List of healthcare providers involved in the care of the patient

The CCR is designed to be technology- and vendor-neutral and uses XML programming. It was designed to achieve more efficiency in communication between providers by assuring a standardized amount of information, enhancing the patient's safety while improving the continuity of care and reducing medication errors and reducing costs.

The Continuity of Care Document (CCD) is "an implementation guide for sharing Continuity of Care Record (CCR) patient summary data" (HL7 2017). It is the result of the joint effort between ASTM International and HL7 and "fosters interoperability of clinical data by allowing physicians to send electronic medical information to other providers without loss of meaning and enabling improvement of patient care … using the HL7 Version 3 Clinical Document Architecture (CDA), Release 2" (HL7 2017).

Vocabulary Standards

Vocabulary standards, a list or collection of clinical words or phrases with their meanings, address the problem of multiple ways to define, classify, and represent language. "Language generally refers to a system of communication using an arbitrary set of vocal sounds, written symbols, signs, or gestures in conventional ways with conventional meanings" (Amatayakul 2017, 289). Medicine has its own language. There are many terms used in medicine that can have multiple synonyms. For example, the terms "medical" and "therapeutic," "curative" and "drug," and "medication" and "pharmaceutical" can be used relatively interchangeably. The use of synonyms can make it difficult to identify patients with a specific disease or condition. Several terms fall into the concept of vocabulary standards, including language, vocabulary, terminology, and nomenclature:

- Language is a system of communication used by a group of people.
- Vocabulary is all the terms that can be used for communication within the area of specialization.
- Terminology means the words used for a specific purpose.
- Nomenclature is a system used to assign names. (Amatayakul 2017, 289–290)

Vocabularies require terms to be evaluated for inclusion. Each term included in the vocabulary should have a unique meaning; however, it should be noted that synonyms are linked within the vocabulary, such as the examples listed above. Terminologies, in general, are a set of terms representing the system of concepts of a particular subject field. A clinical terminology provides the proper context and usage of clinical words as names or symbols. Terminologies, along with classification systems, are necessary to support the EHR, personal health record (PHR), and population health reporting as well as quality reporting (Palkie 2016, 144). Vocabularies and terminologies can have overlapping terms due to synonyms and eponyms. This is one of the challenging aspects of medicine and the application of EHR and diagnostic software to interpret unstructured (and sometimes structured) text from a physician or other healthcare provider.

Systematized Nomenclature of Medicine

As stated previously, nomenclature refers to systems that use established rules that assign the names used in a particular field. The use of a nomenclature allows for comparison and aggregation of data (Amatayakul 2017, 294). The most widely recognized nomenclature in healthcare is the Systematized Nomenclature of Medicine (SNOMED). It was developed in 1975 by the College of American Pathologists, but maintenance was transitioned to the International Health Terminology Standards Development Organization in 2007. The current version, Systematized Nomenclature of Medicine Clinical Terms (SNOMED CT), is the most comprehensive, multilingual clinical healthcare terminology in the world. SNOMED CT contributes to the improvement of patient care by underpinning the development of EHRs that record clinical information in ways that enable meaning-based retrieval.

SNOMED CT is used for the EHR, research, and clinical decisions. The information that SNOMED CT captures includes items such as diagnoses, procedures, signs, symptoms, and cause of injury. SNOMED CT has a concepts table that consists of more than 344,000 concepts, 450,000 medical descriptions, and 700,000 concept interrelations, each of which has a unique meaning and format definition such as 98 degrees versus 98°. It also contains description tables with more than a million language descriptions or synonyms (this allows for flexibility in expressing clinical concepts). A relationships table contains over 1.3 million semantic relationships (ONC 2017f). These relationships are important to data retrieval (Amatayakul 2017, 294). See figure 12.1 for a short example of how clinical information is coded in SNOMED CT.

Figure 12.1. SNOMED CT working behind the scenes in an EHR

In the following excerpt from an EHR, a few of the applicable SNOMED CT codes are noted in parentheses to illustrate what SNOMED CT is doing behind the scenes. It is automatically identifying standard terms and tagging them for future references.

Office visit for a 64-year-old established female patient being seen for review and follow-up of non–insulin-dependent diabetes, obesity, hypertension, and chronic right-sided congestive heart failure. Complains of shortness of breath and admits to dietary noncompliance. Patient's heart failure is assessed (blood pressure measures, level of activity assessed, clinical signs and symptoms of volume overload assessed, respiratory status assessed, and weight recorded). She is counseled concerning diet and current medications adjusted.

- -81531005 | Type II diabetes mellitus in obese (disorder)|
- -59621000 | Essential hypertension (disorder)|
- - 66989003 | Chronic right-sided congestive heart failure (disorder)|
- -26700087 | Dyspnea(finding)
- -129832003 | Noncompliance with dietary regimen (finding)|
- -46973005 | Blood pressure taking (procedure)|
- -398636004 | Physical activity assessment (procedure)|
- -422834003| Respiratory assessment (procedure)|
- -424753004| Dietary management education, guidance, and counseling (procedures)|
- -182838006| Change of medication (procedure)|

Source: Giannangelo 2015.

Logical Observation Identifiers Names and Codes

Logical Observation Identifiers Names and Codes (LOINC) is the preferred standardized terminology for laboratory data in information systems and provides a standard set of codes and names for the electronic reporting of laboratory results (ONC 2017c). It was created in 1994 to assist in the electronic transmission of laboratory data between laboratories, care providers, and third-party payers and is controlled by the Regenstrief Institute for Health Care, an international research organization. LOINC has expanded to include observational data such as vital signs and is also used for standardized assessments and care plans in long-term care and home health. LOINC was not intended to share all data collected about a laboratory test but instead to identify test results. The standardization allows the results from multiple laboratories to be easily understood (Amatayakul 2017, 295).

RxNorm

RxNorm is a clinical drug nomenclature developed by the Food and Drug Administration, the Department of Veterans Affairs, and HL7 to provide standard names for clinical drugs and administered dose forms. It also provides normalized names for drugs and links names to commercial drug databases that are frequently used in pharmacy management and information systems in EHRs. A normalized name is "created by a set of formal rules and logic. In RxNorm, the normalized name allows linking of multiple names at a given level of abstraction"(Nelson et al. 2011). It is nonproprietary and provides the standards for drug ingredients and strength as well as dose formats, drug properties, physiological effects, and therapeutic category (Amatayakul 2017, 296).

Unified Medical Language System

Developed by the National Library of Medicine (NLM), the **Unified Medical Language System (UMLS)** is a program designed to build an automated system that can understand biomedical concepts, words, and expressions and their interrelationships, and it includes concepts and terms from many different vocabularies. To make these links, the UMLS uses more than 100 vocabularies, classifications, and terminologies. To understand how UMLS helps to learn and understand the concepts in medicine, two concepts of how language works must be understood. These two key concepts of UMLS are semantics and syntax. Semantics is a "branch of linguistics dealing with the study of meaning, including the ways meaning is structured in language and how changes in meanings and form occur over time" (Amatayakul 2017, 298). Syntax is described as "the study of patterns of formation of sentences and phrases from words and the rules for the formation of grammatical sentences in a language" (Amatayakul 2017, 298). In other words, how words are sequenced can change the meaning of the phrase. For example, "attending physician" has a very different meaning than "physician attending (to) ..." the former being an adjective describing a type of physician, and the latter being a verb describing the action the physician (of any type) is performing. The UMLS uses knowledge sources to help retrieve data across many databases. These knowledge sources are UMLS Metathesaurus, SPECIALIST Lexicon, and UMLS Semantic Network (Amatayakul 2017, 298).

According to the National Library of Medicine (NLM) the Metathesaurus is "a vocabulary database that contains information about biomedical and health related concepts, their various names, and the relationships among them. It is organized by concept, essentially linking alternative names and views of the same concept and identifying useful relationships between different concepts" (NLM 2017a).

The SPECIALIST Lexicon is "a general English lexicon that includes both commonly occurring words as well as biomedical terms. The purpose of the SPECIALIST lexicon is to support Natural Language Processing. It has over 20,000 entries" (NLM 2017b).

The UMLS Semantic Network is "a set of semantic types that provides a consistent categorization of concepts represented in the Metathesaurus and a useful set of meaningful relationships. Major groupings include anatomical structures, biological functions, chemicals, events, organisms, physical objects and other" (ONC 2017f).

National Drug Codes

National drug codes (NDC) were developed by the Food and Drug Administration to act as a universal unique identifier for human drugs. The NDC identifies the labeler or vendor, product, and trade package size, as shown in table 12.1. This is one of the codes mandated for use by HIPAA. Each code is 10 digits and is divided into three sections. The first section of the NDC identifies the company that manufactures, packages, and distributes the drug. The second section of the code identifies important information about the drug itself such as drug name, strength, form, and formulation for a particular firm. The third and final section identifies the package size (Amatayakul 2017, 297).

Table 12.1.   Examples of national drug codes

Drug	NDC
Fluoxetine	0555-0877
Elocon	54868-2223
Vicodin	12634-129
Glycolax	62175-190
Flonase	0173-0453
Progesterone	0555-0779
Axert	50458-210
Amitriptyline	49999-063
Amoxicillin	0781-6156

Source: FDA 2017.

Current Dental Terminology

The Current Dental Terminology (CDT) is the system used to code dental procedures such as tooth extractions, tooth implants, and such. The CDT was developed by the American Dental Association. It includes diagnostic, preventive, restorative, endodontics, periodontics, and other dental procedures. It is the coding system mandated by HIPAA for reporting dental procedures for billing purposes.

MEDCIN

MEDCIN is a nomenclature and knowledge-based system. It was developed by Peter S. Goltra and is now controlled by Medicomp Systems, Inc. It is the most comprehensive vocabulary for signs and symptoms (ONC 2017f). MEDCIN includes 250,000 clinical data elements that fall into the following categories: symptoms, history, physical examination, tests, diagnoses, and therapy (Amatayakul 2017, 296).

Diagnostic and Statistical Manual of Mental Disorders

Diagnostic and Statistical Manual of Mental Disorders (DSM) is a classification system of mental disorders used by mental health providers. It is published by the American Psychiatric Association. The current edition is known as DSM-5. The purpose of DSM-5 system is to assist physicians in properly diagnosing patients with mental health conditions. It is now linked to the implementation of the *International Classification of Diseases, Tenth Revision, Clinical Modification* (ICD-10-CM) in the United States (Amatayakul 2017, 296). The new format of ICD-10-CM codes was applied to DSM-5 so that its release coincided with the implementation of ICD-10-CM. DSM-5 provides detailed and specific criteria and information in order for physicians to accurately diagnose the mental disorder(s) of the patient. Along with this information, an ICD-10-CM code is provided. ICD-10-CM includes mental disorders and all other diagnoses, but it only provides a list of diagnostic codes and does not provide the detailed information about the diagnosis.

Mapping

To allow for interoperability, a crosswalk between the various terminologies must be created. This crosswalk is called mapping, which is the process of associating concepts from one coding system with concepts from another coding system and defining their equivalence in accordance with a documented rationale and a given purpose. An example of a map is a link between the code for acne in ICD-9-CM and the code for acne in ICD-10-CM. Before the map can be created, there must be an understanding of how the data will be used, because the map must be consistent. Categories, such as the following, can be used in mapping.

- One-to-one: An exact match is made between the systems
- Narrow-to-broad: A more granular term in the starting system maps to a more general term in the receiving system
- Broad-to-narrow: A more general term in the starting system maps to a more granular term in the receiving system
- Unmappable: There is no matching into the receiving system (Palkie 2013, 407)

In order for this mapping to be performed correctly, individuals performing the mapping must have a complete understanding of how the data will be used. Mapping used for a public health case may be different from mapping for a quality improvement case within a hospital. Public health research can involve large databases with decades of hospital discharge data that used ICD-9-CM codes. In order for the research to have continuity with hospital discharge data after September 30, 2015, matching ICD-10-CM to its previous counterpart is imperative.

Use cases are frequently used to create maps. The use case is part of the information system design process. It describes how the user will interact with the system and what the system will do. Use cases are tools that provide very detailed information for programmers to use when developing the system. The health information management (HIM) professional has this knowledge as well as an understanding of classification systems (Palkie 2016, 165). This makes the HIM professional a qualified candidate for this job.

A common mapping system is General Equivalence Mappings (GEMs). GEMs were created by the Centers for Medicare and Medicaid Services (CMS). GEMs are used to convert ICD-9-CM codes to ICD-10-CM or ICD-10-PCS codes or the reverse. Because the two systems are not identical, the user would have to decide which code to select. For example, in ICD-9-CM, obstetrical codes record whether the condition was antepartum, postpartum, and so forth. ICD-10-CM obstetrical codes record trimester rather than antepartum and so forth.

Because of this difference there is no exact match. If everything was an exact match there would not be a need for the new coding system. As a result of the differences GEMs were very important during the transition to ICD-10-CM and ICD-10-PCS and continue to be important for any medical research that must use historical coded data (prior to 2015). Table 12.2 shows an example of mapping between ICD-9-CM and ICD-10-CM.

Table 12.2.   Example of mapping ICD-9-CM to ICD-10-CM

ICD-9-CM	Description	≈ =	ICD-10-CM	Description
742.0	Encephalocele	≈ =	Q01.9	Encephalocele
			Q01.0	Frontal encephalocele
			Q01.1	Nasofrontal encephalocele
			Q01.2	Occipital encephalocele
			Q01.8	Encephalocele of other sites

Some key terms used when mapping ICD-10-CM and ICD-10-PCS are:

- Source code: The origin of the map, or the data set from which one maps
- Target code: The destination map, or the data set in which one attempts to find equivalence or establish the code relationship
- Forward map: A map that translates an ICD-9 code, as source code, to ICD-10 as its target code
- Backward map: A map that links the two coding systems in the opposite direction, moving from ICD-10 to ICD-9
- 1-to-1, cluster, combination, and complex: The types of mapping relations between source and target codes that exist in both forward and reverse directions
  - Cluster map: This is an entry in a GEM where one code from the many target codes can become a map to the source code (OR)
  - Combination map: This is an entry where more than one code is required in the target code set to replicate the complete meaning of the source system (AND)
  - Complex map: This mapping represents multiple code combinations and alternatives that are required to translate a source to a target code (AND and OR) (De 2012)

Messaging Standards

Messaging standards may also be called interoperability standards or data exchange standards. The purpose of messaging standards is to support communication between information systems. With messaging standards, proprietary systems are able to talk to one another, allowing the exchange of data. Standards do this by mapping proprietary forms to other formats. Existing standards have allowed for flexibility, which has caused problems with the interoperability between systems (McKnickle 2012).

The ANSI Accredited Standards Committee (ASC) X12 Insurance Subcommittee develops messaging standards for electronic data interchange (EDI) (Amatayakul 2017, 406). EDI is the exchange of routine business transactions from one computer or information system to another in a standard format, using standard communications protocols. ANSI ASC X12N was adopted by the HIPAA Transactions and Code Sets. This standard is the messaging standard for many of the transactions covered by HIPAA such as claims eligibility inquiry and response, claims status inquiry and response, and payment and remittance advice. ASTM International develops standards for security, health record content, the continuity care record, and the exchange of laboratory data (Abdelhak 2016, 199). Examples of messaging standards include:

- Health Level 7 (HL7)
- Digital Imaging and Communications in Medicine (DICOM)
- National Council for Prescription Drug Programs (NCPDP)

HL7 is the most common application level standard for healthcare; however, there are other standards that are used for special purposes. For example, DICOM is used for medical imaging.

HL7 transfers demographic data, orders, test results, history, and physical examination results (Amatayakul 2017, 402). Whenever an order for a laboratory test or x-ray study is submitted for a patient, the patient's demographic information and health record number from the registration system accompanies the order so that the eventual results will be tied back to that patient's EHR. The use of HL7 standards allows patient care information to be shared across computers while not changing the meaning of the information in the process. HL7 utilizes industry experts to advise and participate in the development of the standards. HL7's **Reference Information Model (RIM)** is a "model of information, or data objects, that is shared and reused between domains of care, such as clinical encounters, laboratory testing, prescriptions, billing, public health reporting, and research" (Orlova 2015). These models and the data specifications make sure that for every data element there is a corresponding relationship or association. Each data element must have a purpose (Amatayakul 2017, 402).

The **Digital Imaging and Communications in Medicine (DICOM)** standard retrieves images and other information from imaging equipment of a variety of different vendors. Areas covered by the standard include message exchange, data dictionary, data structure, and encoding. Although DICOM started out in diagnostic medical imaging, it has broadened to include specialties such as cardiology, dentistry, and radiology. The use of DICOM standards allows images to be transferred between systems from different vendors, ultimately allowing imaging in the picture archival and communication systems to share information with clinical information systems and the EHR. Due to its popularity, DICOM has become an independent SDO and is ANSI-accredited (Amatayakul 2017, 404).

ANSI Accredited Standards Committee X12N (ASC X12N) is responsible for developing the EDI standards used to share information needed for health insurance administrative transactions. These include functions such as benefit enrollment and maintenance and healthcare claim payment and advice. Work continues to increase more applications for the incorporation of health plans and additional privacy and security protocols due to the HIT challenges faced by many healthcare facilities (Amatayakul 2017, 406).

The **National Council for Prescription Drug Programs (NCPDP)** is an independent SDO and is ANSI-accredited. These standards were developed for and used by retail pharmacies and payers for claims, eligibility, and remittance advice. These e-prescription standards, called SCRIPT, control data to be shared for new prescriptions, refills, and other communications between physicians and pharmacies. NCPDP is regulated under the Medicare Modernization Act (MMA) of 2003, Medicare Part D e-prescribing (Amatayakul 2017, 406).

CHECK YOUR UNDERSTANDING 12.1

1. Messaging standards are the same as _____.
   a. EDI
   b. Vocabulary standards
   c. Interoperability standards
   d. UMLS

2. SNOMED is an example of a _____.
   a. Nomenclature
   b. Classification system
   c. Map
   d. Language

3. Which of the following organizations accredits SDOs?

   a. ANSI
   b. HITSP
   c. CCHIT
   d. National Library of Medicine

4. Which of the following is used to identify drugs?

   a. CDT
   b. UMLS
   c. LOINC
   d. NDC

5. What is the term used for a branch of linguistics dealing with the study of meaning, including the ways meaning is structured in language and how changes in meanings and form occur over time?

   a. Semantics
   b. Syntax
   c. Mapping
   d. Metathesaurus

Real-World Case

A local internal medicine and cardiology practice has recently implemented their new EHR system from Company A. Some relatively minor building renovations were required, and additional hardware was installed. Extensive training sessions and onsite support staff spent several months meeting with all users. Superusers and managers were identified and given additional training.

During the testing phases, there were several glitches that needed to be addressed. Because of the practice's long-standing relationship with a local hospital, they had to electronically communicate seamlessly to coordinate ongoing patient care throughout the healthcare continuum. The EHR from Company B is used by the hospital. Technology and software issues had to be addressed to ensure interoperability so that complete patient information was transmitted securely. The application of the HL7 messaging standards were evaluated for each system, and then the firewall and encryption software were adapted to meet data integrity and secure transmission requirements per the required standards. The patient portal for the physician practice had to be coordinated with the hospital's EHR so that patients were able to see information generated from their hospital admission. The cardiologists and internal medicine physicians were incorporating this information into their outpatient treatment plan. These issues have been addressed and care coordination has become more efficient thanks in part to the new electronic processes incorporated into both EHR systems.

REVIEW QUESTIONS

1. Which organization develops messaging standards for EDI?

   a. SDO
   b. ASTM
   c. ANSI ASC X12
   d. ISO

2. Which of the following has standards for the exchanging of digital images electronically?

   a. DICOM
   b. HL7
   c. SNOMED
   d. NDC

(Continued)

REVIEW QUESTIONS (*Continued*)

3. Which standards are used for retail pharmacies and payers for claims?

    a. NDC
    b. NCPDP
    c. RIM
    d. LOINC

4. Which standards are used for the exchange of laboratory data?

    a. NDC
    b. NCPDP
    c. RIM
    d. LOINC

5. Which classification systems, linked with ICD-10, is used by mental and behavioral health providers?

    a. DSM
    b. NDC
    c. DICOM
    d. SNOMED

6. Which terminology is used for dental procedures?

    a. CDT
    b. NDC
    c. DICOM
    d. MEDCIN

7. Which nomenclature has the most comprehensive vocabulary for signs and symptoms?

    a. NLM
    b. DSM
    c. RxNorm
    d. MEDCIN

8. What nomenclature, developed by the FDA, provides standard names for clinical drugs and administered dose forms?

    a. RxNorm
    b. NDC
    c. NCPDP
    d. DICOM

9. What is the most widely recognized nomenclature in healthcare?

    a. ICD-10
    b. MEDCIN
    c. SNOMED-CT
    d. ANSI

10. Which of the following are clear guidelines for the acceptable values of specific data fields and makes it possible to exchange health information using electronic networks?

    a. Data content standards
    b. Messaging standards
    c. Interoperability standards
    d. Vocabulary standards

References

Abdelhak, M. and M. A. Hanken. 2016. *Health information: Management of a Strategic Resource*, 5th ed. St. Louis, MO: Elsevier.

AHIMA Work Group. 2013 (November). Data standards, data quality, and interoperability (2013 update). *Journal of AHIMA* 84(11):64–69 [expanded web version]. http://library.ahima.org/doc?oid=107104.

Amatayakul, M. 2017. *Health IT and EHRs: Principles and Practice*, 6th ed. Chicago: AHIMA.

American National Standards Institute (ANSI). n.d. Standards activities overview. Accessed 1/10/2018. http://www.ansi.org/standards_activities/overview/overview.aspx?menuid=3.

ASTM International. 2015. ASTM Standards for Healthcare Services, Products and Technology. https://www.astm.org/ABOUT/OverviewsforWeb2015/Medical_sector.pdf.

ASTM International. 2018a. Committee E31 on Healthcare Informatics. https://www.astm.org/COMMITTEE/E31.htm.

ASTM International. 2018b. https://www.astm.org/ABOUT/faqs.html.

Biedermann, S. and D. Dolezel. 2017. *Introduction to Healthcare Informatics*, 2nd ed. Chicago: AHIMA.

Centers for Medicare and Medicaid (CMS). 2015. Stage 2 Eligible Professional Meaningful Use Core Measures: Measure 15 of 17. https://www.cms.gov/Regulations-and-Guidance/Legislation/EHRIncentivePrograms/downloads/Stage2_EPCore_15_SummaryCare.pdf.

Conover, K. n.d. Healthcare IT Standards. Accessed 2/24/18. http://ed-informatics.org/healthcare-it-in-a-nutshell-2/healthcare-it-standards/.

De, S. 2012. 8 steps to success in ICD-10-CM/PCS mapping: Best practices to establish precise mapping between old and new ICD code sets. *Journal of AHIMA* 83(6):44–49. http://bok.ahima.org/doc?oid=106975#.WpHQFqinFRY

Duffy, J. 2014. Microsoft HealthVault. https://www.pcmag.com/article2/0,2817,2473749,00.asp.

Food and Drug Administration. 2017. National Drug Code Directory. https://www.accessdata.fda.gov/scripts/cder/ndc/default.cfm.

Health Level 7 (HL7). 2017. About HL7. https://www.hl7.org/about/index.cfm?ref=nav.

International Standards Organization (ISO). 2018. About ISO. https://www.iso.org/about-us.html.

McKnickle, M. 2012. Eight common questions about HL7. http://www.healthcareitnews.com/news/8-common-questions-about-hl7.

National Library of Medicine. 2017a. About the NLM Metathesaurus. https://www.nlm.nih.gov/research/umls/about_umls.html#Metathesaurus.

National Library of Medicine. 2017b. The SPECIALIST Lexicon. https://lsg3.nlm.nih.gov/LexSysGroup/Projects/lexicon/current/web/index.html.

Nelson, S. J., K. Zeng, J. Kilbourne, T. Powell, and R. Moore. (2011). Normalized names for clinical drugs: RxNorm at 6 years. *Journal of the American Medical Informatics Association:*18(4):441–448. http://doi.org/10.1136/amiajnl-2011-000116.

Office of the National Coordinator for Health Information Technology (ONC). 2017a. EHR Functional Model Standards. https://www.healthit.gov/providers-professionals/health-it-curriculum-resources-educators.

Office of the National Coordinator for Health Information Technology (ONC). 2017b. National and International Standards Developing Organizations. https://www.healthit.gov/providers-professionals/health-it-curriculum-resources-educators.

Office of the National Coordinator for Health Information Technology (ONC). 2017c. Standards to Promote Health Information Exchange. https://www.healthit.gov/providers-professionals/health-it-curriculum-resources-educators.

Office of the National Coordinator for Health Information Technology (ONC). 2017d. Standards for Developing Organizations. https://www.healthit.gov/providers-professionals/health-it-curriculum-resources-educators.

Office of the National Coordinator for Health Information Technology (ONC). 2017e. Health Data Interchange Standards. https://www.healthit.gov/providers-professionals/health-it-curriculum-resources-educators.

Office of the National Coordinator for Health Information Technology (ONC). 2017f. Basic Health Data Standards. https://www.healthit.gov/providers-professionals/health-it-curriculum-resources-educators.

Orlova, A. 2015. Overview of health IT standards. *Journal of AHIMA* 86(3). http://bok.ahima.org /doc?oid=107579#.WlbcJ6inFRY.

Palkie, B. 2013. Clinical Classifications and Terminologies. Chapter 15 in *Health Information Management: Concepts, Principles, and Practice*, 4th ed. Edited by K. LaTour, S. Eichenwald Maki, and P. Oachs. Chicago: AHIMA.

Palkie, B. 2016. Clinical Classifications, Vocabularies, Terminologies, and Standards. Chapter 5 in *Health Information Management: Concepts, Principles, and Practice*, 5th ed. Edited by P. Oachs and A. Watters. Chicago: AHIMA.

Learning Objectives

- Educate staff on security issues.
- Discuss federal security regulation.
- Recommend security measures.
- Develop policies and procedures on security practices.
- Control access to protected health information.
- Conduct audit for security violation.

Key Terms

Access controls
Addressable standards
Administrative safeguards
Administrative simplification
Audit controls
Audit reduction tools
Audit trails
Biomedical device
Biometric identifiers
Bots
Business associates
Certified in Healthcare Privacy
    and Security (CHPS)
Certified Information Security
    Manager (CISM)
Certified Information Systems
    Security Professional (CISSP)
Code set
Context-based authentication
Contingency plan
Covered entity (CE)
Data recovery
Degaussing

Designated standard maintenance
    organizations (DSMOs)
Electronic protected health
    information (e-PHI)
Emergency access procedure
Emergency mode operation plan
Encryption
Facility access controls
Firewalls
Forensics
Healthcare clearinghouse
Health Insurance Portability and
    Accountability Act of 1996
    (HIPAA)
Health plan
Information access management
Information system activity
    review
Integrity
Intrusion detection system
Malicious software
Mitigation
Network security

One-factor authentication
Passwords
Phishing
Physical safeguards
Privacy Rule
Protected health information (PHI)
Ransomware
Redundancy
Remote wipe
Required standards
Risk analysis
Risk management
Role-based authentication
Security
Security awareness training
Security event
Security incident
Security management plan
Security official
Security Rule
Spoliation
Spyware
Technical safeguard

Telephone callback	Transmission security	Username
Termination process	Trigger	Virus
Threats	Trojan	Vulnerabilities
Token	Two-factor authentication	Workforce clearance procedure
Transaction and Code Sets rule	User-based authentication	Worm

The security of health information has always been a priority of health information management (HIM) professionals, but it was raised to a new level of importance with the implementation of information systems that document and retain health record information as well as other data that can identify the patient.

Data can be classified in a number of ways. One way is to classify data according to data type—clinical, administrative, financial, and so on. Data can also be classified into categories according to the level of security required. Different terms might be used, but one example is PHI, sensitive, and public. Who has access and how the information is used will be controlled by the classification allocated to it (UAB 2018).

With the paper record, access was limited to the record itself. With the electronic health record (EHR) and other information systems, access is available from anywhere, including outside the healthcare facility.

Historically, security regulations were enacted at the state level, which led to a patchwork of very different laws across the country with no consistency among them. There were, and are, accreditation standards and the Medicare Conditions of Participation that address security, but these standards applied solely to accredited facilities and facilities that treated Medicare patients, respectively. Accreditation standards generally include broad security requirements that vary by accrediting organization. Because of security concerns of healthcare professionals and patients alike, federal laws were enacted. This chapter will address the Health Insurance Portability and Accountability Act of 1996 (HIPAA) and security concepts such as security threats and safeguards.

Introduction to Health Insurance Portability and Accountability Act of 1996

The Health Insurance Portability and Accountability Act of 1996 (HIPAA) is a federal law that impacts many areas of healthcare, including insurance portability, code sets, privacy, security, electronic data interchange (EDI), and national identifier standards. HIPAA is divided into five titles, or sections. This chapter addresses Title II: Fraud and Abuse/Administrative Simplification. The purpose of the administrative simplification title is to improve the efficiency and effectiveness of the business processes of healthcare by standardizing the EDI of administrative and financial transactions. This title was also designed to protect the privacy and security of protected health information (PHI) that is transmitted from one point to another. PHI is individually identifiable health information that is transmitted or maintained in any form or format by an organization subject to HIPAA. A third purpose is to reduce the cost of doing business in healthcare because of antiquated paper systems, nonstandard formats, and lack of accessibility to health records due to loss (45 CFR 160, 162, and 164 2013).

To be subject to HIPAA, an organization must meet the definition of a covered entity (CE). A CE is a health plan, healthcare clearinghouse, or healthcare provider that transmits any health information in electronic form for one of the covered transactions. A health plan pays for the healthcare provided to the individuals covered under the plan. These plans include medical, dental, vision, and other forms of health plans. Healthcare providers include hospitals, physician offices, long-term care facilities, ambulatory surgery centers, pharmacies, and other patient care providers. A healthcare clearinghouse collects billing data and processes it for the healthcare provider. The healthcare clearinghouse then submits the claim to the health plan for payment. The covered transactions that HIPAA addresses are:

- Health plan premium payments
- Enrollment or disenrollment in a health plan
- Eligibility
- Referral certification and authorization
- Claims
- Payment and remittance advice
- Claim status

- Coordination of benefits
- Health claims attachment
- First report of injury (Davis 2003)

Health plans, healthcare clearinghouses, and healthcare providers that do not share patient information for one of these transactions are not CEs and, therefore, are not subject to HIPAA.

HIPAA has greatly impacted healthcare and the HIM profession as a result of changes in processes, emphasis on privacy and security, and patient rights. One of the sections in HIPAA is Administrative Simplification, which includes Transaction and Code Sets Rule, Privacy Rule, and the Security Rule. Although this chapter emphasizes security, as interrelated components of HIPAA, all three of the aforementioned rules are discussed.

Transaction and Code Sets Rule

The **Transaction and Code Sets Rule** was designed to standardize transactions performed by CEs. These standards apply to electronic transactions only, such as claim submission, eligibility queries, and many more insurance-related functions; however, paper submissions are similar. The Department of Health and Human Services (HHS) has assigned the responsibility of developing and maintaining standards for the Transaction and Code Sets rule to six organizations, called **designated standard maintenance organizations (DSMOs)**:

- Accredited Standards Committee X12
- Dental Contact Committee of the American Dental Association
- Health Level 7 (HL7)
- National Council for Prescription Drug Programs
- National Uniform Billing Committee
- National Uniform Claim Committee (45 CFR 160, 162, and 164 2013)

Transaction and Code Sets standards cover the individual data elements and the format of the data for the claim submissions and other functions mentioned earlier in this chapter. The standards enable the use of electronic data interchange (EDI), the transfer of data from one point to another without human intervention, which can significantly improve the efficiency of healthcare. The HIPAA transactions and code sets requirements use ASC X12 standards. These ASC X12 standards mandate the data to be submitted, formatting, and other attributes of the healthcare claims and other financial transactions.

CEs may follow the transaction requirements themselves and send formatted data to the clearinghouse for submission to the third-party payers. The CE also may send unformatted data to a clearinghouse or health plan and have the data converted into the appropriate transaction format.

Designated code sets are also a part of the HIPAA Transactions and Code Set rule. HIPAA defines a **code set** as a set of codes used to encode data elements (45 CFR 160, 162, and 164 2013). These codes record medical diagnoses, procedures, drugs, dental procedures, and other data elements. A code replaces larger pieces of data. For example, the ICD-10-CM code I10 means essential (primary) hypertension. HIPAA mandates the use of certain coding systems in the reporting of diagnoses, procedures, drugs, and more on medical and dental claims. These standards are:

- *International Classification of Diseases, Tenth Revision, Clinical Modification* (ICD-10-CM)
- *International Classification of Diseases, Tenth Revision, Procedural Coding System* (ICD-10-PCS)
- Current Procedural Terminology, Fourth Edition (CPT-4)
- Healthcare Financing Administration Common Procedure Coding System (HCPCS)
- Code on Dental Procedures and Nomenclature, Second Edition (CDT-2)
- National Drug Codes (NDC)

There are also nonmedical codes that can define medical specialties, claim adjustment reasons, reject reason codes, state abbreviations, remittance remarks, and more. See chapter 12 for more information on standards.

Privacy Rule

The HIPAA **Privacy Rule** controls how CEs, defined earlier in the chapter, may use PHI. **Business associates** are individuals or organizations that perform work on behalf of the CE and that require access to PHI. Examples of functions that business associates may perform are coding, release of information, and billing.

Business associates are subject to HIPAA. HIPAA lists the specific data elements that determine whether or not information is PHI. If the information includes any of the data elements in figure 13.1, it is considered PHI and is therefore subject to the HIPAA Privacy Rule.

Figure 13.1. PHI identifiers

1. Name
2. Postal address information, other than town or city, state, and zip code
3. Telephone numbers
4. Fax numbers
5. Electronic mail addresses
6. Social security numbers
7. Medical record numbers
8. Health plan beneficiary numbers
9. Account numbers
10. Certificate/license numbers
11. Vehicle identifiers and serial numbers, including license plate numbers
12. Device identifiers and serial numbers
13. Web universal resource locators (URLs)
14. Internet protocol (IP) address numbers
15. Biometric identifiers, including finger and voice prints
16. Full-face photographic images and any comparable images

Source: 45 CFR 160, 162, and 164 2013.

The Privacy Rule also lists the following PHI-related patient rights:

- Patient must be provided a notice of privacy practices that defines how PHI is used in the CE
- Patient has the right to inspect, copy, and receive a copy of the medical record
- Patient has the right to request an amendment to the health information
- Patient has the right to request communications from the CE through alternative means such as a post office box rather than the home address
- Patient has the right to report violations of the HIPAA Privacy Rule
- Patient has the right to request restrictions on how his or her PHI is utilized by the CE (Rinehart-Thompson 2016, 231)

The CE must have policies in place to allow a patient to claim these rights. Policies and procedures are important to the Privacy Rule compliance program since the rule focuses on processes and the people who develop and follow them rather than on technology. The need for policies and procedures to document security processes is mentioned throughout this chapter. These policies and procedures should be in writing and may be updated at any time. Once the policy and procedure or other required document is updated, replaced, or deleted, the document must be retained for six years from the date it was last in effect. This documentation must be available to members of the workforce responsible for implementing the procedures referred to in the documentation.

Security Rule

Security has two definitions that focus on different aspects of security:

1. The means to control access and protect information from accidental or intentional disclosure to unauthorized persons and from unauthorized alteration, destruction, or loss

2. The physical protection of facilities and equipment from theft, damage, or unauthorized access; collectively, the policies, procedures, and safeguards designed to protect the confidentiality of information, maintain the integrity and availability of information systems, and control access to the content of these systems.

A CE must address all of the aspects included in these definitions as they are all included in the Security Rule. The Security Rule defines the minimum that a CE must do to protect **electronic protected health information (ePHI)**, which is PHI that is "created, received, or transmitted" electronically by CEs (45 CFR 160, 162, and 164 2013). The Security Rule does not apply to PHI in other media such as paper, oral communication, and microfilm. ePHI can be communicated over the Internet or it can be stored electronically, such as on a magnetic drive. Voicemail, fax, and copy machines are not considered to be ePHI.

The Security Rule was developed to be technology neutral and scalable. Technology changes so fast that the Security Rule would need constant revision if specific technologies were mandated; therefore, the rule mandates what needs to be done but not how to do it. For example, the HIPAA Security Rule mandates that physical access to electronic information systems is limited to authorized staff. The rule does not tell the CE how that limitation is to be implemented, so the CE may use card keys, personal identification numbers, keys, biometrics, or other means (described later in this chapter) to control access. Scalable means that the HHS allows CEs to consider the size, complexity, and capabilities of the CE when developing the compliance strategy. The CE can also consider the infrastructure of the CE regarding technology, software, and hardware, as well as the costs of the security measures and the risks to the ePHI (CMS 2007a). Because of scalability, the HHS would expect more rigorous security measures from a 1,000-bed hospital than from a 60-bed hospital or a two-physician practice.

American Recovery and Reinvestment Act of 2009

The American Recovery and Reinvestment Act of 2009 (ARRA) introduced new requirements related to security:

- Certification of EHRs
- Mandated HIPAA audits
- Increased severity of penalties
- Business associates subject to privacy and security regulations

In order to become a certified EHR, the software must meet specified security standards. Vendors apply to have their EHR applications reviewed by one of the Office of the National Coordinator for Health Information Technology–Authorized Certification Bodies and Accredited Testing Laboratories. The benefit to becoming certified is that qualified healthcare providers are able to obtain incentive funds for using the certified EHR in a meaningful way. Refer to chapter 11 for additional information on Meaningful Use.

The increased penalties include prison as well as financial penalties and are discussed later in this chapter. Business associates and their responsibilities related to security are also covered later in this chapter. Refer to chapter 9 for more information about EHRs.

CHECK YOUR UNDERSTANDING 13.1

1. To be subject to HIPAA, an organization must meet the definition of a(n) _____.

   a. CE
   b. Accredited organization
   c. Administrative simplification
   d. Designated standard organization

(Continued)

CHECK YOUR UNDERSTANDING 13.1 (*Continued*)

2. One of the purposes of the administrative simplification title is to _____.

   a. Prevent security incidents from ever occurring in a healthcare facility
   b. Create socialized medicine in the United States
   c. Improve efficiency and effectiveness of healthcare business processes
   d. Establish a prospective payment system

3. Which of the following is an example of the designated standard maintenance organization?

   a. Centers for Medicare and Medicaid Services
   b. HL7
   c. AHIMA
   d. ICD-10-CM

4. ARRA made numerous changes including _____.

   a. Increasing penalties
   b. Changing the definition of ePHI
   c. Changing the definition of a CE
   d. Establishing the concept of business associate

5. Billing Plus is a company that will prepare and submit bill for the hospital. It is a _____.

   a. DSMO
   b. Business associate
   c. Privacy Rule
   d. Code set

Security Threats and Safeguards

Threats are the potential for a vulnerability to be exploited. Vulnerabilities are weaknesses that could be exploited, thus creating a breach of security. Threats come from internal and external sources. Internal threats come from employees, hardware factors, and the environment (water leak, for example). There are five types of human threats to data security, which can be made by current employees, former employees, and hackers:

- Threats from employees who make honest mistakes (human error)
- Threats from employees who exploit their access to data
- Threats from employees who use their access to data for malice or financial gain
- Threats from external individuals who attempt to access data or steal hardware or other equipment
- Threats from angry employees or others who attack the information systems of the CE (Rinehart-Thompson 2016, 256)

Threats due to human error are not intentional and result from mistakes or misunderstandings. Examples of human errors are cutting electricity to a building when digging, destroying the wrong disk, loading data on an Internet server by accident, and entering the wrong configuration setting. Conversely, some threats are classified as intentional activity, including intentional deletion or alteration of data, infecting the information system with viruses, and using data to steal a patient's identity. External threats can be caused by people outside the CE who attempt to gain unauthorized access. External threats also include natural disasters such as floods, tornadoes, and hurricanes, which may cause damage to the CE that destroys the system or temporarily disables access to the system.

The goals of the HIPAA Security Rule are to ensure the confidentiality, integrity, and availability of the ePHI. Confidentiality means providing access to ePHI to only those who need it. Integrity is ensuring that data are not altered, either during transmission across a network or during storage. Integrity is discussed later in this chapter. ePHI must be available when needed for patient care and other uses. Another important term is accessibility, which is ensuring that the ePHI is available to the authorized users whenever it is needed.

The Security Rule is designed to ensure that ePHI remains confidential and is protected from unauthorized disclosure, alteration, or destruction. The Security Rule utilizes administrative, physical, and technical safeguards to protect ePHI. Administrative safeguards are people-focused and include requirements such as training, policies, and assignment of an individual responsible for security. Physical safeguards are mechanisms in place to protect hardware, software, and data. The physical safeguards should protect ePHI from fire, flooding, unauthorized access to hardware, theft, and other hazards. Technical safeguards use technology to protect data and to control access to the data.

Administrative, physical, and technical safeguards are broken down into implementation specifications and standards. The standards tell the CE what must be done, whereas implementation specifications provide direction to help the CE comply with the standards. Each standard is identified as required or addressable. Required standards must be implemented by all CEs to protect the ePHI. Addressable standards must be evaluated by the entity to determine whether or not the standard is reasonable and appropriate. If the standard is reasonable and appropriate, then the CE must implement the standard. If it is not, then the CE has the flexibility to identify an equivalent method of accomplishing the same objective. For example, encryption is an addressable standard, but although the CE does not have to encrypt data, there has to be a method to protect the data from unauthorized use. The CE cannot determine that a standard is not reasonable and appropriate simply because it is expensive. There is no requirement for a standard to be deemed not reasonable and appropriate, but the CE must document the rationale (in case of audit) and what is being done to implement an equivalent method. Each type of safeguard will be discussed later in this chapter.

Administrative Safeguards and the Security Management Process

The Security Rule defines administrative safeguards as

administrative actions, and policies and procedures, to manage the selection, development, implementation, and maintenance of security measure to protect electronic-protected health information and to manage the conduct of the covered entity's workforce in relation to the protection of that information. (45 CFR 160, 162, and 164 2013)

A listing of the administrative safeguards required by the HIPAA Security Rule can be found in table 13.1.

Table 13.1. Administrative safeguards

Standards	Implementation Specifications
Security management	• Risk analysis • Risk management • Sanction policy • Information system activity review
Assigned security responsibility	• None
Workforce security	• Authorization and supervision • Workforce clearance procedures • Termination procedures
Information access management	• Isolating healthcare clearinghouse functions • Access authorization • Access establishment and modification
Security awareness and training	• Security reminders • Protection from malicious software • Log-in monitoring • Password management

(Continued)

Table 13.1. Administrative safeguards (Continued)

Standards	Implementation Specifications
Security incident procedures	• Response and reporting
Contingency plan	• Data backup plan • Disaster recovery plan • Emergency mode operation plan • Testing and revision procedures • Applications and data criticality analysis
Evaluation	• None
Business associate contract and other arrangements	• Written contract or other arrangement

Source: Adapted from 45 CFR 160, 162, and 164 2013.

CEs must create a security plan that "implement[s] policies and procedures to prevent, detect, contain and correct security violations" (CMS 2007a, 3). Some of the ways that this is accomplished is risk analysis, risk management, sanction policy, and information system activity review.

Risk Analysis

Risk analysis is the process of identifying possible security threats to the CE's data and identifying which risks should be promptly addressed and which are lower in priority. The risk analysis process requires the CE to bring staff from across the CE together to identify the data that must be protected. The risk analysis includes estimating the potential costs associated with security breaches and how much it would cost to develop safeguards to prevent these incidents. This analysis must include the risks to data confidentiality and integrity and the availability of the ePHI it controls. To accomplish this, the team has to identify the threats to and vulnerabilities of the CE. Vulnerabilities may be technical or nontechnical. A technical vulnerability would be configuration in the system that allowed inappropriate access. An example of a nontechnical vulnerability is the lack of policies to guide staff (CMS 2007b, 1). Other examples of vulnerabilities would be connection to ePHI through the Internet and lack of detailed security policies, and procedures. The CE also must identify existing security controls such as firewalls, employee termination procedures, and virus protection software. In addition, the team must determine the impact of losing one or more systems owing to malware, sabotage, hardware failure, breach of privacy, or other failure of the CE. The risk analysis must also look for threats such as floods, fire, errors in data entry, viruses, and unauthorized access to ePHI. The Security Rule does not define the steps to be taken for risk analysis. It is left to each CE to develop and maintain its own plan for compliance.

Addressing the threats and vulnerabilities identified during the risk analysis helps prevent failure of information systems. While all information system failures are serious, some have a greater impact on the CE than others. For example, failure of the patient satisfaction database will not be as critical as the failure of the EHR. If the patient satisfaction system is not working for a week, the data entry will be backlogged and the reports may be delayed, but patient care goes on unimpeded. With the EHR, the patient's test results, allergies, past medical history, and other information may not be available, which severely impacts patient care. Not all risks are created equal. Each risk must be evaluated for the likelihood of the event happening. For example, if the CE is located in Alabama, the risk of an earthquake is low, but the risk of a tornado or hurricane will be high. The CE could categorize risks into high, medium, and low based on the impact that the threat would have on the CE. The CE would then need to address the threats—especially the ones deemed to be a high risk. If a vulnerability is activated, the outcome resulting from the vulnerability could take a number of forms. According to the Centers for Medicare and Medicaid Services (CMS), potential impacts include destruction of ePHI, inappropriate access to ePHI, and more.

Based on the likelihood of risk, the impact on the CE, and other findings, the team must recommend controls to reduce the risk to the CE. Examples of controls are sanction policies, firewalls, encryption, and biometrics. These controls will be discussed later in this chapter. These proposals must be in compliance with the HIPAA security rule and be designed to reduce the risk and vulnerabilities to ePHI. The process, findings, and recommendations of the risk analysis process must be documented and retained.

Risk Management

Risk management is a comprehensive program of activities intended to minimize the potential for injuries to occur in a CE and to anticipate and respond to ensuring liabilities for those injuries that do occur. There must be processes in place to identify, evaluate, and control risk. The first step in risk management is the development of a risk management plan. This plan sets the priority for the implementation of the security measure identified in the security assessment. The plan should include a description of the risks, the security measures to be established, and an implementation plan for the security measures, including dates, resources needed (staff, monetary, and others), and ongoing maintenance required (CMS 2007b, 14). Risk assessment and risk management are not one-time events but rather ongoing processes. Although HIPAA does not mandate the frequency of reviews or updates, it does mandate that they must occur as necessary. This time period could be from one to three years, based on the needs of the CE.

In the security management process, the CE must manage security policies. The policies covered under this security management plan must include the policies required to prevent, identify, control, and resolve security incidents (45 CFR 160, 162, and 164 2013). The security management plan should be updated periodically to address changes in law, changes in the CE, and other issues.

Sanction Policy

Each CE must develop a sanction policy that addresses how employees will be penalized for failing to follow security policies and procedures. HIPAA does not require specific employee penalties, but requires the CE to determine how breaches and other violations should be handled. Employees should be notified of the policies and procedures and the penalties that come with violations. They should also sign an acknowledgment of the security requirements to show that they understand that violations may result in disciplinary actions that could include termination of employment. Sanctions should be based on the severity of the failure to comply with the policies and procedures (Burrington-Brown 2003). For example, an employee who fails to log off of a computer during a medical emergency should not be penalized in the same way as an employee who accesses ePHI inappropriately.

CEs are required to conduct an information system activity review, which monitors for the inappropriate use or disclosure of ePHI. HIPAA does not mandate the frequency of this review nor the way this review is to be conducted. These reviews should include logs, access, and incident reporting. The CE should monitor audit logs, the incident log, and other internal and external documentation to identify all successful and unsuccessful attempts to access ePHI (Amatayakul 2017, 377–378).

Assigned Security Responsibility

The Security Rule mandates an individual to be in charge of the security program for the CE. HIPAA calls this individual a security official; however, this position is frequently called chief security officer (CSO) by the CEs. The CSO is responsible for:

- Developing the security goals and objectives for the CE
- Determining how the goals and objectives will be met
- Advising administration regarding information security
- Determining reporting procedures
- Conducting adequate risk assessment and determining the appropriate level of risk acceptance
- Developing and monitoring the overall security program

The CSO works with others who assist in managing the CE's security program. This individual must have a strong understanding of both technology and the business practices of the CE. HIPAA gives little direction as to the role of the CSO, just that the responsibility should be given to a specific individual who is responsible for the overall security program. The CSO may have additional employees assisting. The CSO's role may be a full-time or part-time role, and the CSO may be the same or a different individual from the chief privacy official (CPO). The CPO is in charge of the privacy program for the CE.

Workforce Security

Policies and procedures should be in place to ensure that members of the workforce have the appropriate access to ePHI for their job. Information access management involves implementing policies and procedures to determine which employees have access to what information. One of the ways a healthcare clearinghouse can accomplish this is to isolate PHI from the rest of the clearinghouse's information. Some healthcare clearinghouses are owned and operated by large corporations that conduct business in many different industries. To protect the ePHI, it must be completely separated from the nonhealth clearinghouse segments of the business.

Additionally, each CE workforce member must be given access to data and system functionality, such as accessing the EHR, and then it must be specified what the user can do in the EHR, such as accessing whether or not a patient has an allergy. The CE must have a workforce clearance procedure. The workforce clearance procedure ensures that each member of the workforce's level of access is appropriate. The workforce includes all employees, students, volunteers, members of the board of directors, and others, paid or unpaid, who perform services for the CE. The access determination should be based on risk analysis and each employee's job description. There must be a termination process to eliminate access to the information systems by a member of the workforce when that person's employment with the CE ends—either through resignation or through termination. The termination process should also include review for job-appropriate access levels, to include more or less access to ePHI, as the individual's role in the CE changes.

All workforce members, including administration, board of directors, custodial staff, students, and volunteers, must receive security awareness training, which educates CE employees about the CE's security policies and procedures. Basic training should cover general security policies, physical and workstation security, password management, importance of logging out, and other issues. Many workforce members will require additional security training appropriate to their job functions. For example, management staff will need training on monitoring procedures and security system assessment. HIPAA does not mandate the format that the training takes, but a recommendation is to include it in new employee orientation. Face-to-face training classes should be supported with periodic security reminders, which could take many formats, including:

- Screen savers
- Periodic e-mails
- Articles or statements in an employee newsletter
- Notices posted in public areas

HIPAA requires that documentation of the training, including the following, must be retained for six years:

- Sign-in sheets
- Handouts
- E-mail messages
- Training database identifying training and actions taken (Hjort 2003)

Training should be ongoing and provided whenever there are changes to policies and procedures or to areas related to security.

Managing a Security Incident

No matter how hard a CE strives to eliminate security incidents, they will still occur. The Security Rule defines a security incident as "the attempted or successful unauthorized access, use, disclosure, modification, or destruction of information or interference with system operations in an information system" (45 CFR 160, 162, and 164 2013). Because this definition is broad, the CE should define a security incident for itself. The security incidents should include both information technology incidents and physical security incidents. Examples of security incidents include:

- Someone impersonating an information technology technician asking for a password
- Former employee using old identification and password to access ePHI
- Virus attack that destroyed current files
- Audit trail with evidence that someone misused someone else's password
- Corrupt backup tapes with no ability to restore archived data
- Physical break-in with ePHI copied or stolen

- PHI posted on the Internet from a web portal
- Misdirected e-mail with ePHI
- Terminated employee keeping copies of records with PHI
- CDs containing ePHI found discarded without physical destruction (Amatayakul 2005a)

ARRA requires CEs to actively identify and report security incidents. The security incident policies and procedures should identify how the incidents will be identified and to whom they should be reported. Security incidents throughout the CE should be reported to someone in a centralized role, such as the CSO, and must be addressed quickly because inaction could allow the incident to worsen, such as in the case of a virus (Amatayakul 2005a, 60). Policies and procedures informed by the severity of the security incident should define how the CE will respond. If the incident suggests criminal activity or compromises the safety of an individual, the local law enforcement agency should be contacted.

Forensics "is the process used to gather intact and validated evidence" (Derhak 2003) and is the process that should be used to gather evidence of the security incident. The steps in forensics include:

- Documentation of the investigation conducted
- Protection and preservation of any evidence found, the logs reviewed, and reports
- Documentation of the chain of custody (who had access)
- Use of an exact copy of the media in the investigation (Derhak 2003)

The investigation may require hardware to be confiscated and stored in a secured location, network logs to be printed, data to be backed up, and other investigative steps. Failure to protect data may result in the intentional or unintentional destruction of evidence. "Intentional destruction, mutilation, alteration, or concealment of evidence or alteration of evidence" is called spoliation (AHIMA e-HIM Work Group 2006). During the course of the investigation, a number of steps may be taken such as:

- Recovering deleted files
- Recovering passwords
- Analyzing file access, creation, and modification times
- Analyzing system and application logs
- Determining user and application activity on a system (Derhak 2003)

Once a security incident is identified, the CE must mitigate its harmful effects and document both the incident and the outcome. Mitigation is the process of attempting to reduce or eliminate harmful effects of the breach (45 CFR 160, 162, and 164 2013). Even though it may not be possible to completely mitigate the effects, the CE must do everything possible to protect patients. For example, if a patient's social security number is inappropriately disclosed, the CE may pay for the patient to monitor his or her credit report for a specified period of time.

Security events are poor security practices that have not led to harm, whereas security incidents have resulted in harm or a significant risk of harm (Amatayakul 2005a). Security events may be employee mistakes, many of which result in noncompliance with the CE's security policies, that did not result in disclosure of ePHI.

Examples of security events include:

- Sharing login information with another employee
- Password reminder visible at workstation
- Computer system left logged on and unattended
- System access to patient data down with only paper copies of encounter forms
- Unencrypted or otherwise unsecured e-mail of PHI
- Maintenance personnel fixing equipment with PHI without supervision by the CE's workforce (Amatayakul 2005b)

Although security events do not lead to harm, steps should be taken to prevent the event from occurring again as harm could result in the future. Individual counseling or employee training may be needed. The CSO should monitor trends in the types of security incidents and events that occur. The identification of patterns from this trending yields valuable information regarding threats and vulnerabilities of the CE. These events may result in penalties, as discussed later in this chapter.

Ongoing Security Procedure Evaluation

Implementation of the security safeguards is not enough to comply with HIPAA security regulations. CEs must also critique its security program through ongoing monitoring and evaluation to identify areas for improvement. The evaluation must include both technical and nontechnical processes. Technical processes are those that use technology, such as encryption, access controls, firewalls, audit trails, and other technical tools. Nontechnical processes are the security measures that do not require technology, including policies and procedures, training, evaluations, monitoring, and other administrative responsibilities. The evaluation should address whether or not the CE is meeting the HIPAA security regulations and whether or not the program is still appropriate for the current status of the CE. CEs change over time because of growth (services, employees, and so forth), changes in policies, changes in technologies used, and changes in laws and regulations. The security program must keep up with these changes to ensure that the program is still meeting all HIPAA security regulations.

Contingency and Business Continuity Planning

When information systems are down, CEs must have a plan in place to continue business despite being unavailable to retrieve information, place orders, or perform other key tasks. This plan is called a business continuity plan (BCP). The BCP is a program that incorporates policies and procedures for continuing business operations during a computer system shutdown. The BCP should include when the plan should be implemented, who initiates the plan, which manual processes are to be used, what forms are needed, how to update the database once the system is again operational, and more.

A **contingency plan** is made up of policies and procedures that identify how a CE will react in the event of an information system emergency, such as power failure, natural disaster, a hacker, malware, or a system failure. A CE can take steps to reduce the risk of the EHR or other critical patient care systems from being down or failing, but it cannot eliminate the possibility. Therefore, it is important to back up data so that if the system fails, the data can be recreated from the backups. The contingency plan should include a data-backup plan. The backup plan should address frequency of backups, where the backed up data are stored, testing the backups, and more. The data-backup plan should include all critical sources of information, such as the EHR and clinical information systems.

To help prevent failures due to hardware failure, redundancy is needed. **Redundancy** is duplication of data, hardware, cables, or other hardware components of the information system. As data are entered, it is also saved onto a second computer server, creating a way to access an operational information system with little to no downtime.

There may be a time when disaster strikes and the CE loses data because of flood, fire, tornado, hardware failure, or other failures. The CE must have plans in place to get the information system working again and then to update it with all activities that occurred during the downtime. The **emergency mode operation plan** encompasses procedures necessary to keep the critical business processes of the CE in place during information system downtime. Manual processes such as paper laboratory slips, microfilm of the master patient index, and health record forms must be available in the event that the information system is down. The contingency plan must be tested periodically and revised as areas needing improvement are identified. Not all information systems are equivalent. Some information systems, like the EHR, cause turmoil in a healthcare CE if they are offline. Other information systems, such as a strategic decision-support system, have less impact on the CE because there is no direct impact on patient care. Each information system should be evaluated to determine how critical it is, and a plan of action should be implemented. The plan should also include a prioritized list of applications and data used to determine which information system should be addressed first if multiple systems are down simultaneously. In a healthcare CE, the EHR and other patient care systems would be the top priority, with nonpatient, nonfinancial systems, such as patient satisfaction and chart deficiencies, at the bottom. The priorities would be different for the healthcare clearinghouses and health plans.

Data Recovery

When the information systems are again functional, data recovery must occur. **Data recovery** is the process of recouping any data that has been lost from the information system crash as well as the data that was obtained during the downtime. Data backups may be used to bring the information system back to its original state. Data captured during downtime must be entered into the information system to bring it up to date. Lost data should be recoverable from backup servers or other storage media. Depending on the time since the last backup, little or no data may be lost. The CE must have current backups of the database to be able to re-create the data. Information systems should have a utility to restore data from the backup server or other storage media onto the database. This process should be tested periodically to ensure that the utility is working appropriately.

The CE may want to consider establishing a hot site. A hot site is a remote location that is set-up with an exact duplicate of the information systems and data. With a hot site, a healthcare facility can switch from its local information systems to the hot site automatically preventing downtime and data loss (Dooling et al. 2016, 9).

CHECK YOUR UNDERSTANDING 13.2

1. Addressable standards _____.

   a. Are mandatory as written
   b. Allow an equivalent method to be used
   c. Are optional and can be ignored
   d. Are optional as long as all other requirements are met

2. A healthcare organization can consider size and complexity of the organization when developing the security plan. This flexibility is called _____.

   a. Technology neutral
   b. Administrative safeguard
   c. Scalability
   d. ePHI

3. Identify which of the following is an example of a security event.

   a. A patient is given a copy of health records that belong to another patient.
   b. Two employees have the same sign-in because they share the same position.
   c. ePHI is posted to the Internet.
   d. A hacker accesses ePHI.

4. Ensuring that data are not altered either during transmission across a network or during storage is _____.

   a. Integrity
   b. Accessibility
   c. Confidentiality
   d. Privacy

5. Human errors are _____.

   a. Unintentional
   b. Intentional
   c. Misunderstandings
   d. Threats

Business Associate Contracts or Other Arrangements

Business associates (BA) are organizations that conduct business on behalf of the CE. Examples of BAs are contract coders, application service providers, transcription services, and billing services. These associates require access to PHI (45 CFR 160, 162, and 164 2013) in order to do their jobs. Therefore, BAs are subject to the HIPAA Security Rule. In order for the business associates to gain access to the ePHI, they must assure the CE that they will protect the ePHI and will notify the CE of any failures to do so that result in a breach. There must be a business associate agreement (BAA) between the CE and the BA that meets the requirements established in HIPAA. BAs are liable for noncompliance with the HIPAA privacy and security rules just as if they are a CE.

The BAA spells out the BA's responsibilities and how it should protect PHI. The BAA should also allow the CE to terminate the contract if the BA fails to meet the responsibilities in the BAA.

Technical Safeguards

Technical safeguards are defined by the security rule as "the technology and the policy and procedures for its use that protect electronic protected health information and control access to it" (45 CFR 160, 162, and 164 2013). Technical safeguards use technology, policies, and procedures to protect ePHI from unauthorized access, destruction, or alteration. The policies, procedures, and documentation standards set by the CE define the requirements for the documentation required to show compliance with the technical safeguards. In this section access control systems and authentication, audit controls, and integrity are covered.

Access Control Systems and Authentication

Access controls are a computer software program designed to prevent unauthorized use of an information resource. CEs must define in their policies and procedures who can view, create, and modify data in an information system containing ePHI and use access controls to grant or limit those rights to employees who need them.

Types of Authentication

In **role-based authentication**, the functions and data available to the user are based on the role of the user. For example, a coder in the HIM department needs to review ePHI to properly code the health record; however, the coder would not need to add clinical information to the health record, and access controls would restrict the user from doing so. In role-based authentication, all coders have the same access, and all nurses have the same access. The nurses' functions and data will be different from those of the coders but will be the same for nurses in emergency department, medical-surgery nursing units, and labor and delivery units. Appropriate rights are granted based on role. As the coder's role in the CE changes, there must be a process in place to amend his or her rights.

In **user-based authentication**, the functions and data available are based on the needs of the individual user, not all users with the same job title. For example, some HIM technicians may have the authority to combine duplicate health record numbers, but others would not have access to this function. This method is more accurate than role-based authentication, but it is much more difficult to manage every user individually.

Context-based authentication controls access not only by the role that the employee has in the CE but also by the individual data elements and the context in which the user is working (Amatayakul and Walsh 2001). This is helpful when there are employees, such as nurses, who work in various units or have different roles at different times. For example, a nurse who works full-time in the quality improvement department may work at a nursing unit to earn some extra money for Christmas. As the ePHI and functions needed to perform these roles differ, the access that she has depends on her role at the time.

There may be times when users need to have access to data they are not normally allowed. This is called **emergency access procedure,** or "break the glass." This access usually occurs during a medical emergency and may require a second password or a reason for access. Even in an emergency situation, there must be a way to identify who activated the emergency access and why. The emergency access control system should require a brief note from the user "breaking the glass" to justify why the data were needed. The use of the emergency access procedure must be audited to ensure that the system is not abused (Amatayakul 2005b).

User Authentication Methods

Each user must have unique user identification that tracks that user's actions, although the specific identification technology is not mandated by HIPAA. Some CEs assign a **username**, a type of assigned user identification that may be based on the individual's name. For example, a username for Jane Doe could be jdoe or jane.doe. Others assign a number or other identification information to each user. Social security numbers should never be used for user identification because of concerns about identity theft.

Methods of access control—commonly categorized as something you know, something you have, or something you are—can be used alone or in combination. **One-factor authentication** utilizes one level of access control such as a username and password. There may be two requirements but they are both something you know. A one-factor authentication method could be something you have such as a token (described later in this section) as long as it is not used with another method (something you know or something you are). **Two-factor authentication** combines two different categories of access control, such as something you know and something you have. Common methods of access control—passwords, tokens, biometrics, and telephone callback—are discussed in the following sections.

Passwords are a series of characters that must be entered to authenticate user identity; they are commonly used in conjunction with a username or identifier. Passwords, something you know, are an example of one-factor authentication.

Strong passwords should not be easily guessed. Passwords based on commonly known personal information, such as the user's name, child's name, dog's name, or favorite sports team are examples of passwords that may be easy to crack. Information systems vary in their password requirements. Some require a minimum number of characters such as 7 or 8. The information systems frequently require two or more types of characters such as uppercase letters, lowercase letters, numbers, and symbols. Ideally, passwords should not contain a word found in any language. A strong password might look like Gsge$26Y. Passwords should be changed periodically and reuse of previous passwords should not be allowed at least for a period of time (Amatayakul and Walsh 2001). Many systems force the user to change the password periodically, such as every 30 days or once a year. The CE should establish strict rules for the use of passwords, including the format of the password, the frequency of change, and privacy of the password.

Policies should state that the password is confidential and cannot be shared with anyone else. Some users might write passwords down near the computer so they do not have to remember them. Users might also share their password with other users. For example, if a user forgot her password, she might ask another user to share his password, perhaps even out loud so that it is audible to others in the department and passers-by. Because audit trails, discussed in the next section, record not only what was done but also who did it, the user is responsible for every action under his or her username. Employees who violate policies related to passwords should be disciplined according to the policies of the CE.

One problem with passwords is that users often have too many of them to remember. Information systems throughout a CE frequently require different passwords, thus making it almost impossible for users to remember all of them. One way to overcome this issue is the use of single sign-on systems, which are designed so the user logs in one time. The user is then able to move from one application to another without entering another password. However, this single sign-on makes it even more important to protect the password so that the system is not at risk of unauthorized access.

A token used for security is usually a physical device that an authorized user of computer services is given to aid in authentication. Tokens may be used in conjunction with a password to provide two-factor authentication because a token and a password are two different types of authentications—something you know and something you have. Tokens used by themselves would be a one-factor authentication. Tokens are about the size of a credit card and contain a magnetic strip or chip that identifies the user. An algorithm displays a sequence of numbers in a liquid-crystal display (LCD) window. The characters in the LCD window change at specified intervals, for example, every minute. The user must enter the code on the token in order to access the system. The problem with the use of tokens is that the token may be lost, which will result in the user being unable to access the system and potential unauthorized access.

Biometric identifiers are based on a physical characteristic and are used to access the secure areas such as the data center or an information system. They are categorized as something you have. Retinal scans, fingerprints, facial recognition, and voice prints are biometric identifiers. This method is very secure because it very difficult to forge a person's identity using biometric data; however, biometric identifiers are not without their problems. For example, latex gloves may alter an individual's fingerprint enough to make it unrecognizable, preventing access to the information system.

Another form of entity authentication is telephone callback, which is most commonly used when users access the information system remotely, such as from their home. The user dials into the information system and the information system requests the phone number from which the call originates. If the phone number is an authorized number, the user is allowed into the information system. This method can be used by coders, transcriptionists, and others in the HIM department who work from home. This should not be the only form of entity authentication so that unauthorized users cannot call the phone number.

One of the requirements in the HIPAA Security Rule's technical safeguards is the automated log-off, which automatically logs the user off when a workstation is inactive for a specified period of time, such as five minutes. The amount of time should be a balance between the need for privacy and security and the need to give the user time to review the data. This automatic log-off helps prevent unauthorized users from accessing ePHI when an authorized user walks away from the computer without logging out of the information system. Prior to this log-off, a screen saver that blanks out the screen after a brief period of inactivity should be activated so that passing individuals would not see e-PHI.

Audit Controls

The CE must monitor the security program once it is implemented. One monitoring component required by HIPAA is implementing audit controls, the mechanisms that record and examine activity in information systems. Audit controls serve four purposes:

- Hold individual users personally responsible for their actions
- Use an investigation tool to identify cause of problem, the extent of the problem, and the way to restore the system back to normal operations
- Use real-time monitoring to identify breaches, technical problems, and other security issues quickly
- Watch for intrusions into the system so that the intrusion can be stopped before a breach occurs (Amatayakul 2004a)

Audit trails are the record of these system activities, such as log-in, log-out, unsuccessful log-ins, print, query, and other actions. It also records user-identification information and the date and time of the activity. System-level controls monitor log-on and log-off activity and applications accessed by the user. Application-level controls track what systems were used, what the user saw, and what he or she did. User-level controls record what actions the user initiated, such as resources accessed (Amatayakul 2004a). Review of the audit trail can identify potential security incidents. Audits should be scheduled periodically but can also be performed when a problem is suspected, such as when a patient complains that his or her PHI has been released or in response to a newspaper article or other suspected incidents.

The security audit process should include triggers that identify the need for a closer inspection. These trigger events cannot be used as the sole basis of the review, but they can significantly reduce the amount of reviews performed. Examples of triggers are:

- User has same last name as patient
- Patient is a celebrity, employee, or other public figure
- Access to sensitive diagnoses (psychiatric, acquired immunodeficiency syndrome, and so forth)
- Care providers accessing a patient in whose care they were not involved (AHIMA 2011)

Just because a trigger is activated does not mean that there has been a breach. For instance, with common surnames, such as Smith and Jones, it would be easy for an employee named Smith to care for a patient named Smith who was not related; however, it should be investigated. The patient may or may not be related to the employee—after all, there are many Smiths, and the practice will not catch all relatives, but it is a way to identify something that should be investigated.

CEs choose a variety of strategies for audits. Some turn the audit controls on randomly so that the user never knows if his or her actions are being recorded (Amatayakul 2004a). Others record every action all the time. Whatever the strategy of capture, the data must be audited. This audit should be designed to include a review of the user's actions at different days, times of day, and locations. The security rule does not mandate a specific number of audits, but the CE should base the volume on the size and complexity of the CE. The findings should be reported all the way up the organizational chart to the board of directors.

Audit controls are not without their problems. One is that the audit controls of the various information systems vary in their level of sophistication. Some are only able to record log-ins and not the specific records accessed. Also, recording audit-trail data consumes resources, which may slow down the system and require upgrading the file server. To protect the audit-log data from alteration or destruction, it should be stored on a different server than that for the ePHI. In addition, to prevent alteration or destruction, access to the audit log should be restricted to a limited number of users who have a business need to access the information. Another advantage to the audit-trail data being stored on a separate server is that the increase in storage space will allow longer retention of the data as needed (Amatayakul 2004b). This separation improves the security of the data and provides the necessary storage capability to store the data for long periods of time. HIPAA requires that documentation of the audit activities be retained for six years.

Audit-reduction tools review the audit trail and compare it to criteria specified by the CE, which eliminates routine entries such as the periodic backups (Amatayakul 2004b). This means that backups and other routine maintenance would be removed from the reports from which audits are conducted. The audit-reduction tools can also look for behavior outside the norm. For example, if a nurse works only on the weekend and suddenly logs in on Tuesday, this would be cause for review. There may be a legitimate reason, such as the nurse changed shifts with another nurse, but the nurse could also have been snooping in a neighbor's ePHI. Finally, there are attack signature-detection tools that look for a specific sequence of events that may indicate a security problem, such as multiple failed attempts to log in to the system or an employee who normally accesses the information from the CE accessing it remotely. Actions flagged by the audit-reduction tools should only be viewed as potential problems that should be investigated because there are legitimate reasons for variances and failed log-in attempts. For example, a coder may be coding late at night because he or she may be taking classes during the day.

A review of the audit trail is not the only auditing that should be performed. Another means of auditing is touring the CE to ensure that security policies and procedures are being followed. This would be done by the CSO or a designee. Examples of actions that can be monitored in this way include ensuring that monitors are turned away from public areas, users log out of the system when stepping away from the computer, fax machines with PHI are not in public areas, and no signs of passwords being written down or shared.

Integrity

Technology has advanced to a point at which an unauthorized user can capture data in transit and alter it. Therefore, CEs must confirm the integrity of data passed across a network. Integrity is the security principle that protects data from inappropriate modification or corruption. This includes both unintentional and intentional modifications and destructions. Unintentional modifications and destruction could occur if the wrong data are destroyed, the wrong backup is used to restore data, or an electrical fire destroys the computer. Examples of intentional modification and destruction include intentional deletion of data, induction of virus software, and changing the amount that the employee owes the healthcare facility for treatment provided. Data integrity is preserved when the message received is confirmed as identical to the one sent. Integrity can be validated with checksum validation, defined as a "sum derived from the bits of a segment of computer data that is calculated before and after transmission or storage to assure that the data is free from errors or tampering" (Merriam-Webster 2017a).

Transmission security involves mechanisms designed to protect ePHI while the data are being transmitted between two points. These points can be internal or external to the CE. Encryption is frequently used to protect data as it moves across networks by preventing ePHI from being read by anyone with access to data during transmission. Encryption converts data from a readable form to unintelligible text. This is done with the science of cryptography, using mathematics to convert data into unintelligible data and back again. If encrypted data are intercepted during transmission, the health information is protected because the individual who intercepted the data cannot view it. Only authorized users are able to convert the data back into a readable format.

There are two categories of encryption: symmetric and asymmetric. Symmetric encryption assigns a secret key to data. The computer sending the data uses the key to turn the message into the unintelligible format. The receiving computer uses the same key to revert the data back into its original format. In asymmetric encryption, an extremely popular method also known as public key infrastructure, two keys are used. The sending computer uses a private key to convert the data. The public key is provided to the computer with whom the sender is communicating. This public key converts the data into a readable format. A licensing agency called a certification authority confirms the receiver's identity and relationship to the public key. In doing this, the certification authority issues a digital certificate to the receiver. This digital certificate is part of the integrity process because it ensures that plaintext messages are received without any alterations. This encryption and decryption occurs instantaneously in the background. A public key infrastructure familiar to most people is the secure socket layer (SSL), which is used to transmit protected information when conducting business transactions over the Internet (Rinehart-Thompson 2016, 266). In public key encryption, the user gives the same public key to everyone who should have access to the system.

CEs rely heavily on networks to share information. These networks frequently allow users across the CE's campus and beyond to access ePHI. HIPAA mandates the use of network security methods to protect the ePHI as it travels across the network. Network security uses technology to protect the data transmitted across the network including firewalls and encryption.

A firewall is a computer system or a combination of systems that provide a security barrier or support an access control policy between two networks or between a network and any other traffic outside the network. This gatekeeper is physically located between the routes of a public network like the Internet and those of a private network. All data entering and leaving the CE must pass through the firewall, a process called packet filtering (Novell 2004, 25). The firewall evaluates the data based on user-defined rules. If the data pass the evaluation, the data are allowed in or out of the network. The firewall can be implemented in many ways. It can attach confidentiality messages to all e-mails that leave the CE, limit the size or type of file entering the CE's network, and can limit access to specific websites. The firewall may even scan the data to determine if a virus is attached to prevent a virus from being brought into the CE and spreading.

Another way to protect data as it is transmitting is a virtual private network (VPN). A VPN creates a tunnel through the Internet that allows data to be shared securely. It allows ePHI to be shared over a public network like the Internet and still be protected.

Intrusion detection systems monitor networks and information systems to catch hackers and other intruders. These systems identify security issues. An intrusion detection system is flexible in that it allows the CE to customize the monitoring by adjusting the level of detection that the system is performing (Dill et al. 2016). The intrusion detection system assists the information system staff in monitoring the traffic on the Internet to ensure that it is legitimate and does not contain anything that will harm the ePHI or other data stored in the databases such as malware (addressed later in this chapter). Once a potential threat is identified, then the appropriate steps must be taken to not only protect the data but also keep a similar threat from happening again.

CHECK YOUR UNDERSTANDING 13.3

1. An example of a technical safeguard is _____.

   a. Locked door
   b. Card key
   c. Policy and procedure
   d. Audit control

2. Converting data into unintelligible text is known as _____.

   a. Firewall
   b. Encryption
   c. Mitigation
   d. Intrusion detection system

3. Identify the type of authentication used when all coders have the same access to ePHI and functionality.

   a. User-based
   b. Role-based
   c. Context-based
   d. Both user-based and role-based

4. The access control used in the EHR requires a username and password. This is an example of _____.

   a. Single-factor authentication
   b. Biometrics
   c. Two-factor authentication
   d. Tokens

5. Our computer system just notified us that Mary Burchfield has just looked up another patient with the same last name. This notification is called a(n) _____.

   a. Trigger
   b. Audit reduction tool
   c. Integrity
   d. Audit control

Malicious Software

Malicious software, also known as malware, is designed to harm a computer. Some malware is more of a nuisance, whereas others destroy data or other files that may prevent the computer from operating or can steal data. HIPAA mandates that CEs take steps to protect data and information systems from malware. If malware is introduced into computers in the HIM department, it spreads and can ultimately mean that most, if not all, of the computers in the department are affected. If the computers are unusable, then most of the work in the department would be at a standstill. In this event, the contingency plan discussed earlier would be implemented. HIM professionals can help protect their computers by being cautious when opening attachments to e-mails or when using links within e-mails, by going to a company's website and logging in rather than using links in e-mail, and by otherwise being careful in what e-mails are opened, what software is downloaded, webpages that are visited, and so forth. Malware can also harm biomedical devices. A biomedical device is "an article, instrument, apparatus or machine that is used in the prevention, diagnosis or treatment of illness or disease, or for detecting, measuring, restoring, correcting or modifying the structure or function of the body for some health purpose" (WHO 2017). Examples of biomedical devices are pacemakers and fetal monitoring systems. They pose a significant security risk because they frequently have vulnerabilities such as no antivirus software, no intrusion prevention system, and outdated operating systems (WHO 2017). As discussed in chapter 10, one of the benefits of telehealth is the ability of medical devices to report results to the healthcare provider via the internet. However, this technology also enables device vulnerabilities to be exploited by hacker.

Antimalware and other software packages are designed to identify and stop or clean up malicious software, which includes viruses, worms, Trojans, bots, spyware, phishing, and ransomware.

Virus

A virus "propagates by inserting a copy of itself into and becoming part of another program. It spreads from one computer to another" (Cisco n.d.). The term "virus" is commonly used to indicate malware, but it is technically a specific type of malware. Viruses are designed to do a variety of destructive behaviors. For example, viruses can destroy data or damage the software that starts the computer. Viruses are frequently spread through e-mail through an attachment that is activated when opened. They can spread through the e-mail server and even the user's contact list in e-mail.

Worms

A worm is "standalone software and does not require a host program or human help to propagate" (Cisco n.d.). The worm is programmed to install itself onto a computer attached to a computer network and then moves to all computers on the network. It may harm the system or initiate a denial of service (DoS). The worm frequently spreads through e-mail attachments as well as files downloaded from the Internet. The worm spreads to the e-mail server and then to all of the users listed in the contact list in e-mail.

Trojans

A Trojan is a type of malware that gives the appearance that it is perfectly legitimate software. This tricks the user into accessing it. Once accessed, the Trojan can perform a variety of actions, including pop-ups, deleting data, creating back doors, or other actions (Cisco n.d.).

Bots

Bots perform automated tasks, such as gathering information and instant messaging, thus relieving a person the responsibility of doing it. These actions can be good or bad, depending on who initiates the bots and for what purposes (Cisco n.d.). A bot can be used to locate and access information stored on the computer such as passwords, usernames, credit card numbers, and other information. It can also be used to record keystrokes. The bot can be introduced into the computer by e-mail or social media. The computer can be protected from bots in many ways including the use of firewalls, keeping software up to date, and using antimalware software (Norton n.d.).

Spyware

Spyware may be used to track keystrokes and passwords, monitor websites visited, or other actions and report these actions to the designated person or organization. Spyware is often classified as system monitors, adware, or tracking cookies. Computers are frequently infected with spyware through e-mail and downloaded files. The spyware may slow down the computer system because of its increased activity. It contributes to identity theft and other breaches of privacy by sharing information. Essentially, spyware records computer usage without the user's knowledge and then provides this information to someone with whom the user may not want to share the information. Antimalware software would find and delete the spyware.

Phishing

Phishing is "a scam by which an e-mail user is duped into revealing personal or confidential information which the scammer can use illicitly" (Merriam-Webster 2017b). The e-mail received may look official, but it is not. Its intent is to capture usernames, passwords, account numbers, and any other personal information.

Users should be cautious in giving out confidential information such as passwords, credit card numbers, and social security numbers as many requests for this information received via e-mail is a phishing scam.

Ransomware

Ransomware is a type of malicious software that prohibits access to information systems in an organization. The ransomware programmer may demand money before they will deactivate the ransomware. Unfortunately, this type of malware is gaining in use. Use of ransomware rose by 250 percent in 2017 (Cuthbertson 2017). This can have a major impact on a healthcare provider if it is unable to access the information needed in order to care for its patients. One hospital infected by ransomware paid the ransom in order to regain access to the hospital information system and EHR. It was unable to access the electronic health information for 10 days, causing the return to the paper health record (AHIMA 2017a). When the National Health Service in the United Kingdom was attacked by ransomware in May 2017, patient visits and surgeries had to be canceled (NBC News 2017). Antiransomware software is available to protect computers from ransomware. Other ways of protecting a healthcare facility's computers from ransomware include:

- Employees should use their own devices and use a guest network for personal use (surfing Internet, checking personal e-mail, and so forth).
- Isolate the infected computer immediately to help prevent it from spreading to other computers.
- Store critical data on network drive, not the computer's hard drive. (Butler 2016)

CHECK YOUR UNDERSTANDING 13.4

1. Which type of malware can capture keystrokes?

   a. Spyware
   b. Trojan
   c. Virus
   d. Worm

2. The term used to describe viruses and spyware is called _____.

   a. Malicious software
   b. Spiteful software
   c. Masqueraders
   d. Macros

3. Loss of data due to malware being downloaded onto a computer may be caused by which of the following?

   a. Spyware
   b. Denial of service
   c. Virus
   d. Phishing

4. Identify the type of malicious software that denies an organization access to its own information system.

   a. Ransomware
   b. Phishing
   c. Denial of service
   d. Worm

5. Identify the type of malicious software that appears to be legitimate but then creates pop-ups or other actions.

   a. Ransomware
   b. Trojan
   c. Denial of service
   d. Worm

Physical Safeguards

Physical safeguards are an important part of security. The Security Rule defines physical safeguards as "physical measures, policies, and procedures to protect a CE's electronic information systems, and related buildings and equipment, from natural and environmental hazards and unauthorized intrusion" (45 CFR 160, 162, and 164 2013).

Physical safeguards protect the hardware and software related to the ePHI. The physical plant and equipment must be protected from intentional and unintentional tampering or destruction.

The hardware must be protected from natural disasters such as tornadoes and floods. It must also be protected from fire, theft, and intentional tampering. The policies and procedures should also document how the CE is protecting the equipment from unauthorized access, tampering, and theft. Physical safeguards should include not only the computers and other hardware but also backup tapes. The required physical safeguards and their implementation specifications are listed in table 13.2.

Table 13.2.   Implementation specifications for HIPAA physical standards

Standards	Implementation Specifications
Facility access control	• Contingency operations • Facility security plan • Access control and validation procedures • Maintenance records
Workstation location and use	• None
Workstation security	• None
Device and media controls	• Disposal • Media reuse • Accountability • Data backup and storage

Source: Adapted from 45 CFR 160, 162, and 164 2013.

Facility Access Controls

The CE must implement facility access controls, which limit physical access to the data center and software to only authorized information system staff. Facility access controls must be documented in the policies and procedures. Access to the data center can be controlled by card keys, access codes, or other control methods. The fact that an individual is a member of the workforce does not authorize him or her to be in the data center. Access to the data center should be limited to individuals with a business need, such computer technicians and employees who work in the data center. There must also be policies and procedures regarding the handling of contractors and service technicians. In the event of a system outage, the appropriate staff and contractors must be able to access the system so that the system can be operational as quickly as possible. Individuals with authorized access should wear a picture identification tag at all times. Visitors to the area, such as computer vendors, consultants, and computer technicians, frequently are required to sign in and be escorted while in the data center.

Cameras may be used to record individuals going into the data center and other areas where hardware is located. The video can be used to determine who had access to the data center or other critical areas in the event of a security incident.

Some of the physical safeguards are as simple as locking doors, using an alarm system, bolting the equipment to a desk, and using surge suppressors. Other safeguards include monitoring the temperature of the room so that the computers do not become too hot or too cold because extreme temperatures can damage the computers. There should also be a system in place to extinguish fires.

These physical safeguards will need to be maintained and updated as appropriate to ensure that they continue to protect the ePHI. Examples of this maintenance include installing new security cameras, changing locks, or knocking down walls to expand the size of the data center. The CE must maintain documentation of the preventive maintenance and repairs made. This documentation can be as simple as a logbook or as complicated as a specialized database, depending on the size and complexity of the CE.

Workstation Use

Workstations include not only desktop computers but also handheld devices, laptops, and other pieces of equipment that manage ePHI. Workstations must be protected from unauthorized access. This can be accomplished in a number of ways, such as placing the workstations behind closed doors or other types of barriers. Black-out screens can be used to prevent unauthorized users from seeing the content on the screen when walking by the computer or looking at it over the shoulder of the user. Policies and procedures should be in place to protect the workstations from viruses, breaches of privacy, and other practices. Workstations—including computers, tablets, and laptops that access ePHI—should be used appropriately by the workforce members. It is up to the CE to define what is appropriate.

It is easy for thieves to pick up computers or other pieces of hardware and walk off with them. To protect hardware, security measures can include bolting hardware to desks and locking doors. Security of mobile devices is discussed later in this chapter.

Device and Media Controls

Media, which includes computer hard drives and removable digital storage, must also be protected from loss and destruction. Examples of removable digital storage are external hard drives, thumb drives, CDs, and optical disks. Media that store ePHI must have policies and procedures that control its movement and storage. Because media is small and easily portable, it is easy for employees to move the media and for it to get lost. It is also easily stolen. The CE could create a log to track receipt or removal of the media so that an individual is responsible for the media.

With the advent of portable devices such as tablets and mobile phones, tracking media is becoming more and more difficult because the devices are moved around for use in patient care. The actions, and not the location, of the workstation matter, so the policies should apply to computers at employee's workstations and other locations. It is easy to lose CDs and other media that store ePHI, so CEs must have a policy in place to protect them from loss or destruction. The media must be tracked throughout the CE. This can be done by creating a log that requires staff to check out the media, much like checking a book out of the library or tracking a health record.

Once the media is no longer needed, there should be a formal process for its disposal. Workstations and other media cannot just be thrown away or sold. If ePHI is disposed of improperly, these computers could be found at garage sales and thrift shops still containing this confidential information. Deletion of the ePHI stored on the media does not render it inaccessible; there are utilities, or software programs, that can undelete files. Because of this capability, the media itself needs to be destroyed, or the media should be degaussed. **Degaussing** is application of a magnetic field to the media to render the data on it useless. Degaussing renders data impossible to recover and is not reversible. Another method for sanitizing the hard drive of a computer is overwriting (writing data over the existing data) the data stored on the hard drive. The data may have to be overwritten multiple times in order to prevent recovery. CDs, USB drives, and other media may also be pulverized.

There may be times that the CE wishes to reuse media on which ePHI is stored. For example, workstations frequently may be moved from one location to another to make way for more powerful workstations. The security rule allows this reuse if the ePHI is removed according to policy. Electronic media, computers, and other hardware may be moved within the CE, but there must be a record of where all of the workstations and media are at any given time and who is responsible for the equipment. When a computer has ePHI stored on it, the data should be backed up before the computer is moved. Another method of protecting ePHI when computers are moved is to store the data on a network so that the ePHI is not at risk. If ePHI is stored on the workstation, that data must be removed before the computer is transferred from one location to another or before it is scrapped or sold.

Mobile Security

Mobile devices take many forms, including tablets, smartphones, and thumb drives, and are easily stolen, lost, or misplaced. Every item should have a property control tag attached so that the hardware can be tracked as it moves throughout the CE. This property control tag assigns a unique identifier to the hardware, allowing it to be inventoried. For example, the healthcare facility would know that hardware 12345 is a personal computer that is assigned to Mary Smith in the HIM department. The CE may also want to investigate security options for portable devices such as those that monitor the location of devices. When an inventory is performed, the CE knows exactly where pieces of hardware should be located and what has been moved. Best practices for the use of mobile devices in a CE include:

- Defining who owns the devices—the CE or the user
- Defining who owns the data collected using the mobile device

- Requiring written acknowledgment regarding rules related to mobile devices
- Specifying when mobile devices are the appropriate hardware
- Establishing rules of behavior for authorized use of mobile devices
- Applying appropriate technologies to destroy sensitive information
- Defining what constitutes sensitive information
- Establishing specific procedures for the reporting of device loss or theft
- Using appropriate data management techniques, such as backup and data transfer
- Not storing PHI on mobile devices
- Monitoring mobile devices to ensure safeguards are in place
- Utilizing encryption
- Monitoring of policies, procedures, equipment, and software (AHIMA 2012)

Appropriate steps should be taken to investigate all lost and stolen devices. Staff members who use mobile devices should be trained on the associated privacy and security responsibilities, including physical security, logging off, and other operations.

Some CEs allow healthcare providers to access ePHI on their personal tablet or phone. This practice is known as bring your own device (BYOD). If BYOD is used, there must be policies and procedures in place to address security issues such as encryption and remote wipe. Remote wipe is used when data must be deleted from the mobile device remotely because it has been lost or stolen (Primeau 2017). It could also be used when an employee ceases to work at the healthcare facility.

Fire and Natural Disasters

As discussed earlier, media can be destroyed by natural disaster or fire. Healthcare facilities should have contracts with restoration companies in place in advance of a natural disaster so that efforts to repair the damage from water, fire, mold, chemical spills, and more can occur quickly. These types of events support the need for backups as described earlier. One CE that implemented a document management system properly created a backup file of all of the optical disks. This is a problem because this CE stored the backup file 15 feet from the original disk. The HIM department, where the optical disks were stored, was located in the basement, so if there had been a flood or other disaster both copies would have been lost. Backup files should be stored on an off-site server that would not be at risk for the same disaster. For example, a CE in Georgia could have its data backed up on an information system in Montana. This eliminates the possibility of the same event damaging both the original and the backup databases.

Penalties

The oversight of the HIPAA Security Rule has been given to the Office of Inspector General, which has the right to award civil and criminal penalties. These penalties are awarded when the individual knowingly and willfully violates the security rules. There are four tiers of civil penalties, which are shown in table 13.3.

Table 13.3.   Civil penalties for security rule violations

Violation Category—Section 1176(a)(1)	Each Violation	All Such Violations of an Identical Provision in a Calendar Year
(A) Did Not Know	$100–$50,000	$1,500,000
(B) Reasonable Cause	$1,000–$50,000	$1,500,000
(C) (i) Willful Neglect—Corrected	$10,000–$50,000	$1,500,000
(C) (ii) Willful Neglect—Not Corrected	$50,000	$1,500,000

Source: AHIMA 2013.

Certifications

There are three privacy or security certifications: Certified in Healthcare Privacy and Security (CHPS), Certified Information Security Manager (CISM), and Certified Information Systems Security Professional (CISSP). The CHPS is designed specifically for healthcare, whereas the CISSP and CISM are general security certifications.

Certified in Healthcare Privacy and Security

The **Certified in Healthcare Privacy and Security (CHPS)** credential demonstrates advanced privacy and security skills. These advanced privacy and security skills exceed those in the Registered Health Information Administrator or Registered Health Information Technician examinations. It is sponsored by the American Health Information Management Association (AHIMA). The CHPS examination includes both technical and managerial issues, including a number of topics related to privacy and security. Figure 13.2 shows AHIMA's CHPS competency domains.

Figure 13.2. CHPS domains

Domain 1: Ethical, Legal, and Regulatory Issues/External Environmental Assessment (23–27%)

Domain 2: Program Management and Administration (23–27%)

Domain 3: Information Technology/Physical and Technical Safeguards (23–27%)

Domain 4: Investigation, Compliance, and Enforcement (23–27%)

Source: AHIMA 2017b.

Certified Information Systems Security Professional

The **Certified Information Systems Security Professional (CISSP)** certification is sponsored by the International Information Systems Security Certification Consortium [(ISC)^2]. It is a generic security certification and therefore is not healthcare specific [(ISC)^2 n.d.].

Certified Information Security Manager

The **Certified Information Security Manager (CISM)** is sponsored by ISACA. It is an international examination that is designed for leaders in security who oversee the security programs of organizations (ISACA 2017).

CHECK YOUR UNDERSTANDING 13.5

1. The oversight of the HIPAA security rule is assigned to _____.

    a. AHIMA
    b. Office of the Inspector General
    c. CMS
    d. Business associates

2. Identify a facility access control.

    a. Contingency plan
    b. Backup
    c. Card key
    d. Media controls

3. Remote wipe is used to _____.

    a. Routinely delete ePHI when using BYOD.
    b. Delete ePHI in mobile devices when they are stolen.
    c. Eliminate malicious software.
    d. Prepare an information system for reinstalling data from a backup.

4. A pacemaker is an example of a(n) _____.

    a. Biomedical device
    b. Mobile device
    c. Media control
    d. Remote wipe

5. AHIMA has an advanced certification that covers security. Identify the exam.

    a. Certified information security manager
    b. Certified information systems security specialist
    c. Certified in healthcare privacy and security
    d. Registered health information technician

Real-World Case

Fountain View Hospice is an inpatient hospice that has an EHR. Because of a hurricane, the town, including the hospice, was flooded. Patients had to be evacuated and the data center was underwater. The hospice backs up its files daily and the files are stored at a vendor site across town. The vendor's office was unaffected by the flood, so the backup files are safe. The vendor does not have the EHR application. The flood waters have receded and the building is undergoing renovations. The vendor has stated that there is no way to recreate their application and so a full implementation of the EHR will be necessary and could take a year or more. In the meantime, the hospice will have to operate using paper health records. The hospice will have to pay to select and implement the new information system as well as manage the paper health record.

CHAPTER REVIEW

1. Identify where ePHI is stored.

    a. Voicemail
    b. Paper health record
    c. Fax machines and EHR
    d. EHR

2. A former employee is angry at the CE because he was terminated. He hacked into the EHR and destroyed ePHI. What type of threat is this?

    a. Purposeful
    b. Intentional
    c. Calculated
    d. Premeditated

3. Identify the true statement about integrity.

    a. The CE only has to address data integrity for data stored in the database.
    b. The CE only has to address data integrity for data transmitted across a network.
    c. The CE has to address data integrity for data stored and in transmission.
    d. HIPAA does not require CEs to address data integrity.

(Continued)

4. HIPAA security standards whereby the CE can determine if the standard is reasonable and appropriate is known as _____.

   a. Addressable
   b. Optional
   c. Noncompulsory
   d. Voluntary

5. Administrative safeguards include which of the following?

   a. Emergency access procedure
   b. Mechanism to authenticate ePHI
   c. Security awareness and training
   d. Audit controls

6. Access controls are classified as something you know, something you have, and something you _____.

   a. Are
   b. Choose
   c. Design
   d. Develop

7. A username and password is an example of a _____.

   a. One-factor authentication
   b. Two-factor authentication
   c. Call back
   d. Single sign-on

8. One of the nurses in the quality management department has decided to work a few shifts on the nursing units in order to earn some extra money. When she logs in with her normal sign-in, she has certain functionality; when she logs in differently to work on the nursing unit, she has different functionality. This is known as _____.

   a. Role-based authentication
   b. User-based authentication
   c. Context-based authentication
   d. Emergency access procedure

9. Identify the true statement about audit logs.

   a. Audit logs should be stored on a different server than the ePHI.
   b. Audit logs only capture actions that are outside the norm.
   c. Audit logs monitor only user actions.
   d. Audit logs should be available to a wide range of employees to facilitate audits.

10. Firewalls are part of _____.

   a. Physical security
   b. Network security
   c. Administrative safeguards
   d. Encryption

References

45 CFR 160, 162, and 164. HIPAA administrative simplification regulation text. 2013 (unofficial version, as amended through March 26). https://www.hhs.gov/sites/default/files/hipaa-simplification-201303.pdf.

AHIMA e HIM Work Group on e-Discovery. 2006. New electronic discovery civil rule. *Journal of AHIMA* 77(8). http://bok.ahima.org/doc?oid=106246#.WlKc_uRy5jp.

AHIMA 2007 Privacy and Security Practice Council. 2008. How to react to a security incident. *Journal of AHIMA* 79(1):66–70. http://library.ahima.org/xpedio/groups/public/documents/ahima/bok1_036247.hcsp?dDocName=bok1_036247.

Amatayakul, M. 2001. Selecting Strong Passwords (HIPAA On the Job series). http://bok.ahima.org/doc?oid=59280#.WlKrGORy5jo.

Amatayakul, M. 2004a. Kick starting the security risk analysis. *Journal of AHIMA* 75(7):46–47.

Amatayakul, M. 2004b. The trouble with audit controls. *Journal of AHIMA* 75(9):78–79.

Amatayakul, M. 2005a. Reporting security incidents. *Journal of AHIMA* 76(3):60.

Amatayakul, M. 2005b. Access controls: Striking the right balance. *Journal of AHIMA* 76(1):56–57.

Amatayakul, M. 2017. *Health IT and EHRs: Principles and Practice*. Chicago: AHIMA.

Amatayakul, M. and T. Walsh. 2001. Selecting strong passwords (HIPAA on the job). *Journal of AHIMA* 72(9):16A–D.

American Health Information Management Association (AHIMA). 2012. Practice Brief: Mobile device security (updated). *Journal of AHIMA* 83(4):50–55.

American Health Information Management Association (AHIMA). 2013. Analysis of Modifications to the HIPAA Privacy, Security, Enforcement, and Breach Notification Rules under the Health Information Technology for Economic and Clinical Health Act and the Genetic Information Nondiscrimination Act; Other Modifications to the HIPAA Rules. http://library.ahima.org/xpedio/groups/public/documents/ahima/bok1_050067.pdf.

American Health Information Management Association. 2017a. LA Hospital Pays Hackers After Ransomware Attack. *Journal of AHIMA* 87(4):11.

American Health Information Management Association (AHIMA). 2017b. Commission on Certification for Health Informatics and Information Management (CCHIIM) Candidate Guide. http://www.ahima.org/~/media/AHIMA/Files/Certification/Candidate_Guide.ashx.

American Health Information Management Association. 2011. Security audits of electronic health information (updated). *Journal of AHIMA* 82(3):46–50.

Burrington-Brown, J. 2003. Sorting out employee sanctions. *Journal of AHIMA* 74(6):53–54.

Butler, M. 2016. Tips for Preventing and Responding to a Ransomware Attack. *Journal of AHIMA* http://bok.ahima.org/doc?oid=301485#.WTBYtuQ2xjo.

Centers for Medicare and Medicaid Services. 2007a. Security standards: Implementation for the Small Provider (HIPAA security series). https://www.hhs.gov/sites/default/files/ocr/privacy/hipaa/administrative/securityrule/smallprovider.pdf.

Centers for Medicare and Medicaid Services. 2007b. Security standards: Basics of risk analysis and risk management (HIPAA security series). https://www.hhs.gov/sites/default/files/ocr/privacy/hipaa/administrative/securityrule/riskassessment.pdf.

Centers for Medicare and Medicaid Services. 2007c. Security Standards: Physical Safeguards. (HIPAA security series). https://www.hhs.gov/sites/default/files/ocr/privacy/hipaa/administrative/securityrule/physsafeguards.pdf.

Centers for Medicare and Medicaid Services. 2007d. Security Standards: Technical Safeguards. https://www.hhs.gov/sites/default/files/ocr/privacy/hipaa/administrative/securityrule/techsafeguards.pdf.

Cisco. n.d. What Is the Difference: Viruses, Worms, Trojans, and Bots? Accessed January 7, 2018. http://www.cisco.com/web/about/security/intelligence/virus-worm-diffs.html.

Cuthbertson, A. 2017. Ransomware attacks rise 250 percent in 2017, hitting U.S. hardest. http://www.newsweek.com/ransomware-attacks-rise-250-2017-us-wannacry-614034.

Davis, J. B. 2003. *HIPAA Compliance Manual: A Comprehensive Guide to the Administrative Simplification Provisions for Health Care Professionals*. Los Angeles: PMIC.

Derhak, M. 2003. Uncovering the enemy within: Utilizing incident response, forensics. *In Confidence* 11(9):1–2. http://library.ahima.org/doc?oid=59731#.WoN3deRy5jo.

Dill, M. W., S. Lucci, and T. Walsh. 2016. Understanding cybersecurity: A primer for HIM professionals. *Journal of AHIMA* 87(4). http://bok.ahima.org/doc?oid=301408.

Dooling, J. A., T. Rihanek, D. Warner, and L. A. Wiedemann. 2016. Disaster Planning and Recovery Toolkit. http://bok.ahima.org/PdfView?oid=301964.

Hjort, B. 2003. Practice brief: HIPAA privacy and security training (updated). http://library.ahima.org /xpedio/groups/public/documents/ahima/bok1_048509.hcsp?dDocName=bok1_048509.

International Information Systems Security Certification Consortium [(ISC)²]. n.d. CISSP®—Certified Information Systems Security Professional. https://www.isc2.org/cissp/default.aspx.

ISACA. 2017. Certified Information Security Manager (CISM). http://www.isaca.org/Certification/CISM -Certified-Information-Security-Manager/Pages/default.aspx.

Merriam-Webster. 2017a. Checksum. https://www.merriam-webster.com/dictionary/checksum.

Merriam-Webster. 2017b. Phishing. https://www.merriam-webster.com/dictionary/phishing.

Novell. 2004. Proxy and Firewall Overview and Planning Guide. https://www.novell.com/documentation /nbm38/pdfdoc/overview/overview.pdf.

NBCNews. 2017. Why "WannaCry" Malware Caused Chaos for National Health Service in U.K." https: //www.nbcnews.com/news/world/why-wannacry-malware-caused-chaos-national-health-service-u -k-n760126.

Norton. n.d. What are bots? Accessed January 7, 2018. https://us.norton.com/internetsecurity-malware -what-are-bots.html.

Primeau, D. 2017. How Small Organizations Handle HIPAA Compliance. http://library.ahima.org /doc?oid=302074#.WlgMFeRy5jo.

Rinehart-Thompson, L. A. 2016. Data Privacy and Confidentiality. Chapter 9 in *Health Information Management Technology: An Applied Approach*, 5th ed. Edited by N. B. Sayles and L.L. Gordon. Chicago: AHIMA.

University of Alabama at Birmingham (UAB). n.d. UAB Data Classification Rule. Accessed 1/7/2018. https://www.uab.edu/it/home/data-classification.

World Health Organization (WHO). 2017. Medical Devices. http://www.who.int/medical_devices /definitions/en/.

Information and Data Governance

Learning Objectives

- Compare and contrast information governance (IG) with data governance (DG) and their relative significance.
- Explain the importance of enterprise information management (EIM) and why it has become essential
- Explain the reasons why health information has become a valued strategic asset.
- Summarize the eight key principles of Information Governance Principles for Healthcare (IGPHC).
- Identify tools that can be used to assist a healthcare organization in implementing an IG program.

Key Terms

Big data
Business intelligence (BI)
Charter
Clinical documentation
   improvement (CDI)
Collaboration
Data governance (DG)
Data silo
Data steward
Data stewardship

e-discovery process
Effectiveness
Efficiency
Enterprise information
   management (EIM)
Information asset inventory
Information governance (IG)
Information governance steering
   committee

Information technology
   governance (ITG)
Situation, background,
   assessment, recommendation
   (SBAR)
Stakeholder
Triple Aim
Valued strategic asset

Over the last several decades, the healthcare industry has been collecting and storing massive amounts of data thanks to the electronic health record (EHR). The healthcare industry is also undergoing significant changes in reimbursement, sharing of information through health information exchange, standardization, use of technology, and more. To be successful, the healthcare facility must be able to manage its clinical and administrative data and turn it into useful information that can support the healthcare facility as it undergoes the aforementioned changes. The healthcare facility must have the information needed to make decisions, negotiate contracts, provide quality patient care, and more. Information systems can help turn data into information; however, they too must be managed, as demonstrated throughout this text.

As discussed in chapter 1, the terms "data" and "information" are often used interchangeably, but there are important differences between them that will be illustrated in this chapter as IG and DG are discussed.

As this chapter will show, the control and management—that is, governance—of data and information also have subtle but definitive differences. This chapter will further explain data and information governance, enterprise information management, the Information Governance Adoption Model, and the role of the health information management (HIM) professional in governance activities.

Data and Information Governance

Governance is the establishment of policies for managing organization assets and the continual monitoring of their proper implementation. Data governance (DG) is the overall management of the availability, usability, integrity, and security of the data employed in an organization or enterprise (Data Governance Institute 2013). It is a specific enterprise information management (EIM) function that supports coordination among all other EIM functions. It is the enterprise authority that ensures control and accountability for enterprise data through the establishment of decision rights and data policies and standards that are implemented and monitored through a formal structure of assigned roles, responsibilities, and accountabilities. (EIM will be discussed later in this chapter.) Information governance (IG) is an organization-wide framework for managing information throughout its lifecycle and for supporting the organization's strategy, operations, regulatory, legal, risk, and environmental requirements (AHIMA n.d.a). The American Health Information Management Association (AHIMA) IG infographic, figure 14.1, demonstrates the differences between DG and IG.

DG and IG programs rely on quality data and information for the following reasons:

- To make informed decisions—An informed decision requires a description of the problem at hand; information about the background and circumstances; understanding of any regulatory, legal, and or ethical requirements; and knowledge or creativity to determine solutions. For example, data and information can be used to identify patient care trends, help determine staffing needs, monitor equipment and supplies inventories, and budgetary support for all functions.

- To evaluate patient care and population health—It is important to know how well an individual patient is responding to treatment, if their quality of life has improved because of the treatment, if all of the patients saw their health improve due to a specific therapy, and how that information translates to the local community and possibly state or nation. For example, quality data and information are necessary to evaluate patient treatment outcomes to determine the extent of health disparities and how they compare to state and national levels.

- To evaluate business processes—Efficiency and effectiveness are two buzzwords that are used frequently in healthcare. Effectiveness is the degree to which stated outcomes are attained and efficiency is how the desired outcome is achieved or produced, particularly without wasting resources, such as time, personnel, and money. With the ever-rising costs of therapies, medications, and hospitalizations, healthcare providers must be organized and coordinated to ensure quality services are delivered in a timely and consistent manner. For example, they must evaluate data to determine if utilization management activities, such as discharge planning, are being correctly and appropriately applied.

- To evaluate financial stability—In the United States, healthcare is a competitive market. Profit and positive financial growth must occur in order for the healthcare provider to have a viable future. Quality data is necessary to determine how, where, and why the money generated from treating patients is supporting the healthcare facility, provider, staff, and business functions. For example, healthcare facilities use internal and external data to plan healthcare services to meet the changing needs of their local population.

- To reduce security breaches—Confidentiality and privacy are the cornerstones of HIM. Protecting patient data with security policies, procedures, and training help reduce the opportunity for intentional or unintentional data violations, hacking, and medical identity theft. Security controls on healthcare facility emails, along with staff education, help reduce the risks of opening emails that contain ransomware or other malware, which can significantly disrupt the healthcare facility's operations.

- To control e-discovery costs—This includes the time and effort staff spend on the pretrial identification and investigation of electronically stored data for civil and criminal legal proceedings. The e-discovery process is the pre-trial activities wherein participants acquire and analyze any electronic data that could be used in civil or criminal legal proceedings. Some of the aspects addressed in e-discovery include format of the data, the location of the accumulated data, and record retention and destruction protocols (Rinehart-Thompson 2016, 66). When electronic patient data is subpoenaed, the healthcare facility must guarantee the integrity of the data. Otherwise, the data is considered suspect, which may significantly alter the findings of the case in court.

Figure 14.1. Information governance versus data governance infographic

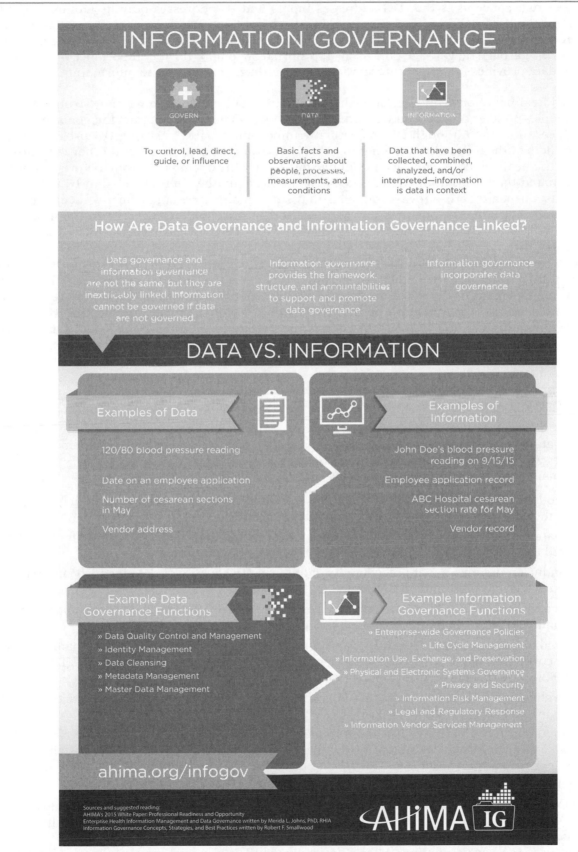

Source: AHIMA n.d.b.

DG is a subset of IG as data is the foundation upon which information is built. A simplistic way of looking at the two concepts is that DG addresses inputs and IG addresses outputs (Johns 2015, xxii). The inputs are the data collected and managed, while the outputs are the reports, statistics and other information that are obtained from the data. Good data is necessary to make appropriate decisions. The acronym GIGO, "garbage in, garbage out," is an appropriate metaphor for the importance of effective DG as "garbage" data provides "garbage" information. This "garbage" or inaccurate information leads to poor decisions.

In today's healthcare environment, a healthcare facility will not survive without strong DG, which addresses people, policies and procedures, and the technology needed to support the goals and mission of the healthcare facility. Although DG is especially important to HIM, a strong DG program requires everyone in the healthcare facility working together. For example, physicians and other care providers document in the health record, coding and billing staff ensure the claim is accurate before submitting it to the insurer, and the information systems department backs-up the data. The goal of IG is to "achieve a state of trust in healthcare information such that safe, quality care and effective decision making are enabled and that patients, business partners, and other stakeholders can rely on the information" (Washington 2015). This trust cannot be established when there is "garbage in," which is why data quality is so important.

DG and IG are examples of the "little picture, big picture" concept. The smaller aspects of DG provide the "little picture" while supporting the "big picture" of IG. IG is the "big picture," the all-encompassing information management of the entire healthcare facility. An example of the "little picture" is a single digit in an International Classification of Disease, Tenth Revision, Clinical Modification (ICD-10-CM) code. If one single digit in the ICD-10-CM code is incorrectly applied on a consistent basis, it could significantly result in the healthcare facility losing hundreds of thousands of dollars in reimbursement and faulty data, which would affect the facility's research. In this way, the "little picture" has significant effects on the "big picture."

Data Governance in Health Information Management

DG and IG are broad concepts that cover many aspects of HIM. These aspects include data quality (chapter 2), databases (chapter 3), data content standards (chapter 11), and security (chapter 12). More DG and IG aspects will be addressed throughout this chapter.

DG is in many ways is the foundation for HIM because it includes:

- Data modeling: The process of determining the user's information needs and identifying relationships among the data. For additional information, refer to chapter 3.

- Data mapping: Allows for connections between two systems. This connection allows for data initially captured for one purpose to be translated and used for another purpose.

- Data audit: An organizational procedure for monitoring the quality of data by analyzing reports for anomalies, inaccuracies, and missing data.

- Data quality controls: Tools such as edits and field types used in information systems that help ensure data quality. Refer to chapter 2 for more information.

- Data quality management: "The business processes that ensure the integrity of an organization's data during collection, application (including aggregation), warehousing, and analysis" (Davoudi et al. 2015). For more on data quality management, refer to chapter 2.

- Data architecture: "The development and maintenance of specifications about data that reside in electronic databases" (Johns 2015, 105).

- Data dictionary: A descriptive list of the names, definitions, and attributes of data elements to be collected in an information system or database whose purpose is to standardize definitions and ensure consistent use (Acker et al. 2017, 10). For additional information on data dictionaries, refer to chapter 3.

Many aspects of DG are not new to HIM professionals. The profession has been involved in data collection, data quality, data storage, data retention, audits, policies, and other DG issues for decades, although how HIM professionals accomplish DG is changing. For example, governance of data collection in the paper health record used to be achieved through form design; in the EHR environment, the same data collection is governed through screen design, the data dictionary, and other tools.

Impact of Data Governance on HIM

DG has a significant impact on healthcare and HIM. A healthcare facility benefits from a strong DG program in many ways:

- Improved data quality
- Reduction of duplication
- Improved trust in data
- Efficiencies
- Cost savings
- Risk mitigations (Reeves and Bowen 2012; Kloss 2013).

Improved data quality and improved trust in data will in turn improve patient care and decision making. DG has also changed the focus of HIM. DG has broadened to include not just patient data but administrative data as well. The skills of the HIM professional must broaden as well in order to provide the leadership and subject matter expertise demanded of them.

Issues to Consider

In order to provide the quality data required by IG, a number of DG issues must be addressed throughout the healthcare facility. These issues include in addition to data quality (discussed in chapter 2) and health informatics (discussed in chapter 1), metadata and data mapping are important factors in DG.

Metadata

Metadata is often referred to as "data about data," but this definition oversimplifies the concept. A better definition is "structured information used to increase the effective use of data" (Johns 2016, 82). It includes the electronic time stamp of when data was created, accessed, or manipulated.

The National Information Standards Organization (NISO) advises that metadata should be used to sustain interoperability. Interoperability is the ability of different information technology systems and software applications to communicate; to exchange data accurately, effectively, and consistently; and to use the information that has been exchanged. Metadata makes it easier to find, acquire, use, and effectively manage the data within the healthcare facility systems. Metadata identifies when an entry was created and who created it, from where it was accessed, and all changes made to the file or document. During an information breach investigation, a single employee's electronic activity or the activity that occurred at a single workstation or terminal can be evaluated. This recommendation is also advocated by the Office of the National Coordinator (ONC) for Health Information Technology in that metadata supports data integrity for health information exchange (HIE) (Dolezel 2015).

Metadata can prove the integrity of a healthcare facility's records by identifying the creation, changes, access, and security of the information to ensure its quality and trustworthiness. There are three types of metadata:

- Descriptive metadata addresses specific data elements acquired and used by the information system. The data dictionary established for all of the datasets within the information system is an example of descriptive metadata. For more on the data dictionary, refer to chapter 3.

- Structural metadata is the process of acquiring, storing, manipulating, and displaying data. Data models, such as entity-relationship diagrams (ERD) and dataflow diagrams (DFD) are diagrammatical or graphic tools used to help program the system and to identify areas of inefficiency. For more on ERD and DFD, refer to chapter 3.

- Administrative metadata is programmed in the information system in order to generate data about the usage of the information system, such as audit trail and activity reports. The audit trail identifies tasks such as who accessed the information system or when and where someone performed a certain data function. For more information about the audit trail, refer to chapter 13. Administrative metadata also includes decision support functions wherein the information system assists in helping to assemble, manipulate, and prioritize data and make recommendations about specific courses of action that can be taken to address an identified issue (Amatayakul 2016, 415). For example, audit trails can identify when a data entry error was made and who made it. Analyzing this type of data entry error activity may show how often it occurs and which employee(s) is(are) responsible. This information could be used in training employees.

There are several data items that are important within the realm of metadata. These items are important because it shows when the data was created and by whom. It alleviates any questions regarding who recorded the information or if any data had been altered, which would call into question the integrity and security of the data. These items are the user name, identification number, patient name, health record number, the name or number of the computer where and when the data was accessed, the date and time information was manipulated, printed, or downloaded, and what documents or reports were accessed or manipulated (Biedermann and Dolezel 2017, 445).

Data Mapping

Sharing data is critical to the healthcare delivery system. In order to be able to use the data to meet the needs of the healthcare facility, semantic interoperability is needed (Maimone 2016). Semantic interoperability is the level of interoperability in which the data within the message can be interpreted between computer systems. One tool used to achieve the semantic interoperability is data mapping. As stated earlier, data mapping supports connections between two systems. This connection allows the data initially captured for one purpose to be translated and used for another purpose.

When mapping data, there is a source and a target. The source is the original data set that is being mapped from. The target is the data set that the source is being mapped to. For example, ICD-10-CM can be mapped to SNOMED CT or the reverse; the mapped data reflects that ICD-10-CM code A00.9 is equivalent to the SNOMED CT code 63650001 (Maimone 2016). The two systems being mapped are not identical, so one entry in the source may map to two, three, or multiple entries in the target. There are three common types of relations between concepts: no match, approximate match, and exact match. The term no match is used when an entry in the source system does not have a similar concept in the target system. Approximate match is when there is a similar concept but it is not identical. The exact match is just that—an exact match between the source and the target (Maimone 2016).

CHECK YOUR UNDERSTANDING 14.1

1. _____ is the processes of what and how data is collected, how to store and protect it, and ensuring its quality and integrity.

   a. IG
   b. DG
   c. GIGO
   d. ITG

2. What acronym is used when expressing that if data are not accurate or complete, any conclusions drawn from them will be incorrect?

   a. IG
   b. DG
   c. GIGO
   d. ITG

3. Which of the following is an organization-wide framework for managing information throughout its lifecycle and for supporting the organization's strategy, operations, regulatory, legal, risk, and environmental requirements?

   a. IG
   b. DG
   c. GIGO
   d. ITG

4. Metadata can be used to ensure _____.

   a. Data quality management
   b. Data architecture
   c. Trustworthiness
   d. "Little picture, big picture"

5. What term is used to describe the degree to how well a goal or an objective is achieved?
   a. Asset
   b. Efficiency
   c. Effectiveness
   d. Stability

Information Governance in HIM

HIM has evolved to include more than health records (which historically has been paper health records). HIM now refers to the all patient content (demographic, clinical, financial, provider, and so forth), and the power of that content to assist in the decision-making processes and delivery of healthcare. Paper health records sat on shelves and were only used when specifically requested. The physical nature of the record meant it was only available in one place at a time, not readily available to help with decision making or managing patients or departments whenever and wherever needed. Abstracted data from these paper health record were placed in secondary files or databases, such as in a physician index or cancer registry. These secondary data sources were useful, but if more detailed information was required, reviewing the paper health record would need to occur again. Research using paper health records was often tedious, requiring the need to sift through pages and pages of data which took a tremendous amount of time. The completeness of the data was also inconsistent; one healthcare facility may be more well-managed and have meticulous records, while another's may be less so. Prior to the Health Insurance Portability and Accountability Act (HIPAA), accessing paper records was also problematic for many providers and patients due to inconsistent application of confidentiality and security practices and policies (Amatayakul 2017, 412). Ensuring the quality, availability, usability, integrity, and security of the health information is a key aspect of information governance.

HIM's professional scope addresses data analytics (chapter 1), health informatics (chapter 1), e-discovery, privacy and security, data quality, and much more. The following section will address how IG views information as a valued strategic asset, the impact of IG, and issues that must be considered.

Valued Strategic Asset

Information is a valued strategic asset and should be managed just like people, processes, money, and other resources. An asset is any resource that is useful and provides a valuable quality. The value comes from its relative worth or importance. Information is a valued strategic asset because of its role in planning for the future of the healthcare facility, making sound clinical and administrative decisions, and managing the financial resources.

In IG, it is not just health information that is valuable, it is all information generated in any capacity by the healthcare facility in the delivery of healthcare services. This includes financial, human resources, accreditation and licensure requirements, clinical, social media, memos and emails, community and business forecasts, and more. (Washington 2015). All of this valuable information can be analyzed, manipulated, and used to determine a course of action designed to produce a desired business outcome. Therefore, data and information have become as valuable to the healthcare facility as its grounds, equipment, and building (Amatayakul 2016, 412).

Impact of IG

Prior to the implementation of EHRs, radiology, lab, and other departments reported results but kept their own information. These "data silos" of information created fragmentation that still haunts some EHR systems. Much like a silo on a farm where each silo holds a different type of grain, a data silo is a separate database or system within a department that does not integrate into the main organizational system nor can others outside of that specific department access it. IG addresses these issues by managing information overall, not just data of one type or in one location. The information can then be used to meet the needs of the healthcare facility.

Issues to Consider

Due to the complexity of IG, there are a number of issues to consider when implementing IG. These include the importance of data quality, business intelligence, IG Steering Committee, leadership, IG charter, IG project plan, SBAR in IG, and inventory assets inventory in IG.

Figure 14.2.   Infographic defining information governance

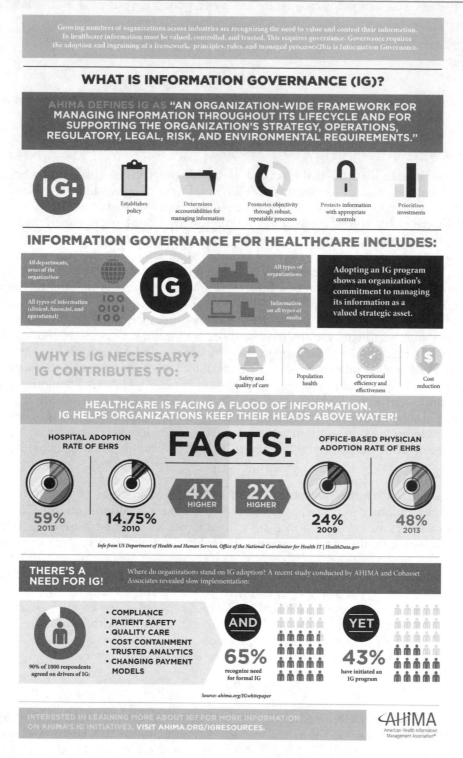

Source: AHIMA 2017.

Importance of Data Quality

Data quality is of utmost importance to IG. Data are like the bricks of a building. Structural integrity relies on high-quality building materials. Well-made bricks provide strength to withstand hurricane winds, driving rain, and other threats. Likewise, high-quality data and information are required to make sound decisions, research health trends, and determine patient care patterns. Data that lack integrity or security will compromise the quality of information, thereby creating potential faults in the decisions and conclusions made based on the compromised materials.

Business Intelligence

Business intelligence (BI) is the end product, or goal, of IG. BI includes information technology and procedures to analyze all aspects of the healthcare facility's performance, including patient care and healthcare services delivery, personnel, clinical applications and outcomes, and all administrative functions (Johns 2015, 229). BI requires quality data, which is ensured and strengthened by DG and IG activities. The executive staff of the healthcare facility must develop the abilities to get quality data and information, apply that information to the situation at hand, and incorporate the knowledge and skills received into the healthcare facility's future processes and decisions. These are functions integral to the IG process of supporting the healthcare facility's strategic mission and daily operations. For example, business intelligence would be used to determine where profits and losses occur and then analyze what contributed to the profit and loss. Administrators and managers, using the data and information generated by the healthcare facility's information systems in DG and IG activities, must also incorporate logic and reasoning, creative problem-solving, as well as self-awareness and emotional knowledge to successfully meet the challenges they face today and in the future.

The term **big data** is mentioned frequently when discussing DG, IG, and BI. In healthcare, big data means "electronic health data sets so large and complex that they are difficult (or impossible) to manage with traditional software and/or hardware; nor can they be easily managed with traditional or common data management tools and methods" (Ragupathi 2014). In order for healthcare facilities to effectively incorporate big data into their strategic and decision-making processes, sophisticated and cutting-edge technologies that address data storage, analytics, and visualization must be applied (Johns 2015, 229). The amount of data generated by the daily operations of just one healthcare facility is enormous. This big data is the foundation from which the BI is created. Big data must be available, must be governed properly to provide quality information, and it must be secure—all of which are DG responsibilities. Only then can it be turned into information from which BI is created.

Information Governance Steering Committee

Because staff throughout the healthcare facility should be involved in IG processes, the healthcare facility should create an **IG steering committee**. This committee could created and dedicated to IG, or the role could be assumed by an existing committee. The IG steering committee is responsible for the oversight of the IG program and it has many roles:

- Identifying the responsible individual or department responsible for IG functions
- Developing relationships between individuals and departments responsible for IG functions
- Creating an IG policy
- Coordinating IG efforts (Blair 2014)

The patient safety and quality of care committee, for example, already uses healthcare facility data to evaluate patient care services to ensure that regulatory, legal, and risk compliance requirements (key aspects of IG) are being addressed and implemented. Therefore, it could feasibly take on the duties of the IG steering committee. If existing committees are utilized, then after the general introduction of the IG concepts within those committees, it may be prudent to develop a subcommittee with pertinent stakeholders such as physicians, nursing and clinical staff, and HIM management personnel. Over time, if IG activities overshadow the scope of the original committee or when timing of activities warrants, a dedicated IG committee may be needed.

Leadership

The IG steering committee is part of the leadership structure of the healthcare facility's IG efforts. Regardless of how the IG efforts begin, IG must have permanent leadership structure, resources (human, monetary, equipment), and executive level commitment. As a crucial resource for the healthcare facility, information requires support and administration at an executive level to ensure efficient and effective use for strategic planning, financial management, and quality and performance improvement applications. Executive level personnel can be referred to as the "C-suite," a jargon term that refers to the positions with titles beginning with "C," such as chief executive officer (CEO), chief financial officer (CFO), and chief information officer (CIO). Rather than dealing with IG's daily operational requirements, C-suite personnel are focused on strategic or conceptual activities—the "big picture" aspects. If IG is not championed by the C-suite, department heads and managers may not feel compelled to engage in or complete required IG or DG processes. Due to the information-centric nature of IG work, HIM and HIT management staff work with the C-suite to establish plans, goals, objectives, policies, and oversight.

Figure 14.3. Organizing for information governance

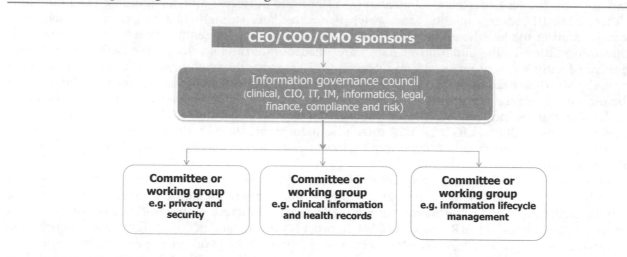

Source: Adapted from Kloss 2015, 38.

Implementing an IG plan is a large undertaking. Initially, it is recommended to start the IG process with existing stakeholder committees within the healthcare facility. These committees already have a formalized structure with assigned personnel. Many of the established committees' existing duties translate directly into many of the functions of IG. For example, an HIM and clinical data and documentation committee is already involved in clinical documentation improvement activities. Once the IG plan is underway, then a IG council (committee) can be created. Additional committees that report to the IG council can be created or supporting activities can continue to be performed by the existing committees. **Clinical documentation improvement (CDI)** is the process an organization undertakes that will improve clinical specificity and documentation, allowing coding professionals to assign more precise disease classification codes. In addition to improving the coding process, CDI also improves and supports data quality, availability, and usability—all key aspects of DG.

Information Governance Charter

As stated earlier, existing committees can be used to lay the groundwork for IG until a formal structure can be created. This groundwork includes many of the activities identified in the IG charter. A **charter** is a document that identifies the purpose, scope, and functions of a program. In combination with the work of existing committees, the IG charter, plan, and personnel can be launched.

AHIMA has developed a charter template (figure 14.4) to assist healthcare facilities in beginning the IG process. Depending on the identified needs and personnel of the healthcare facility, this template can be used to help with the initial start-up of the IG program. This template identifies the purpose, scope and responsibilities, membership and reporting structure, subcommittees, reporting, quorum status, meetings, and date of approval. It also drives the initial discussions regarding the establishment of an IG project plan.

Information Governance Project Plan

AHIMA has developed an IG sample project plan (figure 14.5) to assist healthcare entities with incorporating IG into their work. This five-phased process includes a list of activities for each phase of initiation, planning, execution, control, and close-out. Within each phase, the IG leadership (administrators or steering committee) should consider timeframes, responsible parties, goals and objectives, milestones, and status of the activities. Many of these tasks can be delegated to existing committees or the IG steering committee. The administrator who oversees the IG efforts should oversee the committee(s) engaged in IG. This comprehensive blueprint can be tailored depending on the needs and resources of the healthcare facility.

Figure 14.4.   Information governance charter template

Information Governance Charter Template

Purpose: *(A brief statement of why the group exists and its overall goals)*

Examples: To provide oversight for the use, management, and integrity of information across its lifecycle with a focus on improving patient care, supporting the organization's mission and goals, providing value, minimizing risk and complying with applicable regulations, accreditation, professional practice, and legal standards. To reduce and ultimately eliminate siloed approaches to information management.

Scope and Responsibilities: *(A statement of what the group is expected to do and accomplish, along with identification of boundaries)*

Examples:

1. Guide the development of a formal enterprise IG program
2. Review and approval of information governance policies impacting more than one business unit or department
3. Review and approval of information governance-related strategies and roadmaps
4. Prioritization of information governance-related scope, priorities, and initiatives
5. Establishing information governance-related metrics, evaluation, and oversight of results
6. Coordination of information management responsibilities across the organization
7. Monitor progress and impact

Membership and Reporting Structure: *(a statement of who will participate and contribute to the goals and what leader(s) is/are accountable for assuring the group has appropriate information and resources to accomplish its purpose. May also include subgroups or subcommittees which assist in carrying out the charge. May also include designation of administrative support for meetings and activities)*

Examples of participants:
Medical Staff
Clinical Informatics
Health Information Management
Privacy
IT Security
Quality
Nursing
Legal
Finance
Compliance
Decision support
Research
Risk Management
IG Program Office

Meetings and activities will be coordinated by the executive overseeing the operations of the IG Program Office.

(Continued)

Figure 14.4.   Information governance charter template (Continued)

Sub Committees: *(Examples)*

- *Health Information Management/Medical Record Committee*
- *Privacy and Security*
- *Information Content and Integrity*
- *IT Informatics Steering*
- *Data Governance*
- *Analytics and Business Intelligence*
- *Research*

Reporting:

(Report to the Board on the Committee's activities to include, but not limited to committee minutes, written repo rts and any significant matters under consideration by the Committee.)

Quorum:

Example: Quorum shall be satisfied when at least xxxx (x) members of the Committee are present.

Meetings: *(specifies the frequency and usual time for meetings as well as any attendance and quorum requirements)*

Example: Meetings shall be held no less than _____.

Approval: *(sign off approval of the charter along with date of approval)*

Source: AHIMA n.d.c.

Figure 14.5.   Sample information governance project plan

Information Governance Sample Project Plan

Sample Project Plan for an IG Project

This sample project plan can be used as a starting point for your organization. Engaging project management to assist you in managing this project can help the project move forward.

Task	Start Date	End Date	Responsible	Milestone	Status
Site Information Governance Tasks					
Initiation and Planning					
Create charter for IG program					
Create initial IG project plan					
Create communication plan (include escalation process)					
Determine IG quick wins (cleanup, savings, see note)					
Identify executive sponsors					
Define IG team					
Engage project management team					

Figure 14.5.   Sample information governance project plan (Continued)

Review/create organizational chart for IG					
Regular team meetings for IG team					
Establish budget					
Team training (AHIMA videos)					
Define IG roles as needed					
Site IG project kickoff meeting					
Site IG project planning meeting					
Project Execution					
Approve project plan with team					
Assess status of IG within the organization					
Begin communications per plan					
Senior leadership on board					
IG leader identified					
IG overview education begins					
Team communication begins					
Build value proposition					
Inventory information stores and paper repositories					
Categorize information assets					
Create a compelling story (elevator speech)					
Determine initial IG deliverables					
Determine pain point—first deliverable					
Development of an information classification process for use and valuation of information					
Discuss training needs					
Schedule initial training for core team					
Core team training complete					
Workforce and business partner education begins (IG practices and principles)					
Inventory policies and procedures to be included in IG program					
Begin P&P review					
Schedule P&P updates					
Inventory reports					
Map data flows/information flows					
Review current workflows					
Develop new workflows as needed					
Review job descriptions/role descriptions					
Schedule update of job/roles if needed					
Establish protocols to correct errors in the EHR, PHR, legacy systems, all information systems					
Begin work on IG compliance/monitoring program (to extent possible)					
Project Monitoring					
Publish project status report					
Status meetings and notes					
Project Closure					

(Continued)

Figure 14.5.   Sample information governance project plan (Continued)

Initiation Phase

During initiation you will be setting up the framework for the program. Charter, communications plan, defining the team, and the other initiation steps outline the way the program is organized and how it will be run.

Planning Phase

The planning phase is a rigorous period when you will develop the project plan. First you will create a preliminary scope statement, which is important for evaluating and ad hoc work prioritizing requests. Project plans for information governance will be iterative. The team will define periods for planning and then adjust as the project moves forward.

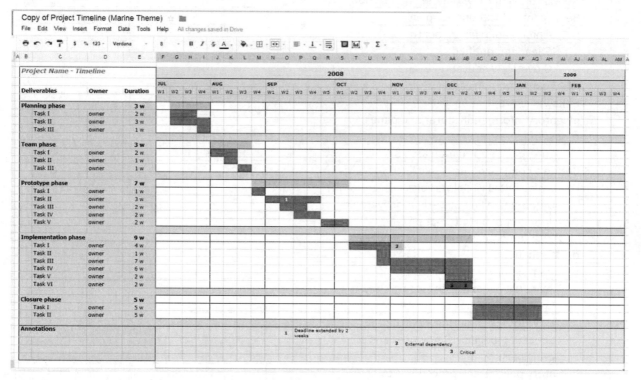

The last step in the planning phase is to present the plan to the project steering committee and receive plan approval.

Execution Phase

Execution for information governance plans can take many forms. Each hospital must define the deliverables, focus, and quick wins for the facility. The team needs to create a compelling story, build a value proposition, and train the team.

Control Phase

During the control phase the project manager must monitor:

- Schedule progress
- Budget
- Scope

Change management is an important piece of the control phase.

Figure 14.5. Sample information governance project plan (Continued)

Change Log Template:

Change Log							
Project:						Date:	
Change No.	Change Type	Description of Change	Requestor	Date Submitted	Date Approved	Status	Comments
Each change request is assigned a reference number.	This may be a design, scope, schedule or other type of change.	The change request should be described in detail.	Who initiated the change request?	When was the request submitted?	When was the request approved?	Is the change request open, closed or pending? Has it been approved, denied or deferred?	This section may describe why the change request was rejected, deferred or provide any other useful information

Close-out Phase

Once the project is complete, the project manager must take steps to appropriately close out the project. The close-out phase is important because it confirms acceptance of the final project deliverables and transfers knowledge gained from the project to operational owners.

- Verify acceptance of final project deliverables
- Conduct post-project assessment and lessons learned
- Conduct post-project review and evaluation
- Recognize and celebrate outstanding project work
- Disburse project resources – staff, facilities, and automated systems
- Complete and archive final product records
- Ensure transfer of knowledge

Summary

Project management is the application of processes, methods, knowledge, skills, and experience to achieve the project objectives. Regardless of the nature of your IG project, the five phases of project management will guide your project to success.

Source: AHIMA n.d.d.

SBAR in Information Governance

SBAR (situation, background, assessment, recommendation) is a process for facilitating communication and resolving problems that has been used by many healthcare facilities in their quest to implement IG. Implementing IG practices is such a complex undertaking that there is bound to be resistance to change, hesitancy, and questioning among administration, the medical staff, clinical personnel, and other stakeholders. See table 14.1 for descriptions of the SBAR components.

Table 14.1. SBAR elements

Element	Description
S = situation	A detailed explanation of the issue or problem
B = background	Concise and significant facts surrounding the issue
A = assessment	Research and analysis of information and suggested options
R = recommendation	Action required to achieve the desired end result

Source: Glondys 2016.

For example, if the healthcare facility has a problem with retention of health information, SBAR can be used to resolve the problem. The process begins with defining the situation or problem that the healthcare facility is having. For example, the healthcare facility has a policy to retain health records for 10 years. The research department plans to undertake some long-term research and needs health information to be retained for a minimum of 20 years. The background identifies facts, such as when the research is starting, what health information is needed, the patients involved, and so forth. During assessment, the healthcare facility analyzes the information collected in the first two steps and comes up with options such as changing the retention of all health information to 20 years and moving the health information needed for research to another database for the extended retention period. The recommendation identifies the action to take from the options identified in the assessment component.

Information Asset Inventory for Information Governance

An information asset inventory is a list of information resources throughout the healthcare facility; it includes all of the types of information identified earlier in the chapter. The inventory should be stored in a spreadsheet or other tool to facilitate access to and ongoing maintenance of the list. This inventory should include both paper and electronic records, reports, medical imaging, and both structured and unstructured data. The inventory is critical to the creation of an IG program because all of the data and information to be managed must known. The responsibility for maintaining the inventory must be assigned (Downing et al. 2017). It could be assigned to the steering committee, the HIM director, the HIM department, or other individual or group.

Once the inventory is created, it should be used to classify information by its importance to the healthcare facility. The information asset inventory will be used in a number of functions, including creation of a retention schedule, identifying redundancies (duplication), and compliance with laws and regulations (Downing et al. 2017).

Strategic Alignment

Strategic alignment is "the process and the outcome of linking your organizational structure and resources with your strategy and business environment to achieve performance improvement" (Washington 2017). IG is not a one-time project to fix a specific issue. It is a method of addressing how the healthcare facility is managed so that it will sustain itself in the healthcare marketplace and how it will continue its role as a valuable member of the community. These efforts should be based on the healthcare facility's goals and objectives. The healthcare facility's plans, goals, and activities cannot be monitored and implemented without trustworthy organizational data. Yearly performance evaluations are performed on all staff members; the same can be done with the healthcare facility. When evaluating a facility, one of the questions that should be asked is whether or not the healthcare facility achieved its identified annual goals. This is one way that BI comes into play. The information needed to answer this question and more can be generated from the healthcare facility's information systems and used to assess each goal to determine if the healthcare facility met the mark. IG and the healthcare facility's strategy for success must align to achieve those goals.

Information Governance Principles for Healthcare

AHIMA took an assertive and proactive role in the acceptance and promotion of IG concepts and has worked with ARMA International (formerly known as Association of Records Managers and Administrators) and other key healthcare stakeholders to develop IG best practices. ARMA International is a professional association and a recognized authority on IG in most areas, such as information technology, legislative and regulatory bodies, and finance, that utilize information as a strategic asset (ARMA 2017). The result of their collaboration was Information Governance Principles for Healthcare (IGPHC). IGPHC applies to all aspects of information and subsequent business transactions across all areas of the healthcare industry organizations (Washington, 2015). A stakeholder is someone who has a concern about the identified issues and the healthcare facility's data. These individuals or groups can be internal or external customers of the healthcare facility. These customers would include employees and managers, executive staff, clinical and medical staff, accrediting agencies, and local/state/federal government.

AHIMA used the Generally Accepted Recordkeeping Principles from ARMA International to develop the founding eight key principles for IG (Amatayakul 2016, 413). Ensuring the trustworthiness of a healthcare facility's information is the ultimate goal for IG. AHIMA, in collaboration with ARMA International and major healthcare leaders and stakeholders, reconfigured the Generally Accepted Recordkeeping Principles into a set of guidelines to meet the needs of the healthcare industry's information explosion.

The key IG principles, which are defined in table 14.2, are based on "accuracy, timeliness, accessibility, and integrity" (Bass et al. 2014, 3). The application of the principles can be adjusted based on the needs of the healthcare facility (Bass et al. 2014).

Table 14.2. IGPHC principles defined and exemplified

Principle	Definition	Example
Accountability	Designation or identification of a senior member of leadership responsible for the development and oversight of the IG program	Chief data officer (CDO)—executive-level personnel with power and authority to administer program
Transparency	Documentation of processes and activities related to IG are visible and readily available for review by stakeholders	Minutes of IG meetings; clear hierarchy reporting; established lines of communication to all levels of workforce
Integrity	Systems evidence trustworthiness in the authentication, timeliness, accuracy, and completion of information	Data quality management program, clinical documentation improvement activities; data stewardship relationships
Protection	Program protects private and confidential information from loss, breach, and corruption	Security and privacy policies and training; risk and breach analysis; mitigation protocols
Compliance	Program ensures compliance with local, state, and federal regulations, accrediting agencies' standards and healthcare organizations' policies and procedures and ethical practices	Chief compliance officer; Joint Commission surveys and activities
Availability	Structure and accessibility of data allows for timely and efficient retrieval by authorized personnel	Authorization, access, and authentication procedures
Retention	Lifespan of information is defined and regulated by a schedule in compliance with legal requirements and ethical considerations	Federal and state regulations; healthcare facility's legal counsel and chief compliance officer
Disposition	Process ensures the legal and ethical disposition of information including, but not limited to, record destruction and transfer	Retention guidelines; reputable and verifiable destruction/deletion procedures

Source: Adapted from Davoudi et al. 2015.

Information Technology Governance

It is difficult to think about IG or DG without thinking of information technology. To clarify, information technology is the computer technology (hardware and software) combined with telecommunications technology (data, image, and voice networks) and is also a term that encompasses most forms of technology used to create, store, exchange, and use electronic information. Almost all administrative functions are performed on a computer using various software applications. The hardware and software are the tools used in DG and IG. These tools can be used to facilitate budget analysis, regulatory compliance review, medical research on patient care outcomes, and many other purposes. The analysis relies on data gathered and secured within the scope of DG. Decisions based on the results of the budget analysis or patient outcomes research reflects the scope of IG. At times, it is difficult to separate the tool from the activity, as hardware and software are necessary to perform most healthcare functions. The information technology need must not only be available but appropriate to meet the needs of the healthcare facility (AHIMA n.d.a).

Information technology governance (ITG) is a subdomain of IG and is essential for any organization using information technology. ITG is the management of all information technology investments, including the selection, implementation, maintenance, evaluation and its coordination. For more on these topics refer to chapters 4 and 5. ITG also encompasses every aspect of the information technology infrastructure, such as hardware, software, communication, and technology tools, policies and procedures to provide efficient processes for all electronic activity within the healthcare facility. ITG is typically led by the chief information officer (CIO).

DG and ITG work very closely together to advance IG. ITG focuses on the tools for acquiring and manipulating data and information. DG focuses on quality, integrity, and security of the data and information. Neither DG or ITG is more important than the other as both are critical to the process. See figure 14.6 for a conceptual diagram of these relationships.

Figure 14.6.   Diagram of DG and ITG roles related to IG

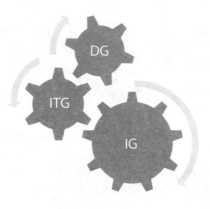

CHECK YOUR UNDERSTANDING 14.2

1. The founding principles of IG are based upon what other organization's principles for recordkeeping?

   a. AMA
   b. AMIA
   c. AHIMA
   d. ARMA

2. What IGPHC principle identifies the trustworthiness of the information?

   a. Transparency
   b. Integrity
   c. Compliance
   d. Availability

3. What concept describes the management of hardware, software, and all technology components of a healthcare facility?

   a. DG
   b. IG
   c. ITG
   d. IGPHC

4. What concept describes the newly established importance of health information as a requirement to help a healthcare facility provide the best possible patient care and remain a vital aspect to its community for the future?

   a. Sustainability
   b. Compliance
   c. Disposition
   d. Valued strategic asset

5. What term is used to describe the process and the outcome of linking the organizational structure and resources with the strategy and business environment to achieve performance improvement?

   a. Strategic alignment
   b. IG
   c. DG
   d. HIM

Enterprise Information Management

Enterprise information management (EIM) is the set of functions used to plan, organize, and coordinate people, processes, technology, and content for managing information as a corporate asset that ensures data quality safety, and ease of use. It is ensuring that the processes are in place to generate trust in the information being used (AHIMA n.d.a).

The concepts of EIM and IG are intertwined. IG establishes the direction for information resources while EIM identifies the issues, policies, and more that the IG steering committee or appropriate person must address (Kloss 2015, 45). Since these concepts are intertwined, the same committees and individuals can address both. It is important to understand that IG is a paradigm shift. A paradigm is a philosophical or theoretical framework within which a discipline formulates its theories and makes generalizations. A paradigm shift can be thought of as a new and significantly different way of thinking about how to perform a function or make decisions. In this case, IG offers a significantly different way of viewing and using information to benefit the healthcare facility. IG, much like quality and performance improvement, is a continuous program that facilitates the Triple Aim of healthcare, which is to improve population health, enhance the patient's experience within the healthcare field, and to reduce the per capita cost of healthcare services (Washington 2015). To evaluate whether those goals have been achieved, reliable information is required. An example of this is using the data gathered from patient satisfaction surveys to evaluate how patients felt about how they were treated and how they perceived the quality of their care. Tracking positive and negative perceptions of the quality of care could lead to quality and performance improvement activities. In this section, the building blocks of EIM and its degree of impact on HIM will be addressed.

Building Blocks of EIM

There are five building blocks that are identified as essential foundation pieces for successful EIM. These building blocks are the following:

- Privacy, security, and confidentiality
- Integrity and quality
- Design and capture
- Content and records management
- Access and use

Each of these building blocks should be addressed in terms of "policy, process, procedures, people, and technology" (Kloss 2015, 49). See table 14.3 for a description of these building blocks.

Table 14.3.   Building blocks of EIM

Building Block	Description
Privacy, security, and confidentiality	Compliance metrics; security assessments and liabilities; monitoring non-authorized access; policies, procedures, and training
Integrity and quality	MPI maintenance and integrity, error prevention/correction, DQM functions application
Design and capture	Data templates, redundancy checks, accuracy training, standardization
Content and records management	Retention and disposition policies and procedures for all healthcare facility business and clinical records, legal and regulatory requirements
Access and Use	Authorization processes, release of information, patient portals, research and population health studies

Source: Czarkowski and Clark 2015.

Impact of EIM on HIM

The five building blocks of EIM outline many HIM skills thus making the HIM professional the perfect individual to lead EIM efforts. With the adoption of the EHR and other technologies, HIM is becoming more and more involved throughout the healthcare facility not just in the traditional HIM department. This decentralization of HIM is due to embedding the management of information within the business processes of the healthcare facility (Kloss 2015, 160). Many of the resulting HIM roles are requiring advanced degrees in specialized areas (Kloss 2015, 163).

Information Governance Adoption Model

Knowing that the implementation of an IG program will be a daunting task, AHIMA developed a prototype plan, referred to as the information governance adoption model (IGAM), to assist healthcare facilities when attempting to implement IG. The functions or skills that are necessary to build an IG program are identified and diagrammatically presented in an easy to understand format in figure 14.7.

The model provides a way for healthcare facility to evaluate their IG efforts, and determine where their efforts should focus (Downing 2015). There are 10 core competencies in the IGAM. These core competencies have performance measures that a healthcare facility can use to guide them through their implementation of IG (Butler 2016):

1. IG structure: Creates the information governance program including executive sponsorship, IG committee, and policies and procedures to support the program

2. Strategic alignment: Ensures that the information governance program strategy aligns with the organizations strategy, mission, vision and goals

3. Privacy and security: Protects information across all types of information, all media, throughout the lifecycle

4. Legal and regulatory: Verifies a proper, accurate, reliable, efficient response to regulatory audits, information requests, and e-discovery

5. Data governance: Ensures usable and reliable data through comprehensive and proven data management practices

6. IT governance: Strives for risk reduction through an integrated approach to technology selection, evaluation, and use

7. Analytics: Proves the value of information governance and contributes to a data-driven decision-making culture in the organization through use of advanced tools and technologies

8. IG performance: Measures the performance and impact of the IG program

9. Enterprise information management: Guides practice for information through the information lifecycle across the healthcare ecosystem

   a. Ensuring the value of information assets, requiring an organization-wide perspective of information management functions; it calls for explicit structures, policies, processes, technology, and controls

   b. The infrastructure and processes to ensure the information is trustworthy and actionable

10. Awareness and adherence: Creates a path for trusted information and safe use of health IT through consistent behavior with respect to information use, sharing, handling, access, storage, retention, and disposition (AHIMA 2014)

While it is best to start the IGAM process with the IG structure competency, healthcare facilities can enter the IGAM at other points depending on their needs, current status, and resources available. The healthcare facility may decide to start at the legal and regulatory competency and evaluate its processes to ensure compliance efforts facility-wide. Alternately, the healthcare facility may decide to evaluate all technology used within the facility to determine needs, resources, and solutions to any IT issues, before progressing to the next competency.

Figure 14.7. AHIMA's Information Governance Adoption Model (IGAM)

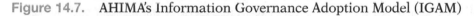

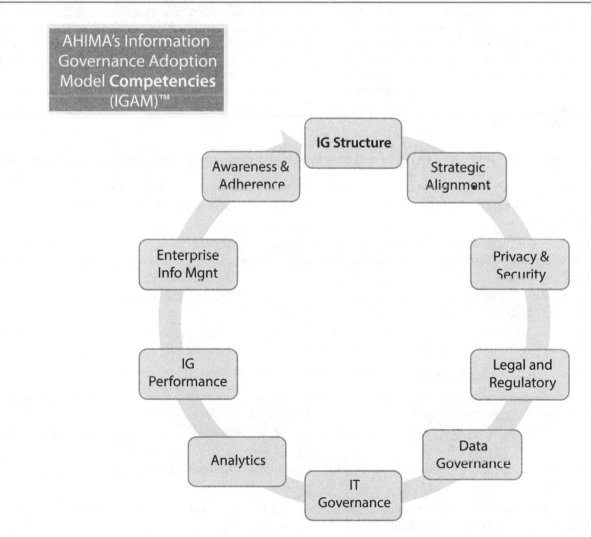

Source: Downing 2016.

Generally, it takes approximately 12 to 18 months to implement an IG program, depending on size of healthcare facility, personnel involved, budget, and other resources (Washington 2015). Many of the IG activities, while not difficult, can be very time consuming to organize and complete. Because the overarching concepts of IG reach into many administrative and clinical activities, IG must be overseen by C-suite personnel, such as a CIO. This person must have the authority and responsibility to be able to direct all IG-related activities.

Collaboration is the key imperative "people-skill" for the IG leader because employees throughout the healthcare facility must be involved. This collaboration involves bringing various people and departments together, finding common ground and solutions, and coming to a consensus for a plan of action. As IG champion, the CIO can delegate specific DG activities to the responsible individuals.

HIM professionals are ideally suited as key players in the IG implementation efforts due to their education in HIM principles and experience with managing and protecting health information. Many HIM professionals have experience in various management positions and providing HIM to other department managers to evaluate that unit's performance. A 2015 study showed that HIM professionals led the IG initiatives at 73 percent of the surveyed healthcare facilities (Washington 2016). HIM professionals are adept at educating healthcare facility employees about the benefits of IG implementation. This training would start with the executive level, then move to key department managers, and then to non-management staff. This can education can be achieved in workshops and seminars or hiring of an IG consultant. In addition to understanding the concepts of IG, all management personnel must understand the amount of work that this new effort will need in order to be implemented successfully as well as the benefits. The implementation of an EHR for most healthcare facilities was a monumental task. Implementing and executing an IG plan is just as monumental, if not more so since it impacts the entire healthcare facility. Executives must understand that IG is not about information technology, or HIM, or the EHR, but about the use of acquired information and subsequent knowledge for decision making across all areas, clinical or administrative, of the healthcare facility. Once the IG plan is operational, then healthcare facility data and information can be used aggressively by the C-suite to more efficiently and effectively manage the healthcare facility and all activities. Then, decisions and actions of the healthcare facility can truly be data-driven (Washington 2016).

Roles for the HIM Professional in Data Governance and Information Governance

Regardless of the HIM professional's role in DG and IG, two sets of skills are necessary for HIM professionals—hard skills and soft skills. Hard skills deal with basic areas of technology. These hard skills include:

- Informatics skills involve basic computer literacy; programming basics and languages (SQL and HL7); use of basic office application software including databases, graphics, and spreadsheets; and decision support systems
- Data analytic skills including healthcare statistics and research fundamentals; trend analysis and predictive modeling; financial data and budget analysis
- Data use skills encompass the application of secondary data; data visualization (display) techniques; and the ability to use any technology to collect, store, analyze, and report a wide variety of information

Soft skills refer to more subjective traits that involve perception and more analysis:

- Communication skills not only involve verbal and written forms but also interpersonal skills, collaboration, and understanding what was meant in addition to what was said
- Critical thinking uses logic and reasoning to interpret situations and people, apply principles to processes, and creating new ideas
- Decision making and judgement aid the ability to choose the best options based upon some type of cost benefit analysis

New graduates and HIM professionals must be assertive in trying to obtain the soft skills, in particular, as experience is the best teacher (Dooling et al. 2016).

There are a number of roles for the HIM professional in DG and IG due to their knowledge of data management, privacy and security, and other areas. Many of these roles include data collection, data retention, and other traditional roles which have been broadened thanks to the EHR, DG, and IG. The HIM professionals may work throughout the healthcare facility including working in information technology, research, data analysis and other areas. This chapter focuses on three HIM roles related to IG and DG—data steward, clinical data improvement coordinator, and data analyst.

Data Steward

IG processes ensure the integrity (that is, having sufficient reliability, honesty, and dependability to merit confidence) of the healthcare facility's data. One objective of IG is "stewardship of information that supports compliance and risk management" (Washington 2015). Meeting this objective requires at least one data steward, an individual appointed with responsibility and accountability for data, usually in a specific domain (Johns 2016, 92). Data stewards serve as liaisons between designated IG personnel and the healthcare facility's staff whose duties are associated with ITG, DG, or EIM. Data stewardship is the formalization of accountability and a continuum of stewardship responsibilities across the data life cycle and across the enterprise. Data stewardship is carried out by a network of designated employees who are responsible for managing, collecting, viewing, storing, sharing, disclosing, and otherwise making use of personal health information. Health data stewardship is the management and responsibilities of an activity according to its established goals and objectives, regulatory and accreditation conditions, and other organizational obligations to guarantee that health information is used appropriately (Johns 2016, 92). HIM professionals can easily transition into data stewardship positions because they have always been intimately involved in the collection, quality evaluation, maintenance and storage, and security of patient data. They understand not only the what, where, when, and how, but also the why of health information (Downing 2016).

Clinical Documentation Improvement Coordinator

The ultimate goal of CDI is to provide comprehensive and unambiguous communication about a patient's medical condition, course of treatment, and care. Historically, CDI's initial focus was to provide clear documentation of diagnostic and procedural coding, but it has evolved to include the DG aspects of availability and usability so that quality data and information can be used for any purpose within the healthcare facility. HIM professionals are instrumental in devising the CDI plan for the healthcare facility. The CDI plan is a program in which the CDI coordinator reviews health records for incomplete documentation, prompting clinical staff to clarify ambiguities, which allows coding professionals to assign more precise disease classification codes. To prove competence in this realm, an HIM professional (or other) can become a certified clinical document improvement practitioner (CDIP). CDIP is an AHIMA credential awarded to individuals who have achieved specialized skills in clinical documentation improvement.

Health Data Analyst

The transition to heavy use of technology and EHR systems in healthcare over the last decade has led healthcare facilities to consider what to do with all of the data they have collected and stored and how to use it to improve services and better manage patient care. The role of health data analyst has emerged to help healthcare facilities leverage this data. A health data analyst uses application skills to manage, analyze, interpret, and transform health data into accurate, consistent, and timely information. HIM professionals can apply their knowledge and skills of data analytics (discussed in chapter 1) to facilitate the transition to IG.

The certified health data analyst (CHDA) credential identifies practitioners who have the knowledge to acquire, manage, analyze, interpret, and transform data into accurate, consistent, and timely information while balancing the healthcare facility's strategic vision with day-to-day details. CHDA-credentialed professionals exhibit broad organizational knowledge and the ability to communicate with individuals and groups at multiple levels, both internal and external (AHIMA 2018).

Future of Data and Information Governance in Health Information Management

With the continued adoption of the EHR and the associated data and information that it creates, the need for DG and IG is expected to continue. The IG and DG efforts will mature, and healthcare facilities will benefit from the efficiencies, cost savings, and risk mitigations that result from the DG and IG initiatives (Kloss 2013).

CHECK YOUR UNDERSTANDING 14.3

1. Which of the following is a reason a HIM professional should be a leader in IG?

   a. Knowledge of data management
   b. Knowledge of soft skills
   c. Their role in the C-suite
   d. Their understanding of ITG

2. Which of the following is a building block of EIM?

   a. Work plan
   b. Strategic mission
   c. Design and capture
   d. Goals and objectives

3. HIM professionals' role in the business of healthcare has always included which concept of the management of health information?

   a. Reliability
   b. Timeliness
   c. Comprehensiveness
   d. Stewardship

4. Which of the following is a "hard skill" regarding technology?

   a. Computer literacy skills
   b. Communication skills
   c. Critical thinking skills
   d. Decision-making skills

5. What credential indicates that a person is skilled and knowledgeable about the analysis of acquired data to interpret and apply to the healthcare facility's strategic mission, goals and objectives, and performance improvement initiatives?

   a. RHIA
   b. CDIP
   c. CHDA
   d. RHIT

Real-World Case

Lewis-Beck Medical Center (LBMC) is a 650-bed acute care hospital in north Florida. In the last decade, this geographic area has experienced a significant increase in the number of persons moving to here who are 60 years and older. It has become a popular destination due to a reasonable cost of living, temperate weather, close to the Gulf of Mexico, quality schools and healthcare facilities, and many university-sponsored cultural events. There are currently 17 assisted living and memory care facilities approved or being built to address this need. LBMC recognized this trend early on. Using data analytics software and statistical predictions, C-suite personnel were able to identify trends and patterns in patient care for this age group. A concerted effort was made to recruit and/or train physicians and nurses specializing in geriatric medicine. Additional staffing and locations were added to provide physical, occupational, and speech therapy. Physician group practices associated with the hospital have increased the number of physicians with specialty training in cardiology, oncology, and internal medicine. LBMC strengthened or established relationships with the organizations building the assisted living communities and memory care centers. Working with local universities and a community college, education and training programs were identified and implemented to meet the employment demand. The local senior center, an organization providing education, health screening, entertainment, and cultural programs for active seniors, was identified as a key stakeholder and gateway to this population. LBMC regularly evaluates internal and external data to monitor trends to meet the need of this fast-growing segment of the local population.

CHAPTER REVIEW

1. What term is used to describe the process and the outcome of linking the healthcare facility structure and resources with the strategy and business environment to achieve performance improvement?

   a. Valued strategic asset
   b. Efficiency
   c. CQI
   d. Strategic alignment

2. What organization has been a leader in the promotion and application of information governance principles to improve healthcare?

   a. AMA
   b. ARMA
   c. AHIMA
   d. AMIA

3. _____ deals with collection, security, and integrity, or the input of data and _____ is the result of data manipulation within an information system resulting in information or knowledge, in whatever form, or the output of data used to make decisions, strategic plans, and performance improvement activities.

   a. DG, IG
   b. IG, DG
   c. ITG, IG
   d. ITG, DG

4. Which of the eight key principles of IG deals with the documentation that can be accessed and used at any point in time by authorized personnel?

   a. Transparency
   b. Integrity
   c. Compliance
   d. Availability

5. What term is used to describe the degree to which stated outcomes are attained?

   a. Effectiveness
   b. Efficiency
   c. Evaluation
   d. Strategic

6. What is the name of the process that has the pre-trial activities where the participants acquire and analyze any electronic data that could be used in civil or criminal legal proceedings?

   a. IG
   b. DG
   c. IGAM
   d. e-discovery

CHAPTER REVIEW (*Continued*)

7. What document identifies a five-step process that describes all the activities that are needed in order to implement an IG program in a healthcare facility?

   a. CDI
   b. Charter
   c. ITG
   d. IG project plan

8. Which of the EIM building blocks refers to the retention and disposition policies and procedures for all healthcare facility business and clinical records and the legal and regulatory requirements of health information?

   a. Content and record management
   b. Privacy, security, and confidentiality
   c. Integrity and quality
   d. Design and capture

9. What is the term used to identify a separate database or system within a department that does not integrate into the main organizational system and cannot be accessed by others outside of that specific department?

   a. Data silo
   b. Information system
   c. Information technology
   d. Data architecture

10. What term is used to describe the process an organization undertakes that will improve clinical specificity and documentation that will allow coding professionals to assign more concise disease classification codes?

    a. IG
    b. CDI
    c. ITG
    d. DG

References

Acker, B. M., P. Bankowski-Petz, S. Costello, S. Crabb, K. Fahy, B. Glondys, S. Goodell, et al. 2017. Information Governance Toolkit. http://bok.ahima.org/PdfView?oid=302242.

American Health Information Management Association (AHIMA). n.d.a. Information Governance Glossary. Accessed March 4, 2018. http://www.ahima.org/topics/infogovernance/ig-glossary.

American Health Information Management Association (AHIMA). n.d.b. Information Governance. Accessed February 18, 2018. http://www.ahima.org/topics/infogovernance/igbasics?tabid=resourceshttp://www.ahima.org/topics/infogovernance/igbasics?tabid=resources.

American Health Information Management Association (AHIMA). n.d.c. Information Governance Charter Template. Accessed February 18, 2018. https://library.ahima.org/doc?oid=301383.

American Health Information Management Association (AHIMA). n.d.d. Information Governance Sample Project Plan. Accessed February 18, 2018. http://bok.ahima.org/PdfView?oid=301384.

American Health Information Management Association (AHIMA). 2018. Certified Health Data Analyst. http://www.ahima.org/certification/chda.

American Health Information Management Association (AHIMA). 2017. What is Information Governance (IG)? http://library.ahima.org/doc?oid=300851#.WonfdORy5jo. http://www.ahima.org/~/media/AHIMA/Files/HIM-Trends/IG_Infographic.ashx.

American Health Information Management Association (AHIMA). 2014. Information Governance Principles for Healthcare. www.ahima.org/~/media/AHIMA/Files/HIM-Trends/IG_Principles.ashx.

Amatayakul, M. K. 2016. Health Information Systems Strategic Planning. Chapter 13 in *Health Information Management: Concepts, Principles, and Practice*, 5th ed. Edited by P. and A. Watters. Chicago: AHIMA.

ARMA International. 2017. FAQ: General ARMA. http://www.arma.org/r1/faq.

Bass, D., B. Bigelow, G. Datskovsky, S. Empel, D. K. Green, A. Goel, L. Hamilton, M. Martin, G. Tegethoff, M. G. Reeves, L. M. Washington, and S. Wolfskill. 2014. Information Governance: Principles for Healthcare (IGPHC). www.ahima.org/~/media/AHIMA/Files/HIM-Trends/IG_Principles.ashx.

Biedermann, S. and D. Dolezel. 2016. *Introduction to Healthcare Informatics*, 2nd ed. Chicago: AHIMA.

Blair, B. T. 2014. Information Governance: Healthcare and Beyond. http://bok.ahima.org/doc?oid=300858#.Wojk5-Ry5jo.

Butler, M. 2017. Three Practical IG Projects You Should Implement Today. http://bok.ahima.org/doc?oid=302031#.Wony1uRy5jo.

Butler, M. 2016. Cultivating Healthcare Information Governance: How to Grow Your Program Maturity. http://bok.ahima.org/doc?oid=301341#.Woi82eRy5jo.

Czarkowski, L. and J. Clark. 2015. Drafting a Blueprint for Information Governance. http://bok.ahima.org/doc?oid=107798#.Wonz3-Ry5jo.

Data Governance Institute. 2013. Defining Data Governance. http://www.datagovernance.com/defining-data-governance/.

Davoudi, S., J. Dooling, B. Glondys, T. L. Jones, L. Kadlec, S. M. Overgaard, K. Ruben, and A. Wendicke. Data Quality Management Model (2015 Update). http://bok.ahima.org/doc?oid=107773#.WnPe7qinFRY.

Dolezel, D. Metadata Offers Roadmap to Structured Data. http://bok.ahima.org/doc?oid=107555#.WnPfH6inFRY.

Dooling, J., S. Houser, R. Mikaelian, and C. Smith. 2016. Transitioning to a Data-Driven, Informatics-Oriented Department. http://bok.ahima.org/doc?oid=301903#.WnPfUqinFRY.

Downing, K., K. Fahy, K., M. Foster, M. Hermann, A. Meehan, L. Washington, L., J. Woebkenberg. Information Asset Inventory for Information Governance. http://bok.ahima.org/doc?oid=302048#.Woipx-Ry5jo.

Downing, K. 2016. Importance of Data Stewards in Information Governance. http://bok.ahima.org/doc?oid=301584#.WnPf7ainFRY.

Downing, K. 2015. AHIMA's IG Maturity and Adoption Model Turns the Corner. http://journal.ahima.org/2015/09/28/ahimas-ig-maturity-and-adoption-model-turns-the-corner/.

Glondys, B. 2016. Getting Started with Information Governance: Applying SBAR to IG. http://bok.ahima.org/doc?oid=301346#.WnPgXqinFRY.

Johns, M. 2016. Data Governance and Stewardship. Chapter 3 in *Health Information Management: Concepts, Principles, and Practice*, 5th ed. Edited by P. Oachs and A. Watters. Chicago: AHIMA Press.

Johns, M. 2015. *Enterprise Health Information Management and Data Governance*. Chicago, IL: AHIMA.

Kloss, L. L. 2015. *Implementing Health Information Governance: Lessons from the Field*. Chicago: AHIMA Press.

Kloss, L. L. 2013. Leading Innovation in Enterprise Information Governance. http://bok.ahima.org/doc?oid=106902#.Wom9puRy5jo.

Maimone, C. 2016. Data Mapping Best Practices (2016 update). http://bok.ahima.org/PB/DataMapping#.WoZIIsORy5jo.

Raghupathi, W., and V. Raghupathi. 2014. Big data analytics in healthcare: promise and potential. *Health Information Science and Systems*, 2, 3. http://doi.org/10.1186/2047-2501-2-3.

Reeves, M. G. and R. K. Bowen. 2012. Governing Healthcare's Most Valuable Asset—Data. http://bok.ahima.org/doc?oid=105688#.WonM6uRy5jo.

Rinehart-Thompson, L. 2016. Legal Issues in Health Information Management. Chapter 2 in *Health Information Management: Concepts, Principles, and Practice*, 5th ed. Edited by P. Oachs and A. Watters. Chicago: AHIMA.

Washington, L. 2017. Strategic Alignment: The Driving Force for Information Governance. http://bok.ahima.org/doc?oid=302023#.WnOADqinFRY.

Washington, L. 2016. Early Learning from AHIMA's IG Pilots. http://bok.ahima.org/doc?oid=301648#.WnOAmqinFRY.

Washington, L. 2015. Information Governance Offers a Strategic Approach for Healthcare (2015 update). http://bok.ahima.org/doc?oid=107796#.WnOAaqinFRY.

Chapter 15

Role of HIM Professionals in Information Systems

Learning Objectives

- Compare various technology-driven roles performed by health information management (HIM) professions.
- Identify information technology tasks performed by HIM professionals in traditional and nontraditional settings.
- Explain why HIM professionals are qualified for the various technology-driven roles.

Key Terms

Analytics
Chief clinical informatics officer (CCIO)
Chief security officer (CSO)
Chief technology officer
Clinical informatics coordinator
Commission on Accreditation for Health Informatics and Information Management Education (CAHIIM)

Commission on Certification for Health Information and Information Management (CCHIIM)
Content analyst
Data analyst
Data architect
Data integrity analyst
Data quality manager
Director of clinical informatics
HIM Reimagined (HIMR)

Informatics researcher
Information system trainer
Mapping specialist
Registered Health Information Administrator (RHIA)
Registered Health Information Technician (RHIT)
Research and development scientist
Vice president of information technology

Health information management (HIM) is an allied health profession that is responsible for ensuring the availability, accuracy, and protection of the clinical information that is needed to deliver healthcare services and to make appropriate healthcare-related decisions. A closely related field, health informatics, is the scientific discipline "that concerns itself with the cognitive, information processing, and communication tasks of medical practice, education, and research, including the information science and the technology to support these tasks" (Greenes and Shortliffe, 1990).

With the advent of the electronic health record (EHR), the role of the HIM professional has changed. As the data they manage are digitized, health information managers are becoming increasingly involved in information systems, automated systems that use computer hardware and software to record, manipulate, store, recover, and disseminate data (that is, a system that receives and processes input and provides output). Many HIM skills have transferred to this digital environment, such as understanding the content of the health record, coding systems, documentation, and statistics. Other HIM skills have had to evolve, such as to the management of databases rather than the physical paper health record or managing the data dictionary rather than creating a form. It is important for the HIM profession to position itself as the central player in the EHR, data analysis, health information exchange, and other roles created by the digitizing of health information. The combination and depth of these skills make HIM professionals uniquely qualified for the roles discussed in this chapter and a valuable asset to the information technology staff, administration, researchers, and others. As a result, HIM professionals frequently serve as liaisons between the technical information system staff (programmers, network administrators, and so forth), who are skilled in technology but may not understand healthcare, and the clinicians who provide excellent patient care but may not understand technology.

As the legal health record becomes more electronic, it is important that HIM professionals lead the transition to the EHR. The legal health record comprises the documents and data elements that a healthcare provider may include in response to legally permissible requests for patient information. If the HIM professional is not involved in this transition, issues related to retention, data quality, security, release of information, and other data management topics may be ignored or incorrectly implemented, thus increasing the risk of Health Insurance Portability and Accountability Act (HIPAA) violations, reimbursement denials, state licensing problems, lawsuits, and more. These changes are creating new career opportunities for HIM professionals. These opportunities are seen in the roles that HIM professionals are fulfilling today. The skills possessed by HIM professionals, roles by setting, and roles by functions are discussed in this chapter.

Health Information Management and Technology Competencies

Education is critical in preparing new and current HIM professionals for the roles found in the electronic environment. The Commission on Accreditation for Health Informatics and Information Management Education (CAHIIM) is responsible for establishing the content that accredited master's, bachelor's, and associate's programs must teach their students. The entry level competencies are updated periodically to remain current. These documents define the content that the accredited HIM programs must cover. Topic areas covered in both the associate level and bachelor level in HIM curriculum include the following:

- Health data structure, content, and standards
- Information protection: access, disclosure, archival, privacy, and security
- Healthcare privacy, confidentiality, legal issues, and ethical issues
- Information and communication technologies
- Data, information, and file structures
- Data storage and retrieval
- Informatics, analytics, and data use
- Revenue management
- Compliance
- Leadership (CAHIIM 2014)

A recent study of HIM job postings found many of the job postings focused on "documentation, standards, data, health information technology and analytics" (Marc et al. 2017, 25). Analytics is analyzing data (in this case healthcare data) and turning it into information and knowledge that can be used in decision making. Figure 15.1 shows a word cloud of the top 100 terms used in the job postings. The more often the word or phrase is used, the larger it appears in the word cloud. A review of the word cloud shows many of the concepts and terms covered in this textbook.

The entry-level competencies are developed based on research that identifies what HIM professionals are currently doing in the field and what the profession is expected to do in the future. This research is conducted about every five years in order to keep up with the changes in the HIM profession, technology, and healthcare. Many of the CAHIIM competencies required are technological in nature, whereas many others, although not technological themselves, are important for working with the EHR. For example, although reimbursement itself is not an information system topic, technology is valuable to coding, chargemaster, compliance, and other reimbursement-related functions. The next sections will address the skills that the HIM professional possesses, HIM Reimagined, HIM roles by employer type, and HIM roles by function.

Figure 15.1.   Top 100 terms used in job posting

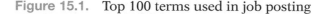

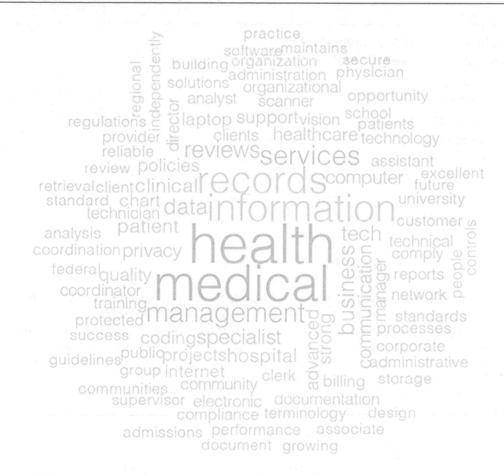

Source: Marc et al. 2017.

Skills Required of HIM Professionals

The HIM professional must have a broad range of skills in areas including data management, data analysis, system analysis, system implementation, health data structure, documentation requirements, data quality, information system management, privacy and security, coding, and reimbursement. There are other professions that require some of the same skills a HIM professional holds, but there is no other profession that requires the same mix, depth and breadth of these skills.

Most, if not all, of these skills depend on technology in some way. Some of these skills involve the development or usage of the information system; others rely on the output from the information system to provide the data needed to conduct analysis. A Workforce Study conducted by the Caviart Group on behalf of the American Health Information Management Association (AHIMA) identified the top 10 HIM skills needed for the future (figure 15.2.). These top 10 HIM skills show the direction of the profession and where HIM professionals need to focus their attention.

It is expected that over the next 10 to 20 years, the HIM professional will continue to need skills in information systems, data analysis, security, and other information system–related areas (Caviart Group 2015). The connection to information systems may not be obvious as first glance. For example, the clinical documentation skills are enhanced through the use of good screen design, a good data dictionary, edits, reminders, and alerts. Another example is problem-solving skills. If a problem occurs in the implementation of an information system, the HIM professional must be able to identify the root cause of the problem, identify options for resolving the problem, select an option, and take the necessary steps to resolve the problem. This information will continue to impact the educational programs across the country.

Registered Health Information Administrator (RHIA) and **Registered Health Information Technician (RHIT)** certification examinations are based on the same domains (topic areas) used by

Figure 15.2.   Top 10 HIM skills of the next 10 to 20 years

1. Electronic health records management skills
2. Skill in managing information privacy and security
3. Analytical thinking skills
4. Critical thinking skills
5. Skill in ensuring data integrity
6. Problem solving skills
7. Communication skills (written, spoken, and/or presentation)
8. Clinical documentation improvement skills
9. Leadership skills
10. Skill in analyzing big data

Source: Adapted from the Caviart Group 2015, 10.

CAHIIM; however, the exams are written by the **Commission on Certification for Health Information and Information Management (CCHIIM)**, the independent body within AHIMA that establishes and grants professional certifications in health informatics and HIM professions. The RHIA is for those who graduate from an accredited bachelor in HIM program. The RHIT is for those who graduate from an accredited associate's-degree–level HIM program. These examinations are both entry-level certifications over the entire scope of HIM skills. With additional education and work experience, the HIM professional may earn specialty certifications, many of which are related to the content of this text. Some of the specialty certifications offered by AHIMA are:

- Certified in Healthcare Privacy and Security (CHPS): The CHPS is an advanced certification that focuses on privacy and security.
- Certified in Health Data Analytics (CHDA): The focus of the CHDA is statistics, data visualization (graphs and charts), data collection, data analysis, and more.
- Certified Professional in Health Informatics (CPHI): The CPHI covers information systems, database management, data analysis, and more.
- Certified Coding Specialist (CCS): The CCS is an advanced coding certification for both inpatient and outpatient coding.
- Certified Documentation Improvement Professional (CDIP): The CDIP's focus is on improving the documentation of the health record to improve patient care, decision making, and more.

Roles by Setting

HIM professionals work in a number of different healthcare settings (hospitals, home health, long-term care facilities, and so forth), some of which are discussed in this chapter:

- Healthcare facilities
- Information system vendors
- Consulting firms
- Government agencies
- Standards developmental organizations
- Educational facilities

The importance and level of various information systems skills that a HIM professional needs depend on the setting in which he or she works. These are the types of organization where HIM professionals work. Later in the chapter, some specific HIM roles related to information systems in these settings are covered.

Healthcare Facilities

In a healthcare facility, the HIM professional may be employed in the traditional HIM department in roles such as cancer registry, HIM director and other supervisory and management staff, and coder. HIM professionals are also employed in other departments throughout the healthcare facility, such as information systems department, finance department, revenue cycle management, or quality improvement department. HIM professionals are found in roles such as system implementation, privacy and security officer, project management, and more.

Vendors

HIM professionals work in many different types of vendor environments, such as HIM equipment and supplies and information systems. In the information systems vendor environment, the HIM professional can be found in system development, customer service, system implementation, training, and other roles. In many of these roles, the HIM professional works with hospitals and other clients around the country to support their information system needs such as help with project management, system selection, and system implementation. Many vendor roles require the HIM professional to travel and to telecommute when not traveling.

Consulting Firms

Many of the vendor roles mentioned in the vendor section may also be found in consulting firms. The consultants are contracted by the healthcare facilities to assist in various HIM roles, such as interim management, coding, information systems training and implementation, and other projects the healthcare facility does not have time or expertise to handle alone. The specific role will be defined by the needs of the healthcare facility and the contract signed between the two parties. As with the vendor environment, the HIM professional may spend a lot of time traveling to client sites.

Government Agencies

The roles in government agencies will vary by the agency in which the HIM professional operates. Examples of government agencies where HIM professionals might work at the federal level include the Centers for Medicare and Medicaid Services, National Centers for Health Statistics, Agency for Healthcare Research and Quality, and Veterans Administration, to name a few. HIM professionals also frequently work at the state or local health department. Roles can be traditional HIM roles, such as director of the HIM department at a Veterans Administration hospital, or may include nontraditional roles in agencies across local, state, and federal government levels, such as data collection, data analysis, standards development, monitoring compliance with regulations, public health agencies, and research. These tasks will require information systems and someone to manage them and the data collected. With the focus on quality of care, the EHR, fraud and abuse, and other HIM responsibilities, there is a need for HIM professionals to assume development and oversight roles in these areas.

Standards Development Organizations

In standards development organizations, HIM professionals assist in the development, implementation, and testing of standards; educating the public; and ensuring that sound HIM principles are used. They can also participate in data modeling, data warehousing, development of a data dictionary, and data mapping. The HIM professionals' input is important because of their knowledge of data quality, data collection, data content, and other related areas. Again, the HIM professional is a valuable part of this team because of the wide range of skills he or she possesses.

Educational Facilities

In colleges and universities, HIM educators play an important role in the future of HIM as they prepare students and established HIM professionals for the information systems roles that they will encounter. Educators should have professional experience in the HIM field and must continually educate themselves on changes in the profession in order to formally educate the student. Not only do HIM educators need to know about current HIM practices, but they also need to know about learning styles and teaching strategies. The CAHIIM entry level curricula provide a guide for educators as they prepare students for the roles in HIM. Frequently, students decide on an HIM career path while earning their associate's or bachelor's degree in HIM. In order to reach their career goal, they may have to obtain more education and work their way into the role that they want. For example, if a HIM graduate wants to work as a consultant assisting in the selection and implementation of information systems, the graduate should work in a healthcare facility with the information systems, then gain experience with system selection and implementation at the healthcare facility prior to becoming a consultant. Another example is the role of educator; HIM professionals in colleges and universities must have the necessary education in order to teach. HIM educators should generally hold at least a degree higher than the level at which they are teaching. Thus, in an associate's-degree–level HIM program, the HIM educator should have at least a bachelor's degree; likewise, an HIM educator in a bachelor's-degree–level in HIM program should have at least a master's degree. HIM educators must be prepared to teach courses on the CAHIIM competencies, including those related to information systems. The HIM educator needs to teach hard skills—the skills related to information systems—and soft skills, such as problem solving and critical thinking (the ability to look at a situation from multiple perspectives and be able to apply knowledge and skills to assess the situation).

CHECK YOUR UNDERSTANDING 15.1

1. The organization that accredits HIM educational programs is _____.

   a. AHIMA
   b. CAHIIM
   c. The Joint Commission
   d. CMS

2. The credential for someone who graduates from an accredited associate-level HIM program and passes the national examination is _____.

   a. RHIA
   b. CDA
   c. CHPS
   d. RHIT

3. Which of the following healthcare settings hires out HIM professionals to healthcare facilities?

   a. Standard development organization
   b. Vendor
   c. Consultant
   d. Government agencies

4. Identify the skill that an HIM professional has _____.

   a. Computer programming
   b. System analysis
   c. Installing the physical network
   d. Building a computer

5. True or false? Entry-level competencies are based on current practices only.
   a. True
   b. False

Roles by Function

HIM professionals have been active in many information system roles for a number of years, although the variety of these roles is expanding with the evolution of technology and informatics. This section discusses both the traditional and contemporary jobs related to information for HIM professionals.

Traditional HIM Information Systems Job Titles and Descriptions

Many HIM positions are related to technology in one way or another. HIM professionals have long worked in information technology roles within healthcare facilities and vendor sites, including the more traditional information technology roles of systems analyst, system implementation, project manager, system development, technical support, training, and sales. A brief description of these HIM professionals' roles follows:

- Systems analyst—Identifies the stakeholders of an information system as well as the functionality required of a system. Tasks include data collection, data analysis, and developing data flow diagrams. The systems analyst would assist in the reengineering of business processes that would take advantage of the benefits of the system being implemented.

- System implementation—Assist in many aspects of the process, such as systems analysis, developing the request for proposal, selecting systems, setting configurations, training, reengineering, and other steps in the process.

- Project manager—Controls the budget, staff, and other resources allocated to ensure the goals of the system are met.

- System development—Adds value to the programming staff because they know the HIM functions and processes needed. HIM professionals are not computer programmers; however, they frequently help design the system that the programmers will create. For example, a HIM professional assisting in the development process would know that amendments to the EHR or other clinical system must be documented as such, and the original information must be retained and available only with specific access rights. Their HIM knowledge allows them to determine if the needs of the facilities and regulatory and accreditation demands are being met.

- Technical support—Assists with technical problems that are encountered with an information system. They identify the source of the problems and take the necessary steps to resolve them. These problems could be inability to access an information system or a function that is not working.

- Information system trainer—Responsible for the development and implementation of the training plan discussed in chapter 13.

- Vendor sales team member—Talks to the HIM purchasers of information systems with an understanding of the daily HIM issues.

Contemporary HIM Information Systems Job Titles

HIM professionals are going beyond the traditional information system roles they have occupied for years. They are now working in roles such as data integrity analyst, data analyst, and other new and evolving roles. Some of these roles include:

- The chief clinical informatics officer (CCIO) works with clinical providers, such as physicians and nurses, to lead them in the use of technology to improve quality of care, medical education, and healthcare research (AHIMA 2017a). The CCIO role is a "big picture" role in that the CCIO works to ensure that the technologies needed by the healthcare providers are identified and ultimately implemented.

- The director of clinical informatics is the leader in the implementation of the EHR as well as the post-implementation services described in chapter 6. The director is the champion for the EHR and works with the implementation team to ensure they have the resources needed (AHIMA 2017a).

- The research and development scientist works to create new abilities in health information technology. These roles may be found in colleges and universities (AHIMA 2017a). The research and development scientists invent the technologies that are used in healthcare, such as telehealth applications.

- A mapping specialist creates maps between systems such as vocabularies and classification systems (AHIMA 2017a). The mapping specialist must be an expert in both systems so that they can correctly create the maps. For example, in *International Classification of Diseases, Ninth Revision, Clinical Modification* the diagnosis code for pneumonia, unspecified is 486. The code for the same condition is J18.9 in *International Classification of Diseases, Tenth Revision, Clinical Modification*. Not only do the codes from both systems have to be correct when mapping, but also the rules of both systems have to be followed. These codes can be built into information systems facilitating the mapping and the use of the maps for reports, studies, and more.

- The **data integrity analyst** is responsible for ensuring the quality of the data in HIM information systems, as discussed in chapter 2. Data integrity analysts must be able to apply data and content standards to data collection and data storage. They must be able to maintain the information systems, ensure compliance with legal and accreditation requirements, and be able to analyze data (AHIMA n.d.a).

- The **clinical informatics coordinator** requires knowledge of clinical information systems such as those described in chapter 8. They are experts in the data retrieval needed by healthcare providers while conducting patient care (AHIMA n.d.a).

- An **informatics researcher** is responsible for ensuring the availability of data needed. This role also develops the data collection methods needed for the various types of data. The focus is to identify best practices in providing healthcare (Nelson and Staggers 2018).

- The **data analyst** applies his or her skills to manage, analyze, interpret, and transform health data into accurate, consistent, and timely information.

- The **content analyst** designs the clinical information system that will be implemented. Their work is directed by the needs of the users. They are also advocates in the usage of health information technology in healthcare (AHIMA n.d.a).

- The **chief technology officer** assists in the development of the healthcare facility's strategic business plan in relation to information systems and technology. Their goal is to ensure the healthcare facility operates effectively and that they are competitive with other healthcare facilities within their community (AHIMA n.d.a).

- A **vice president of information technology** will develop and implement a strategy for the healthcare facility that ensures that the healthcare facility has the technology needed to grow and improve. The strategy should ensure that the needs of the healthcare facility are met into the future (AHIMA n.d.a).

- The **data quality manager** works with physicians and other healthcare providers to assist them in the achievement of the healthcare facility's data quality goals as needed for coding and reimbursement as well as general documentation throughout the healthcare facility. This role is responsible for the quality management functions at the healthcare facility (AHIMA n.d.a; AHIMA n.d.b).

- The **data architect** contributes to the development of the data models covered in chapter 3. They are also involved in the information governance activities discussed in chapter 13 and data management. Data management is the combined practices of HIM, information technology, and health informatics that affect how data and documentation combine to create a single business record for a healthcare organization (AHIMA 2017).

- The **chief security officer (CSO)** is responsible for protecting data from unauthorized access, alteration, and destruction. This role is responsible for

  o Developing and establishing a compliance program (refer to chapter 13)

  o Monitoring state, federal, and local laws as well as proposed regulations

  o Monitoring trends related to security and updating policies

As discussed in chapter 13, among the CSO's specific responsibilities are performing or delegating the responsibility for audits to ensure that policies are being followed and that breaches have not occurred. This individual would also be responsible for risk assessment and ensuring that the current security plans are working.

New HIM graduates have learned many of the skills required for these roles in college and will learn more through on-the-job training. Current HIM professionals prepare for these roles in a number of ways, such as going back to school, on-the-job training, and in continuing education programs.

HIM Reimagined Initiative

As discussed previously, the role of the HIM professional is changing dramatically. The knowledge of what the future holds is important to ensure that the skills of the HIM professional meet the needs of the employers. AHIMA has been researching the needs of the healthcare delivery system in order to identify what the future of the HIM profession should be. In addition to the changes discussed already, the HIM profession must address changes in "approaches to medicine, increased automations, and aging of the population" (Sandefer et al. 2017, 4). Failure to meet the needs of the healthcare delivery system may result in the HIM professional becoming obsolete. If the HIM profession does not address the changes, other professions will. There are three areas that must be addressed:

- Healthcare environment: There are significant changes in reimbursement, patient treatment, consumer informatics, and more. The HIM profession and HIM professionals must adapt to these changes to ensure that health information documentation, information systems, data collection and usage, and other skills/tools are available to meet the needs of the healthcare delivery system.

- Trends at colleges and universities: Education costs are escalating at the same time that state funding is decreasing. To address these changes, higher education is investigating new options as well as expanding others. In addition to the traditional certificates and degrees, college and universities are expanding education options to apprenticeships, digital badges, e-portfolios, and more.

- Needs of workforce: Many employers are looking for specific credentials and education for their employees in order to reduce the training that the employee needs to become productive. Employers are expecting lifelong learning from their long-term employees in order to help ensure that employees continue be productive in the evolving environment. Employers are also using apprenticeships to help new graduates bridge the gap between college and employment. (Sandefer et al. 2017)

The result of the research into the future of HIM is the HIM Reimagined (HIMR) vision, which identifies four recommendations:

- Increasing the number of AHIMA members holding graduate degrees
- Increasing the research related to HIM and health informatics
- Increasing opportunities for specialization in HIM
- Revising the RHIT certification to become RHIT (+Specialty)

With the RHIT (+Specialty) certification, new graduates would be eligible to sit for not only the RHIT exam but a specialty exam, too. The speciality certification would depend on the specialty tracks that the student takes during his or her associate's degree program. At the time this textbook was written, the specialty tracks have not been published. The purpose of these four HIMR recommendations is to support the transition to technology-focused skills.

Increasing the number of HIM professionals with graduate degrees is important, as many of the new skills HIM professionals need require more advanced education than has been available at the associate's or bachelor's degree levels. In order to increase the number of members holding graduate degrees, HIMR recommends increasing scholarships, increasing the number of faculty qualified to teach HIM at the graduate level, and implementing a formal HIM graduate curriculum. The recommendation for increasing research related to HIM and health informatics will be met through research grants, dissertation scholarships, research on the HIM skills needed, and data analytics. HIMR proposes a major revision to the associate's degree in HIM. The general HIM skills content will be reduced, allowing students to choose a specialization. These specializations will be based on present and future speciality certifications such as the CHDA or CDIP. The bachelor's degree will be a generalist degree and therefore will cover many different areas of the profession. The master's degree, like the associate's, will reduce the general health information content to allow for specializations. This would allow specializations for lower-level and higher level positions within the profession. These changes, based on both industry and educational needs, are drastic changes and will not happen overnight. The rollout of these changes began in 2017 and will continue through 2027.

CHECK YOUR UNDERSTANDING 15.2

1. What is the role of a data architect?
   a. Health information resource management and innovation
   b. Information governance and stewardship
   c. Managing the technology
   d. Data model development

(Continued)

CHECK YOUR UNDERSTANDING 15.2 (*Continued*)

2. What role designs information systems based on the needs of the user?

   a. Vice President, Information Technology
   b. Data analyst
   c. Data quality manager
   d. Content analyst

3. Which HIM job title includes the development of the request for proposal?

   a. Resource manager
   b. Data translator
   c. Data analyst
   d. Systems analyst

4. The HIM role that ensures that data are available is known as _____.

   a. Resource manager
   b. Data translator
   c. Data analyst
   d. Informatics researcher

5. HIMR has several recommendations including _____.

   a. Increasing the number of AHIMA members earning graduate degrees
   b. Eliminating the RHIT certification
   c. Increasing the content covered by the RHIT certification
   d. Eliminating graduate level education programs in HIM being accredited

Real-World Case

Marie earned her bachelor's degree in HIM. After working in traditional HIM roles for a few years, she decided that she wanted to be involved in the selection and implementation of the EHR and other healthcare information systems. Marie went back to school and earned her master's degree in health informatics. After graduation, Marie worked for an information system vendor for several years. She decided to take another turn in her career path and become a professor in an accredited HIM program. She took a position as a faculty member in a bachelor's-level HIM program. Marie now teaches the information system courses for the HIM program and is able to give the students real world examples from her experience in the traditional HIM departments and the information system vendor. Marie enjoyed her position so much that after teaching for a while, Marie went back to school again to earn her doctorate degree in adult education.

CHAPTER REVIEW

1. The RHIT exam requires students to graduate from a(n) _____.

   a. Accredited associate's degree in HIM
   b. Bachelor's degree in HIM (accredited or nonaccredited)
   c. Accredited bachelor's degree in HIM
   d. Associate's degree in HIM (accredited or nonaccredited)

2. A HIM professional would like to work for an organization that hires HIM professionals to work in system development and customer service. Identify this type of setting.

    a. Vendor
    b. Consulting firm
    c. Standards development organization
    d. Government agency

3. Entry level curricula for accredited HIM programs is set by _____.

    a. Healthcare providers
    b. CCHIIM
    c. Individual colleges and universities
    d. CAHIIM

4. The healthcare facility needs to collect data, perform data analysis, and create data flow diagrams. This task would be assigned to which of the following roles?

    a. Project manager
    b. System development
    c. Systems analysis
    d. Technical support

5. Data and content standards are applied by which role?

    a. Mapping specialist
    b. Data integrity analyst
    c. Clinical informatics coordinator
    d. Content analyst

6. HIMR identified three areas to be addressed. They are healthcare environment, the needs of the work force, and _____.

    a. Lifelong learning
    b. Technological changes
    c. Trends in higher education
    d. Level of specialization

7. Increasing opportunities for specialization in HIM is a recommendation of _____.

    a. CAHIIM
    b. Colleges and universities
    c. CCHIIM
    d. HIMR

8. The role that is involved in the development of data models is _____.

    a. Informatics researcher
    b. Content analyst
    c. Data quality manager
    d. Data architect

9. The field that uses information science and technology to support information-processing and communication of healthcare practice is known as _____.

    a. Health information management
    b. Health informatics
    c. Health information technology
    d. Privacy and security

(Continued)

CHAPTER REVIEW (*Continued*)

10. Failure of the HIM professional to be involved in EHR implementation may lead to _____.
    a. Errors in programming
    b. Data quality not being addressed
    c. Lack of training
    d. CAHIIM competencies not being met

References

American Health Information Management Association. n.d.a. Career Map. Accessed January 14, 2018. http://hicareers.com/CareerMap/.

American Health Information Management Association. n.d.b. Data Quality Manager. Accessed 14 January 2018. http://library.ahima.org/PdfView?oid=22988.

American Health Information Management Association. 2017. Sample Job Description: Data Architect. http://bok.ahima.org/doc?oid=301375#.WUHnbuQ2xjo.

Caviart Group. 2015. Results of the AHIMA 2014 Workforce Study. http://library.ahima.org/PdfView?oid=300801.

Commission on Accreditation for Health Informatics and Information Management (CAHIIM). 2014. CAHIIM Curriculum Report—AHIMA Entry Level Competencies for Health Information Management (HIM) at the Associate Degree Level. http://www.cahiim.org/documents/AS%202014%20Competencies%20Report.xlsx.

Greenes R. A. and E. H. Shortliffe. 1990. Medical informatics: an emerging academic discipline and institutional priority. https://jamanetwork.com/journals/jama/article-abstract/380818?redirect=true.

Nelson, R. and N. Staggers. 2018. *Health Informatics: An Interprofessional Approach*. St. Louis, MO: Elsevier.

Marc, D. T., J. Robertson, L. Gordon, Z. Green-Lawson, D. Gibbs, K. Dover, and M. Dougherty. 2017. What the data say about HIM professional trends. *Journal of AHIMA* 88(5): http://bok.ahima.org/doc?oid=302104&utm_source=Real%20Magnet&utm_medium=email&utm_term=CareerMinded_July17_m&utm_content=HIM%20Career%20Resources%20and%20News%20-%20Fighting%20the%20Robots%20with%20Education&utm_campaign=Newsletters_Career%20Minded#.Weyt5uRe7IV.

Sandefer, R., M. Millen, M. Sharp, K. Abrams, S. Carlon, A. Chenoweth, M. B. Haugen, et al. 2017. HIM Reimagined: Transformation Starts with You. http://www.ahima.org/about/him-reimagined/himr?tabid=whitepaper.

Source: American Health Information Management Association. 2010. RFI/RFP template (Updated). http://library. ahima.org/xpedio/groups/public/documents/ahima/bok1_047959.hcsp?dDocName=bok1_047959.

The request for information/request for proposal (RFI/RFP) process is vital to procuring a system that meets organizational and user needs. Because of this, it is imperative that adequate time be allotted for the process.

This template is provided as a sample tool to assist healthcare providers as they issue an RFI or an RFP for electronic health record (EHR) or component systems. It is meant to be used in conjunction with the practice brief titled "The RFP Process for EHR Systems."

Healthcare providers should customize this sample template by using the components that are applicable for their needs, adding components as necessary, and deleting those that are not.

Sections 1 and 2 should be completed by the facility.

1. Introduction (introducing the facility to the vendor)
   a. Brief Description of the Facility
   b. Facility Information
      i. Complete Address
      ii. Market (acute, ambulatory, long-term care, home health)
      iii. Enterprise Information. The organizations should provide all relevant information including whether the facility is a part of a healthcare delivery system, the facilities that are included in the project, and their locations.
      iv. Size. The organization should provide any information that will be relevant to the product such as the number of discharges, visits, beds, etc.
      v. General Description of Current Systems Environment. The organization should provide general information regarding current information systems structure (i.e., hardware and operating systems).
   c. Scope
      The organization should provide a brief narrative description of the project that the RFP covers and the environment sought (e.g., phased approach, hybrid support).

2. Statement of Purpose
   a. Overall Business Objectives/Drivers
      The organization should list high-level business goals it is looking to achieve by implementing the software.

b. Key Desired Functionality
When requesting information for the facility-wide solution (e.g., EHR), the organization should list the various features and functions of the system desired, as well as any pertinent details.

    i. Clinical Repository

    ii. Clinical Documentation

    iii. Computerized Physician Order Entry (CPOE)

    iv. Ancillary Support (e.g., laboratory, radiology, pharmacy, etc.)

    v. Picture Archiving Communication System (PACS)

    vi. Electronic Document Management/Document Imaging

    vii. Customizable Workflow Management

    viii. Interoperability (e.g., for health information exchange)

    ix. Patient Portals

    x. Other

c. HIM Department Operations
When requesting information for the HIM solution, the organization should list the various processes and functions of the system it is looking for, as well as any pertinent details.

    i. Chart Analysis/Deficiency Management

    ii. Coding/Abstracting

    iii. Patient Identity Management/Electronic Master Patient Index (e-MPI)

    iv. Health Record Output and Disclosure Management

    v. Release of Information

    vi. Screen Input Design

    vii. Support for Mandated Reportable Data Sets

    viii. Other

d. System Administration—Records Management and Evidentiary Support
This functionality is applicable to or used for all components or modules of an application. Facility requirements for this functionality should be specified in the detailed system requirements.

    i. User Administration

    ii. Access Privilege Control Management

    iii. Logging/Auditing Function

    iv. Digital Signature Functions

    v. Records Management Function

    vi. Archiving Functions

    vii. Continuity of Operations (e.g., support for backup, recovery)

    viii. Maintenance of Standardized Vocabularies and Code Sets

e. Future Plans
General description of long-term plans, including identified future systems environment and projected timetables.

Sections 3 and 4 should be completed by the vendor.

3. Requirements
Vendors should provide availability and timelines for development of software to fulfill requirements not available at this time.

a. User Requirements
Each functional area is expected to have its own set of user requirements.

Sample questions related to HIM functional user requirements and features are provided below. This table is a sample only. Organizations must customize this RFP template to meet their needs.

Functional User Requirements/Features (Also refer to certification requirements and Health Level Seven (HL7) EHR System Functional Model (EHR-S FM) for other key requirements/features.)	Available	Custom Developed	Future Development	Not Available
Chart Completion/Deficiency Analysis				
Can the organization define the intervals for aging analysis (e.g., 7 days, 14 days, 21 days, etc.)?				
Does the system allow for standard and ad-hoc reporting for chart deficiency/delinquency analysis?				
Can delinquency reports be sent to physicians/clinicians in electronic (e.g., e-mail or fax) and paper formats (letters)?				
Does the system allow you to define or detail all deficiencies by provider, by area of deficiency, or other combinations (e.g., group practices, etc.)?				
Does the system allow the organization to list all records (charts) by the deficiency type?				
Can deficiency analysis be conducted at the time the patient is prepared for discharge from the facility?				
Does the system support most industry standard dictation systems to allow transcribed reports to be easily and efficiently completed?				
Does the system allow for end-user notification when information identified as incomplete/missing is completed?				
Coding Completion/Analysis				
Does the system support automation of coding work flow (e.g., computer-assisted coding)?				
Does the system support automated case assignment to work queues?				
Can the user assign cases based on special attributes (e.g., VIP, dollars, or case type such as cancer or trauma, etc.)?				
Does the system support online communication between employees and managers?				
Does the system support most industry standard encoders/groupers?				
Does the system support both on-site and remote coding activities?				

(Continued)

Functional User Requirements/Features (Also refer to certification requirements and Health Level Seven (HL7) EHR System Functional Model (EHR-S FM) for other key requirements/features.)	Available	Custom Developed	Future Development	Not Available
Does the system support assignment of high-risk coding to supervisory staff or allow coding verification as staff complete cases?				
Does the system contain tools for monitoring and evaluating the coding process?				
Does the system support electronic query capabilities?				
Coding/Transaction Standards (see also Section 4.k)				
Does the system support ICD-10-CM and/or ICD-10-PCS in addition to ICD-9-CM?				
Does the system use General Equivalence Mappings (GEMs), such as between ICD-10-CM/PCS and ICD-9-CM or SNOMED CT and ICD-9-CM?				
Is the system compliant with the Version 5010 transaction standard?				
Health Record Output and Disclosure				
Does the system allow a unified view of all component subsystems of the EHR at the individual patient level and at the date of service encounter level for purposes of disclosure management (including the ability to print and generate electronic output)?				
Does the system provide the ability to define the records or reports that are considered the formal health record for a specified disclosure or disclosure purposes?				
Does the system allow VIP patients to be flagged and listed confidentially on corresponding reports (i.e., census)?				
Does the system produce an accounting of disclosure, reporting at a minimum the date and time a disclosure took place, what was disclosed, to whom, by whom, and the reason for disclosure?				
Does the system provide the ability to create hard copy and electronic output of report summary information and to generate reports in both chronological and specified record elements order?				
Does the system provide the ability to include patient identifying information on each page of electronically generated reports and provide the ability to customize reports to match mandated formats?				

Does the system allow for redaction and recording the reason, in addition to the ability to redact patient information from larger reports?

Release of Information (Note: Administrative release of information functionally may or may not be an integral component of an EHR system.)

Does the system support HIPAA management of non-TPO disclosures?

Does the system track and report the date/time release of information requests are received and fulfilled?

Does the system allow the ability to track whether the release of information consent/authorization was adequate, in addition to a corresponding disposition?

Does the system generate invoices with user-defined pay scales?

Does the system allow tracking of payments received?

Does the system generate template letters for standard correspondence (e.g., patient not found, date of service not valid, etc.)?

Does the system allow information to be released electronically?

Authentication

Does the system authenticate principals (i.e., users, entities, applications, devices, etc.) before accessing the system and prevent access to all nonauthenticated principals?

Does the system require authentication mechanisms and can the system securely store authentication data/information?

If user names and passwords are used, does the system require password strength rules that allow for a minimum

number of characters and inclusion of alphanumeric complexity, while preventing the reuse of previous passwords, without being transported or viewable in plain text?

Does the system have the ability to terminate or lock a session after a period of inactivity or after a series of invalid log-in attempts?

(Continued)

Functional User Requirements/Features (Also refer to certification requirements and Health Level Seven (HL7) EHR System Functional Model (EHR-S FM) for other key requirements/features.)	Available	Custom Developed	Future Development	Not Available
Access Controls				
Does the system provide the ability to create and update sets of access-control permissions granted to principals (i.e., users, entities, applications, devices, etc.) based on the user's role and scope of practice?				
Does the system inactivate a user and remove the user's privileges without deleting the user's history?				
Does the system have the ability to record and report all authorization actions?				
Does the system allow only authorized users access to confidential information?				
Does the system prevent users with read and/or write privileges from printing or copying/writing to other media?				
Does the system define and enforce system and data access rules for all EHR system				
resources (at component, application, or user level, either local or remote)?				
Does the system restrict access to patient information based on location (e.g., nursing unit, clinic, etc.)?				
Does the system track restrictions?				
Does the system have the ability to track/audit viewed records without significant effect on system speed?				
Does the system allow for electronic access to specified patients/encounters for external reviewers?				
Emergency Access Controls				
Does the system allow emergency access regardless of controls or established user levels, within a set time parameter?				
Does the system define the acceptable circumstances in which the user can override the controls for emergency access, as well as require the user to specify the circumstance?				
Does the system require a second level of validation before granting a user emergency access?				
Can a report be generated of all emergency access use?				

Does the system provide the ability to periodically review/renew a user's emergency access privileges?			
Does the system provide the ability to generate an after-action report to trigger follow-up of emergency access use?			

Information Attestation

Does the system provide the ability for attestation (verification) of EHR content by properly authenticated and authorized users different from the author (e.g., countersignature) as allowed by users' scope of practice, organizational policy, or jurisdictional law?			
If more than one author contributed to the EHR content, does the system provide the ability to associate and maintain all authors/contributors with their content?			
If the EHR content was attested to by someone other than the author, does the system maintain all authors and contributors?			
Does the system provide the ability to present (e.g., view, report, display, access) the credentials and the name of the author(s) and the attester, as well as the date and time of attestation?			

Data Retention, Availability, and Destruction

Does the system provide the ability to store and retrieve health record data and clinical documents for the legally prescribed time or according to organizational policy and to include unaltered inbound data?			
Does the system provide the ability to identify specific EHR data for destruction and allow for the review and confirmation of selected items before destruction occurs?			
Does the system provide the ability to destroy EHR data/records so that data are not retrievable in a reasonably accessible and usable format according to policy and legal retentions periods, and is a certificate of destruction generated?			

Record Preservation

Does the system provide the ability to identify records that must be preserved beyond normal retention practices and identify a reason for preserving the record?			

(Continued)

Functional User Requirements/Features (Also refer to certification requirements and Health Level Seven (HL7) EHR System Functional Model (EHR-S FM) for other key requirements/features.)	Available	Custom Developed	Future Development	Not Available
Does the system provide the ability to generate a legal hold notice identifying whom to contact for questions when a user attempts to alter a record on legal hold or an unauthorized user attempts to access a record on legal hold?				
Does the system provide the ability to secure data/ records from unauditable alteration or unauthorized use for preservation purposes, such as a legal hold?				
Does the system provide the ability to merge and unmerge records?				
Does the system allow a record to be locked after a specified time so no more changes may be made?				
Minimum Metadata Set and Audit Capability for Record Actions				
Does the system capture and retain the date, time stamp, and user for every object/data creation, modification, view, deletion, or printing/export of any part of the medical record?				
Does the system retain a record of the viewer?				
Does the system retain a record of the author of a change?				
Does the system retain a record of the change history?				
Does the system retain a record of the source of nonoriginated data?				
Does the system retain the medical record metadata for the legally prescribed time frame in accordance with the organizational policy?				
Does the system include the minimum metadata set for a record exchanged or released?				
Pending State				
Does the system apply a date and time-stamp each time a note is updated (opened/ signature event)?				
Does the system display and notify the author of pending notes?				
Does the system allow the ability to establish a time frame for pending documents before administrative closing?				

Does the system display pending notes in a way that clearly identifies them as pending?				
Does the system allow the author to complete, edit, or delete (if never viewed for patient care) the pending note?				

Amendments and Corrections

Does the system allow the author to correct, amend, or augment a note or entry?				
Does the system allow the author to indicate whether the change was a correction, amendment, or augmentation?				
Does the system record and display the date and time stamp of the change?				
Does the system provide a clear indicator of a changed record?				
Does the system provide a link or clear direction to the original entry/note?				
Does the system retain all versions?				
Does the system disseminate updated information to providers that were initially autofaxed?				

Documentation Succession Management and Version Control

Does the system manage the succession of documents?				
Does the system retain all versions when a change is made?				
Does the system provide an indicator that there are prior versions (when appropriate)?				
Does the system indicate the most recent version?				

Retracted State

Does the system allow for removing a record or note from view?				
Does the system allow for access of a retracted note or record?				
Does the system allow the user to record the reason for retraction?				
Does the system allow for notification of the viewers of the data to present correct information (if applicable)?				

(Continued)

Functional User Requirements/Features (Also refer to certification requirements and Health Level Seven (HL7) EHR System Functional Model (EHR-S FM) for other key requirements/features.)	Available	Custom Developed	Future Development	Not Available
Data Collection and Reporting				
Does the system allow for real-time data collectionand progress measurement against preset targets?				
Does the system produce reports on turnaround days, dollars pending, costs per chart by process, days to billing, and so on, as related to AR?				
Does the system have the ability to track clinical decision-making alerts (e.g., when they were added to the system or discontinued, used, ignored, etc.)?				
Does the system comply with meaningful use reporting requirements?				
Patient Financial Support				
Is your proposed solution fully integrated (or able to interface with the patient financial system), offering users an electronic form of the business office?				
Can patient information be placed in folders to easily identify those details that refer to the patient (guarantor) account(s)?				
Can you electronically capture, store, and retrieve computer-generated documents and reports, such as the UB-04 or the CMS 1500, which are HIPAA transaction standard compliant?				
Patient Portals				
Does the system allow for electronic patient access (e.g., Web portal)?				
Health Information Exchange				
Does the system enable participation in local health information exchange initiatives?				

b. System Requirements

Organizations should provide a list to vendors of what current technology needs to be supported. Vendors should then provide information on their system's available requirements.

Sample questions related to system requirements and features are provided below. This table is a sample only. Organizations must customize this RFP template to meet their needs.

System Requirements/Features (*Also refer to certification requirements and Health Level Seven (HL7) EHR System Functional Model (EHR-S FM) for other key requirements/features.)	Available	Custom Developed	Future Development	Not Available
General System Requirements				
Is the system integrated or interfaced?				
Does the system provide the ability to archive via tape, CD, or DVD? Describe any other options.				
Are the COLD (computer output to laser disc) data streams available in ASCII (American Standard Code for Information Interchange)?				
Does the system support audit trails at the folder level for managing access, editing, and printing of documents?				
Does the system make audit trail logs available to the organization, including the date, time, user, and location?				
Does the system support an online help function/feature?				
Is the proposed solution scalable (e.g., can it support 50 to 800 workstations, concurrent users, etc.)?				
Does the system have the capability of recording change management logs related to platform upgrades and patches?				
Can the system identify or distinguish the facility location in a multi-entity environment?				
Can the system support a centralized database across multiple facilities?				
How compliant is your product with the HL7's EHR-S FM and EHR profiles? (Please provide us with your HL7 EHR-S FM and profile conformance statements.)				
System Security				
Does the system monitor security attempts for those without user rights and those logged in the audit trail/log?				
Does the system track all activity/functions, including where they change the database, and can they be managed through the audit trail/log?				

(Continued)

System Requirements/Features (*Also refer to certification requirements and Health Level Seven (HL7) EHR System Functional Model (EHR-S FM) for other key requirements/features.)	Available	Custom Developed	Future Development	Not Available
Does the system use encryption methods that render protected health information unreadable in compliance with the latest industry approaches and guidelines?				
Technical Requirements				
Do communication components include TCP/IP (transmission control protocol/internet protocol)?				
Does the system use CCITT Group III, IV for compression schemes?				
Does the system support standard HL7 record formatting for all input and output?				
Does the system support SQL for communication?				
Does the system support thin client PCs?				
Is the system sized for capacity to allow for planning? Describe your recommendations.				
Does the system support disk shadowing and system redundancy provisions? Please describe.				
Can your solution be supported as an Application Service Provider (ASP) hosted model?				
Does the system support browser-based options?				
Integration of Narrative Notes				
Does the system support HL7's Clinical Document Architecture Release 2 (CDA-R2) standard for the encoding of narrative, text-based clinical information?				
Does the system receive, display, transform, and parse CDA-encoded clinical documents as described in the HL7 CDA-R2 Implementation Guides for document types, such as History and Physical Note, Consultation Note, Operative Note, and Diagnostic Imaging Report?				
Does the system receive, display, transform, and parse CDA-R2-compliant documents with encoded headers (Level 1 encoding)?				
Does the system process CDA-R2-compliant documents that include Level 2 encoding?				
Does the system process CDA-R2-compliant documents that include Level 3 encoding?				

c. Interfaces

Organizations should provide a list of existing interfaces that will need to be supported, as well as new interfaces that will have to be created and supported, including any pertinent interoperability information that exists and will be needed in the future. Vendors should provide information regarding their system's ability to meet the organization's interface requirements.

4. Vendor Questionnaire

The organization should request information about the vendor and the product to assist with decision making.

a. Vendor Background and Financial Information
   i. Company Name and Geography. The organization should request an address of a branch close to the facility, as well as the headquarters. Staff may want to visit both.
   ii. Company Goals
   iii. Year the Company Was Established, Significant Company Merges, Acquisitions, and Sell-offs
   iv. Whether the Vendor Is Public or Privately Owned
   v. Bankruptcy/Legal Issues (including under which name the bankruptcy was filed and when, or any pertinent lawsuits, closed or pending, filed against the company)
   vi. Research and Development Investment (expressed in a total amount or percentage of total sales)
   vii. Status of Certification

b. Statement of Key Differentiators

The vendor should provide a statement describing what differentiates its products and services from those of its competitors.

c. Customer Base and References
   i. Customer List (or total number of customers per feature or function, if a list of customers cannot be provided owing to confidentiality/privacy concerns)
   ii. References That Can Be Contacted. The vendor should provide references the facility can contact/visit based on product features and functions most suitable to the facility, as well as those using the latest versions of the software.

d. Qualifications
   i. The vendor should provide a list of qualifications and resume, including a sample list of similar projects and clients.

e. User Participation
   i. User Groups

      Organizations should provide a list of the user groups and ask whether it can attend a meeting or a call for review purposes.
   ii. Requirements Gathering

      The vendor should request information regarding customer participation in requirements-gathering stages of system development. How is customer feedback, such as requests for new requirements, handled?

f. Technology

The vendor should provide technology specifications that support the product (e.g., database, architecture, operating system, ASP versus in-house, etc.).

g. Services

The vendor should describe the services offered and corresponding fees (if applicable).
   i. Project Management
   ii. Consulting
   iii. MPI Cleanup
   iv. Integration
   v. Legal Health Record Definition

      vi. Process Reengineering

     vii. Other

h. Training

The vendor should outline the training provided during and after implementation.

i. Product Documentation. The vendor should specify the product documentation that is available and its formats.

j. Implementation/Migration. The vendor should provide detailed information about the implementation such as the timelines and resources required.

k. Data Conversion

    i. If the system is not currently ICD-10-CM/PCS or Version 5010 compliant, describe plans for becoming compliant by regulatory required dates.

    ii. How will the system handle both ICD-9-CM and ICD-10-CM/PCS data?

    iii. How long will the system support both ICD-9-CM and ICD-10-CM/PCS codes?

    iv. If the system uses General Equivalence Mappings (GEMs), such as between ICD-10-CM/PCS and ICD-9-CM, describe how the integrity of the maps is maintained.

    v. Describe other data conversions (e.g., document imaging, platform conversions).

l. Maintenance

    i. Updates/Upgrades

    The vendor should provide information on how the system is maintained, including how often the updates/upgrades are applied, methods used (e.g., remotely, on-site), and by whom.

    ii. Compliance with Meaningful Use Incentive Requirements

    The vendor should provide its plan for addressing meaningful use on an ongoing basis, including plans for achieving corresponding certification requirements.

    iii. Expected Product Lifetime

    The vendor should outline the expected time frame for the next version requiring a different platform or operating system upgrade

    iv. Customer Support

    The vendor should outline the types of customer support packages offered (e.g., 24/7, weekday only), methods of support (e.g., help desk or tickets), and the tools used (e.g., 800 number, e-mail, web-based, etc.).

    v. Expected Facility Support

    The vendor should outline the number of full-time employees expected to support the product at the facility.

m. Pricing Structure

    i. Product Software Pricing

       1. Price

       The vendor should provide the price of the proposed solution, broken down by application/module, including licensing fees.

       2. Cost of Ownership (breakdown over a certain number of proposed contract years)

       3. Other Costs (maintenance, upgrades, consultation and support fees, post-implementation training and services, travel, etc.)

       4. Discounts (available discounts such as those based on participating as a beta site)

    ii. Invoicing (fee schedule and terms)

    iii. Return on Investment

    iv. Acceptance Period

    The vendor should outline the terms for validating the product after implementation and the refund policy

n. Warranty

The organization should request a copy of the warranty, as well as how it is affected by maintenance and support agreements after the implementation period

Sections 5 and 6 are to be completed by the facility.

5. Vendor Requirements and Instructions

a. RFP Questions

The facility should provide the name and contact information of one person to whom all questions concerning the RFP should be directed. Generally, questions about the RFP must be submitted in writing within a given time frame, and the questions and answers are distributed to all vendors responding to the RFP. Provide the preferred method of contact, such as fax number or e-mail.

b. Response Format, Deadline, and Delivery

c. Contract Duration

The facility should request that the vendor to disclose how long the returned information will be considered valid.

6. Terms and Conditions

a. Confidentiality

State confidentiality rules in regard to the information the facility disclosed in the RFP as well as the rules pertaining to the information provided by the vendor).

b. Information Access

The facility should describe who will have access to the returned RFP and for what purpose.

c. Bid Evaluation and Negotiation

The facility should briefly describe the evaluation process and the deadlines and provide the appropriate information if vendors are allowed to negotiate after the evaluation is complete.

d. Formal Presentation

The facility should describe process and format requirements if the vendor is invited to present the software product suite.

e. Acceptance or Rejection

The facility should describe how the vendor will be notified regardless of whether the product is selected or not.

f. Contract Provisions

The facility should note the sections of the RFP response that can be included in the final contract.

g. Type of Contract

The facility should let the vendor know if this will be firm fixed price, cost plus fixed fee, a time and materials, or other type of contract.

Check Your Understanding Answer Key

Chapter 1

1.1.

1. b. Extranets are used to access the healthcare facility's systems by those outside of the organization.
2. b. Cloud computing is a system that operates on a computer that is owned and maintained by a vendor.
3. b. The American Recovery and Reinvestment Act of 2009 encouraged the implementation of the EHR through Meaningful Use.
4. b. Computers in healthcare began in the 1960s with the use of financial systems.
5. b. The intranet uses Internet technologies to store information for employees. It is not the Internet.

1.2.

1. a. The CHDA certification covers data analysis which is a component of data analytics.
2. d. Dashboards provide current status on key indicators.
3. c. Applied informatics works to improve processes.
4. b. Many HIM professionals are able to work from home and some HIM departments are now virtual.
5. c. Health informatics is a multidisciplinary field that strives to improve healthcare.

Chapter 2

2.1.

1. d. Data integrity tools include edit checks and required fields.
2. c. Hot spots provide additional information about the data element.
3. c. Radio buttons are good for a small number of entry choices such as with gender.
4. b. Health records are a primary data source.
5. a. Drop down boxes are good to limit entries but allows a number of options from which to choose.

2.2.

1. d. Authorship is identifying who created an entry.
2. c. Data cleansing is looking for duplication of data, missing data, and outliers.
3. a. Documentation integrity issues include copy and paste, authorship, amendments, and more.
4. d. Data granularity ensures the level of detailed required is collected.
5. c. Data accessibility ensures that data is available when it is needed.

Chapter 3

3.1.

1. c. Autonumbering provides a unique number that will never be assigned again.
2. a. Normalization is breaking the data elements into the level of detail desired by the healthcare facility.
3. b. A record is data collected on a single patient.
4. a. Words such as "and," "or," and "not" are used to restrict queries.
5. c. The data dictionary specifies the metadata including the length of a field.
6. c. A mask allows the user to enter characters without the formatting. The information converts the data into the correct format.

3.2.

1. a. An entity is a person, location, thing, or concept that is to be tracked in the database.
2. c. A data flow diagram shows how data flows within an information system.
3. b. An attribute is a fact about an entity.
4. a. A relational database stores data in rows and columns—in other words, a table.
5. b. A use case is used to show developers how users will use the information system.

Chapter 4

4.1.

1. b. A project lasts for a finite period of time and has a specific outcome. Implementing an EHR is a project.
2. a. The project definition is indicates what you plan to accomplish.
3. d. The critical path shows the steps that must stay on track to prevent the implementation date from slipping.
4. b. The design plan spells out the details required to implement an information system.
5. a. Scope creep occurs when the definition of the project expands during the project.

4.2.

1. a. Functional requirements are a list of functions or tasks that the IS must be able to perform.
2. d. Flowcharts show the steps in a work process.
3. a. The RFI requests basic information on an information system.
4. b. The design stage is where the required functionality is identified.
5. d. Alpha sites partner with the IS vendor in order to design an IS.

4.3.

1. **b.** Spreadsheets can be used to compare responses to RFPs.
2. **b.** Force majeure prevents a party in the contract from being responsible for penalties due to an act of God.
3. **c.** Contracts should always be a win-win.
4. **a.** Escrow occurs when a software is held by a third party. The third party provides the healthcare facility with the software in the event that the vendor goes out of business.
5. **b.** A weighted decision matrix is a method used to compare and select the information systems.

Chapter 5

5.1.

1. **d.** Setting configurations populate tables, control when bills drop, and more.
2. **c.** Reengineering forces you to rethink processes to make them more efficient and to include the new information system.
3. **a.** Site preparation is ensuring there is space, electrical sockets, and anything else needed to add computers to an area.
4. **a.** Data conversion is changing data from one format to another.
5. **a.** GUIs utilize icons and other tools to interact with the computer.

5.2.

1. **b.** Updates to software should be loaded into the test environment to ensure it works.
2. **d.** The parallel go-live model operates the old information system and the new information system to ensure the new information is working as expected.
3. **a.** Adults like to have a say in their education, and they have a need to see the relevance of what they are learning.
4. **b.** Integration testing ensure that printers, scanners, computers, and other components work together.
5. **c.** Support and evaluation include day to day maintenance and determining what you could do better with the next implementation.

Chapter 6

6.1.

1. **c.** The encoder is specialty software used by coders to select the appropriate code for the diagnosis(es) and procedure(s) supported by the health record.
2. **c.** The automated codebook encoder is an encoder that lists diagnoses and procedures in alphabetic order much like the alphabetic index located in the International Classification of Diseases, Tenth Edition, Clinical Modification (ICD-10-CM) and Current Procedural Terminology (CPT) codebooks.
3. **a.** The grouper is a computer program that uses specific data elements to assign the diagnostic and procedural codes entered into the encoder into the appropriate Medicare severity diagnosis-related groups (MS-DRG) or other diagnosis-related group (DRG).
4. **b.** The ROI system is designed to manage the processing of requests for protected health information (PHI) received and processed by the HIM department. Use of the information system begins when a new request is entered into it. It continues to track the request as it is processed and acts as a historical database of all requests processed and ultimately used to generate reports.

5. c. A disclosure management system tracks the disclosures made throughout the healthcare facility for reporting purposes. This tracking is required by the Health Insurance Portability and Accountability Act (HIPAA). The covered entities must provide the patient with an accounting of disclosures upon request.

6.2.

1. d. One of the data elements unique to the cancer registry include ICD-O codes.

2. a. A registry is a collection of care information related to a specific disease, condition, or procedure that makes health record information available for analysis and comparison.

3. b. The chart locator system, also called chart tracking system, is designed to identify the current location the paper health record or information.

4. d. The cancer registry information system tracks information about the patient's cancer TNM (tumor, node, metastasis) stage.

5. a. Trauma registry software tracks patients with traumatic injuries from initial trauma treatment to death.

6.3.

1. c. CDI is the process a healthcare entity undertakes that will improve clinical specificity and documentation that will allow coders to assign more concise disease and procedural classification codes

2. a. The physician uses the dictation system to dictate, but the HIM department uses the system to transcribe the report.

3. d. The healthcare quality indicator system is an abstracting system that records information about the patient and the care provided to the patient.

4. a. Birth certificate software will capture the minimum data set established by the National Center for Health Statistics (NCHS) and any state-required data.

5. c. Expanders allow transcriptionists to type an acronym such as "CHF" and the full phrase "congestive heart failure" will automatically be spelled out, thus saving keystrokes and time.

Chapter 7

7.1.

1. c. The financial information system is critical to the fiscal health of the healthcare facility. The healthcare facility must receive accurate financial information in a timely manner to monitor and manage the finances of the healthcare facility.

2. a. The encoder is a specialty software that helps the coders determine the most appropriate diagnostics and procedural codes which in turn are used to determines reimbursement for the healthcare facility.

3. c. The human resources information system (HRIS) tracks employees within the organization. This tracking includes promotions, transfers, terminations, performance appraisal due dates, and absenteeism.

4. a. HIM professionals should be involved in the development and management of the chargemaster. The codes and charges must be updated at least annually.

5. d. Both ICD-10 and CPT classification codes are updated on a regular basis. These changes must be implemented and verified within the facility's chargemaster.

7.2.

1. c. It is a patient-identifying directory referencing all patients related to an organization and which also serves as a link to the patient record or information, facilitates patient identification, and assists in maintaining a longitudinal patient record from birth to death.

2. d. An EIS dashboard report gives administration-structured information to make intelligent decisions for the future.

3. c. Algorithms are used by organizations to determine the "probability of a duplicate in order to identify potential duplicate MPI entries."

4. b. Advantages of the EIS include assistance in making strategic decisions about the facility.

5. a. An IDS is an organizational arrangement of a network of health providers that may include hospitals, physicians, and health maintenance organizations (HMOs) that provide coordinated services along the continuum of care from ambulatory, acute, and long-term care and may extend across a geographical region.

7.3.

1. b. With the practice management system, scheduling, patient accounting, patient collections, claims submission, appointment scheduling, human resources, and other functions all are built into a single system.

2. b. The R-ADT system generates some key reports used by many departments within the facility. These include the daily admission list, discharge list, census report, transfer list, and bed utilization reports. The facility may also generate monthly, quarterly, yearly, and ad hoc reports to show type of patient treated, number of discharges, number of admissions, occupancy rates, and other information needed.

3. a. The scheduling system can help with this by scheduling tests, beds, operating rooms, staff, and other resources wisely.

4. a. With the focus by the Joint Commission on patient safety, the physical plant is focused on providing equipment and a healthcare environment that is vital to the well-being of the guests, staff, and ultimately the patients within the facility.

5. d. The R-ADT system issues the health record number assignment to the patient folder.

Chapter 8

8.1.

1. c. OCR is defined as a method of encoding text from analog paper into bitmapped images and translating the images into a form that is computer readable.

2. a. Target sheets are blank pages, except for a barcode, that will tell the scanner and ultimately the computer the content of the pages that follow.

3. c. Indexing is the abstracting of data that will be used to retrieve the image.

4. c. There must be an electronic or computerized print tracking log, similar to an audit log, that indicates who requested or submitted the print order, where the printing occurred (which printer was used and in what area of the healthcare facility), date and time of printing, what forms or reports were printed, and any other pertinent information the healthcare facility deems appropriate.

5. c. Annotation is the ability to alter the image in some way. The highlighting tool highlights important sections of text, much like a highlighter pen on paper.

8.2.

1. d. In a PACS, x-rays, MRIs, mammograms, and other radiological examinations are stored digitally, thus eliminating the need to store and manage the physical film.

2. d. A radiology information system (RIS) is used to collect, store, and provide information on radiological tests such as x-rays, ultrasound, magnetic resonance imaging (MRI), computerized tomography (CT), and positron emission tomography (PET).

3. b. The ability of these images to be viewed from any location by the radiologist and other users is called teleradiology.

4. a. Currently, LISs involve many interfaces since they are still typically stand-alone systems, separate from the EHR. It is important for these interfaces to work seamlessly with the specified EHR system to ensure integration with the clinical and communications needs of the healthcare facility (Biedermann and Dolezel 2017, 84).

5. c. Picture archival communication system (PACS) is an integrated computer system that obtains, stores, retrieves, and displays digital images.

8.3.

1. c. A nursing information system will document the nursing care provided to a patient. Clinical documentation is any manual or electronic notation or recording made by a physician or other healthcare clinician related to a patient's medical condition of treatment.

2. b. The PIS can be stand-alone or integrated with other systems in the healthcare facility such as CPOE.

3. b. Smart cards enable portable storage of health and insurance information.

4. d. Telehealth, also known as telemedicine, is the use of telecommunications and networks to share medical and nonclinical information between a patient and a healthcare provider located at different sites.

5. d. The HIM professional is typically not a direct user of the various CISs discussed throughout this chapter; however, the HIM professional accesses the information through either the CIS or the EHR.

Chapter 9

9.1.

1. b. With its seminal publication, *To Err Is Human: Building a Safer Health System*, the Institute of Medicine, now the National Academy of Medicine (NAM), advocated for the use of health information technology (HIT) to help prevent many of mistakes that regularly occur in the delivery of healthcare that lead to the injuries and deaths of tens or thousands of patients (NAM 2000, 1).

2. b. Reminders can notify physicians of screenings that should be performed based on the patient's age and gender.

3. b. A personal health record (PHR) is an electronic or paper health record maintained and updated by an individual for himself or herself.

4. d. A longitudinal health record is a permanent record of significant information listed in chronological order and maintained across time, ideally from birth to death.

5. a. An EHR is designed to not only be used by the originating healthcare entity but be able to be referred to and transmitted to authorized and authenticated users at other healthcare entities.

9.2.

1. b. The PHR contains health information that comes from both the physician and the patient, but the PHR is controlled by the patient.

2. c. The CPOE system notifies clinical departments, such as the laboratory, radiology, physical therapy, and dietary departments, of orders made by the physician.

3. c. As of 2015, approximately 97 percent of hospitals had certified EHR technology.

4. c. The Affordable Care Act (ACA) and the Healthy People 2020 campaign support monitoring population health to create social and physical environments that promote good health.

5. b. EMAR, also referred to a bar-code medication administration record (BC-MAR) automates many of the medication administration processes in a healthcare facility.

9.3.

1. **a.** One of the primary barriers to EHR implementation is cost.
2. **a.** The EHR enables quick access to patient records for more coordinated, efficient care.
3. **c.** There is variation between inpatient and outpatient EHR systems.
4. **a.** Limited health information technology (IT) workforce and training programs is a barrier to EHR implementation. Through and repetetive training and communication can counter this.
5. **a.** HIT has a significant role in improving the health of not only a medical practice's population, but the population on the community level.

9.4.

1. **a.** Drop-down lists, checkboxes, radio buttons, and other forms of controlled data entry are used in structured data entry.
2. **a.** Interoperability is the ability of different information systems and software applications to communicate and exchange data.
3. **b.** The hybrid record is a combination of paper and electronic health records; a health record that includes both paper and electronic elements.
4. **c.** Unanticipated consequences that have arisen with the use of the EHR include increased work for clinicians, unfavorable workflow changes, ongoing demands for system changes, conflicts between electronic and paper-based systems, unfavourable changes in communications, and negative user emotions.
5. **d.** Natural language processing (NLP) is the conversion of unstructured data into structured data through the use of computer algorithms or statistical methods.

Chapter 10

10.1.

1. **c.** Health literacy includes everything that would influence their ability to make healthcare decisions—which would include their ability to read and understand discharge instructions.
2. **a.** Jargon is specialized terminology used by a specific group.
3. **d.** The patient portal is where patients can communicate with healthcare provider, access information, schedule appointments and more.
4. **b.** The personal health record allows patients to add and control information.
5. **c.** Social media is a great way for a patient to keep family members updated on his condition.

Chapter 11

11.1.

1. **d.** The practice of pharmacies receiving electronic prescriptions from hospitals, physician practices, and health departments is called e-prescribing.
2. **b.** HIE is defined as the formal agreed-upon process for the seamless exchange of health information electronically between providers and others with the same level of interoperability, according to nationally recognized standards, typically through a HIO that serves as an intermediary to facilitate access and retrieval of clinical data to provide safer, timelier, efficient, effective, equitable, patient-centered care.
3. **d.** Interoperability is defined as the capability of different information systems and software applications to communicate and exchange data.

4. **c.** The Office of the National Coordinator (ONC) for Health Information Technology (ONC) was established in 2004 as a result of an executive order by President George W. Bush calling for the healthcare industry to implement an electronic system for health records and to have an interoperable communication system between all HCOs by 2014.

5. **b.** Based on the hardware and equipment connectivity used in the exchange, this type of interoperability allows any computer or device to exchange data with another computer or device without corrupting the data or creating errors.

11.2.

1. **a.** LHIOs and RHIOs are groups of healthcare organizations in specific geographic areas that share electronic health information according to accepted standards.

2. **b.** Equity of treatment and services with improved health outcomes leading to a reduction of health disparities.

3. **a.** In 2016, follow-up research from Johns Hopkins University School of Medicine indicated that that number may well be above 250,000 deaths per year, making medical mistakes the third leading cause of death in the United States.

4. **a.** The eHealth Exchange Sequoia Project is a group of "federal agencies and non-federal organizations that came together under a common mission and purpose to improve patient care, streamline disability benefit claims, and improve public health reporting through secure, trusted, and interoperable health information exchange."

5. **c.** BYOD (bring your own device) refers to healthcare providers using their personal smart phones and other devices and the increase in mobile technology.

11.3.

1. **b.** Meaningful use (MU) is a regulation that was issued by the Centers for Medicare and Medicaid (CMS) on July 28, 2010, outlining an incentive program for eligible professionals (EPs), eligible hospitals, and critical access hospitals (CAHs) participating in Medicare and Medicaid programs that adopt and successfully demonstrate meaningful use of certified EHR technology.

2. **a.** CEHRT must be evaluated independently of the vendor by the ONC or designee that the EHR in question must meet identified criteria and standards for functionality and interoperability in order to qualify for the MU incentive program.

3. **d.** They CQMs are criteria and tools to measure or quantify healthcare processes, outcomes, patient perceptions, and organizational structure and/or systems that relate to one or more of the quality goals for health care: effective, safe, efficient, patient-centered, equitable, and timely.

4. **a.** Population health, or public health, focuses on preventing, diagnosing, and treating an entire group of people rather than one person at a time.

5. **d.** Query-based exchange is a find-and-seek request for information that is sent through the HIO to find any health information on a specified individual.

11.4.

1. **a.** Identity or patient matching is the process in which the HIO identifies the right person within the database to exchange information between HCOs.

2. **c.** Consent management has nothing to do with the consent for treatment but rather consent or approve the HIO to transmit health information between two or more authorized entities.

3. **b.** A biometric is a physical characteristic of the patient or users (such as fingerprints, voiceprints, retinal scans, iris traits) that systems store and use to authenticate identity of the patient or before allowing the user access to a system.

4. **b.** The *opt-out with exceptions* model sets the default for health information for patients to be included, but the patient can opt-out completely or allow only select data to be included.

5. **a.** Opt-in consent means that the patient must specifically agree to have the personal health information accessible for the HIE.

Chapter 12

12.1.

1. **c.** Messaging standards may also be called interoperability standards or data exchange standards.
2. **a.** The most widely recognized nomenclature in healthcare is the Systematized Nomenclature of Medicine (SNOMED).
3. **a.** The American National Standards Institute (ANSI) is the SDO for the United States and is a representative to the ISO.
4. **d.** National drug codes (NDC) were developed by the Food and Drug Administration to act as a universal unique identifier for human drugs.
5. **a.** Semantics is a "branch of linguistics dealing with the study of meaning, including the ways meaning is structured in language and how changes in meanings and form occur over time."

Chapter 13

13.1.

1. **a.** Only covered entities are subject to HIPAA.
2. **c.** One of the purposes of administrative simplification is to improve the efficiency and effectiveness of healthcare business processes such as claims submission.
3. **b.** HL7 is a designated standard development organization.
4. **a.** ARRA made numerous changes to HIPAA, including increasing penalties that are awarded for noncompliance with the Security Rule.
5. **b.** Business associates do work on behalf of the CE that requires access to ePHI.

13.2.

1. **b.** These standards allow the CE to use an equivalent alternative if the addressable standard is a hardship.
2. **c.** HIPAA allows CEs to consider the size of the organization and other factors when developing their security plan.
3. **b.** Each employee should have their own sign-in but it is unlikely that there will be a security incident as a result.
4. **a.** Integrity is ensuring that data are not altered either during transmission across a network or during storage.
5. **a.** A human error, such as deleting the wrong file, is unintentional.

13.3.

1. **d.** Audit controls are an audit control along with access controls and more.
2. **b.** Encryption is turning data into unreadable text.
3. **b.** This methodology controls access to an information system based on the user's role in the organization. All individuals with that same role will have the same capabilities.
4. **c.** The user name and password is only a single factor authentication as it utilizes only the "what you know" methodology.
5. **a.** Triggers can be used to flag suspicious activities for further review.

13.4.

1. **a.** Both bots and spyware can capture keystrokes.
2. **a.** Viruses and spyware are two types of malicious software, also known as malware.
3. **c.** Viruses can do a lot of damage to an information system including loss of data.

4. a. Ransomware can be used to block access to an information system.

5. b. Trojans appear to be legitimate but instead cause some types of harm to a facility such as pop-ups.

Chapter 14

14.1.

1. b. Data governance (DG) is the overall management of the availability, usability, integrity, and security of the data employed in an organization or enterprise.

2. c. The acronym GIGO, "garbage in, garbage out," is an applicable metaphor for the importance of effective DG. If the data or information is incorrect, changed due to transmission issues, or used in the wrong context, then anything built upon this faulty foundation may be incorrect, invalid, or unreliable.

3. a. Information governance is defined as an organization-wide framework for managing information throughout its lifecycle and for supporting the organization's strategy, operations, regulatory, legal, risk, and environmental requirements.

4. c. Metadata can prove the integrity of a healthcare facility's records by identifying the creation, changes, access, and security of the information to ensure its quality and trustworthiness.

5. c. Effectiveness is the degree to which stated outcomes are attained and efficiency is how the desired outcome is achieved or produced, particularly without wasting resources such as time, personnel, and money.

14.2.

1. d. ARMA International is a professional association and a recognized authority on information governance in most areas, such as information technology, legislative and regulatory bodies, and finance, that utilize information as a strategic asset.

2. b. Integrity: Systems evidence trustworthiness in the authentication, timeliness, accuracy, and completion of information.

3. c. ITG also encompasses every aspect of IT infrastructure such as hardware, software, communication, and technology tools, policies and procedures to provide efficient processes for all electronic activity within the healthcare facility.

4. d. Information is a valued strategic asset because of its role in planning for the future of the healthcare facility, making sound clinical and administrative decisions, and managing the financial resources.

5. a. Strategic alignment is "the process and the outcome of linking your organizational structure and resources with your strategy and business environment to achieve performance improvement."

14.3.

1. a. HIM professionals should be a leader in DG and IG due to their knowledge of data management, privacy and security, and other areas.

2. c. The five building blocks of EIM includes design and capture.

3. d. Health data stewardship is the management and responsibilities of an activity according to its established goals and objectives, regulatory or accreditation conditions, and other organizational obligations to guarantee that health information is used appropriately.

4. a. The "hard skills" deal with basic areas of technology. Informatics skills involve basic computer literacy; programming basics and languages (SQL and HL7); use of basic office application software (other than word processing) for databases, graphics, and spreadsheets; and decision support systems.

5. c. The certified health data analyst (CHDA) credential identifies practitioners who have the knowledge to acquire, manage, analyze, interpret, and transform data into accurate, consistent, and timely information, while balancing the "big picture" strategic vision with day-to-day details.

Chapter 15

15.1.

1. b. CAHIIM is the accreditation organization for HIM educational programs.
2. d. To be eligible for the RHIT exam, the candidate must earn an associate degree from a CAHIIM accredited program.
3. c. Consultants are hired by healthcare facilities for special programs, act as HIM director temporarily and more.
4. b. System analysis is one of the many skills listed that an HIM professional has.
5. b. Entry level competencies look at current and future practices.

15.2.

1. d. The data architect assists in the data model development.
2. d. The content analyst designs information systems based on the needs of the users.
3. d. An HIM professional involved in systems implementation would be involved in many implementation tasks including development of the request for proposal.
4. d. The informatics researcher is responsible for ensuring the data needed is available by managing the data collection process.
5. a. There were four HIMR recommendations Including Increasing the number of AHIMA members earning graduate degrees.

Glossary

Acceptance testing: A type of testing that occurs after the go-live date

Access controls: A computer software program designed to prevent unauthorized use of an information resource

Addressable standards: Must be evaluated by the entity to determine whether or not the standard is reasonable and appropriate

Administrative information system: A system that manages the business of healthcare; is the first information systems to be used in healthcare. The data collected in this system are mainly financial or business-oriented in nature, rather than clinical

Administrative safeguards: Administrative actions, and policies and procedures, to manage the selection, development, implementation, and maintenance of security measure to protect electronic-protected health information and to manage the conduct of the covered entity's workforce in relation to the protection of that information. (45 CFR 160, 162, and 164)

Administrative simplification: Improves the efficiency and effectiveness of the business processes of healthcare by standardizing the EDI of administrative and financial transactions and protects the privacy and security of protected health information (PHI) that is transmitted from one point to another

Alpha site: The first healthcare facility to implement the information system

American National Standards Institute (ANSI): The SDO for the United States and a representative to the ISO

American Recovery and Reinvestment Act (ARRA): Enacted to stimulate the US economy during a recession that started in 2007. A significant portion of ARRA was dedicated to expanding the use of HIT to improve the business efficiency and effectiveness of HCOs while increasing patient safety and positive health outcomes. It also enacted an incentive program known as Meaningful Use

Anesthesia information system: A system that collects information on preoperative, operative, and postoperative anesthesia-related clinical information. This system follows the patient through the surgical process

Annotation: The ability to add to the image in some way; because the image may be a legal document, the image itself cannot be altered; however, an overlay to the document will show the annotation

ANSI Accredited Standards Committee X12N (ASC X12N): Responsible for developing the EDI standards used to share information needed for health insurance administrative transactions

Audit controls: The mechanisms that record and examine activity in information systems

Audit log: Or audit trail, an electronic footprint of the actions that occurred in a particular file in an information system or that were performed by a specific individual

Audit trails: The record of information system activities, such as log-in, log-out, unsuccessful log-ins, print, query, and other actions

Audit-reduction tools: Tools that review the audit trail and compare it to criteria specified by the CE, which eliminates routine entries such as the periodic backups

Authorship: The origination or creation of recorded information attributed to a specific individual or entity acting at a particular time

Automated codebook encoder: An encoder that lists diagnoses and procedures in alphabetic order much like the alphabetic index

Back-end speech recognition (BESR): A speech recognition technology in which the physician dictates in the traditional manner and an editor listens to the audio and reviews the document created

Backscanning: The process of scanning past health records into the DMS so there is an existing database of patient information, making the DMS valuable to the user from the first day of implementation

Backward map: A map that links the two coding systems in the opposite direction, moving from ICD-10 to ICD-9

Barcode medication administration record (BC-MAR): See Electronic medication administration record (EMAR)

Best of breed: Choosing the ISs based on functionality rather than by vendor

Best of fit: The decision to purchase software from a single vendor

Beta sites: The healthcare facilities who subsequently implement the information system

Bidder's conference: A meeting for vendors to come to the healthcare facility to ask questions about the request for proposal, the healthcare facility, and other important points

Biomedical device: An article, instrument, apparatus, or machine that is used in the prevention, diagnosis, or treatment of illness or disease, or for detecting, measuring, restoring, correcting, or modifying the structure or function of the body for some health purpose

Birth certificate information system: A state-approved system in which the birth certificate data are entered, after the HIM staff interviews the mother or other parents or guardians and reviews the health record. This software reports births occurring in the healthcare facility to the state health agency

Blue Button: A campaign that was established by The Office of the National Coordinator for Health IT (ONC). It is a consumer-motivated method to improve healthcare by having the patient or caretaker actively involved in decisions and planning by having direct access to personal health information

Bots: Perform automated tasks, such as gathering information and instant messaging, thus relieving a person the responsibility of doing it

Bring your own device (BYOD): Healthcare practitioners using their personal smartphones or other devices rather than devices provided by the HCO, the personal device must meet specific encryption and other security protocols to protect PHI as required by the HCO

Cancer registry information system: An information system that tracks information (including very detailed information regarding diagnosis and treatment) about the patient's cancer from the time of diagnosis to the patient's death

Certified EHR technology: An EHR that has been evaluated by a member of the Office of the National Coordinator–Authorized Certification Bodies (ONC-ACBs) and verified that it meets the criteria set by the MU incentive programs

Certified health data analyst (CHDA): Advanced certification sponsored by AHIMA that covers data management, data analytics, and data reporting

Certified in healthcare privacy and security (CHPS): Credential that demonstrates advanced privacy and security skills. These advanced privacy and security skills exceed those in the RHIA or RHIT examinations. It is sponsored by AHIMA

Certified information security manager (CISM): Sponsored by ISACA; an international examination that is designed for leaders in security who oversee the security programs of organizations

Certified information systems security professional (CISSP): Certification sponsored by the International Information Systems Security Certification Consortium. It is a generic security certification and therefore is not healthcare specific

Change management: The formal process of introducing change, getting it adopted, and diffusing it throughout the healthcare facility

Chargemaster: A financial management form or software that contains information about the healthcare facility's charges for the services it provides to patients (also called a charge description master [CDM]); it automates the coding process for routine procedures

Chart deficiency system: A system that track and record documentation omission due to deficiency in the health record that comes to the HIM department. Deficiencies can be in paper, imaged, or electronic records depending on the information system used

Chart locator system: A system is designed to identify the current location of the paper health record. This tracking is important because paper records are moved from place to place for patient care, quality reviews, coding, and many other purposes

Chart tracking system: See Chart locator system

Clinical data repository (CDR): A centralized data repository

Clinical decision support (CDS) system: The process in which individual data elements are represented in the computer by a special code to be used in making comparisons, trending results, and supplying clinical reminders and alerts

Clinical document architecture (CDA): Standards developed by HL7 for the electronic exchange of clinical documents, such as discharge summaries and progress notes

Clinical documentation improvement (CDI) system: The recognized process assists in identifying ways to improve clinical documentation in the health record

Clinical documentation improvement (CDI): The process an organization undertakes that will improve clinical specificity and documentation that will allow coding professionals to assign more concise disease and procedural classification codes

Clinical documentation: Any manual or electronic notation or recording made by a physician or other healthcare clinician related to a patient's medical condition or treatment

Clinical informatics coordinator: Individual who requires knowledge of clinical information systems. They are experts in the data retrieval needed by healthcare providers while conducting patient care

Clinical information system (CIS): A system that collects and stores medical, nursing, clinical ancillary areas (such as radiology and laboratory), and therapy department information related to patient care

Clinical messaging: A tool that connects the medical staff and hospital by providing access to information systems such as order entry and results reporting and DMS

Clinical pathways: A tool designed to coordinate multidisciplinary care planning for specific diagnoses and treatments

Clinical practice guidelines: A tool that provides a detailed, step-by-step guide used by healthcare practitioners to make knowledge-based decisions related to patient care and issued by an authoritative organization such as a medical society

Cloud computing: A computer system that is owned and maintained by a vendor

Cluster map: An entry in a GEM where one code from the many target codes can become a map to the source code

Cluster, combination, and complex: The types of mapping relations between source and target codes that exist in both forward and reverse directions

Code set: A set of codes used to encode data elements

Combination map: This is an entry where more than one code is required in the target code set to replicate the complete meaning of the source system

Commission on Accreditation for Health Informatics and Information Management Education (CAHIIM): Board responsible for establishing the content that accredited masters, bachelor, and associate programs must teach their students

Commission on Certification for Health Information and Information Management (CCHIIM): The independent body within AHIMA that establishes and grants professional certifications in health informatics and HIM professions

Complex map: This mapping represents multiple code combinations and alternatives that are required to translate a source to a target code

Computer on wheels (COW): A computer used at the point of care, which involves a wireless computer mounted on a mobile cart that can be moved from patient to patient

Computer-aided software engineering (CASE): A tool designed to create many of the diagrams and other tools used in the data model

Computer-assisted coding (CAC) system: A software program used to analyze the clinical data found in an electronic health record

Computer-assisted instruction (CAI): A software program designed to use multimedia and interactive technology to teach a topic

Computerized provider order entry (CPOE): Preprogrammed clinical decision support designed to assist the user through making an entry appropriately

Conceptual data model: Model that is not tied to a particular database model, but rather defines the requirements for the database to be developed. It is the basis for the logical and physical data models

Consent management: A component of identity management within HIE; because of HIPAA, patients have the right to refuse to participate in the HIE and to limit who can view their information. Consent management has nothing to do with the consent for treatment but rather the patient consents or approves the HIO to transmit health information between two or more authorized entities

Consolidated (centralized) model: Many independent HCOs connected with the HIE and aggregate data was stored and shared within a central repository managed by the HIE

Consumer engagement: A diverse set of activities that can include interacting with healthcare providers, seeking health information, maintaining a PHR, and playing an active role in making decisions in regard to personal healthcare

Consumer health applications: Healthcare-based applications designed for use by the patient or provider on smart phones, tablets, and other computers

Consumer informatics: Also known as consumer health informatics; the field devoted to informatics from multiple consumer or patient views

Consumer-mediated exchange: A type of HIE that is controlled by patients who want to control the use and access of their health information

Content analyst: Individual who designs the clinical information system that will be implemented. Their work is directed by the needs of the users. They are also advocates in the usage of health information technology in healthcare

Context-based authentication: Controls access not only by the role that the employee has in the CE but also by the individual data elements and the context in which the user is working

Contingency plan: Plan that is made up of policies and procedures that identify how a CE will react in the event of an information system emergency such as power failure, natural disaster, or a system failure

Continuity of Care Document (CCD): An implementation guide for sharing continuity of care record (CCR) patient summary data

Continuity of care record (CCR): A core data set, which is the most relevant administrative, demographic, and clinical information about a patient's healthcare, covering one or more healthcare encounters

Core data set: A data set that contains the most relevant administrative, demographic, and clinical information about a patient's healthcare

Covered entity (CE): A health plan, healthcare clearinghouse, or healthcare provider that transmits any health information in electronic form for one of the covered transactions

Critical path: The sequence of stages that takes the longest amount of time to complete the project

Current Dental Terminology (CDT): The system used to code dental procedures such as tooth extractions, tooth implants, and such

Dashboards: Reports of process measures to help leaders follow progress to assist with strategic planning. The dashboard provides the status on key measures

Data accessibility: Data items can be easily obtainable by authorized users

Data accuracy: Data that are free of identifiable errors

Data analyst: Individual who applies his or her skills to manage, analyze, interpret, and transform health data into accurate, consistent, and timely information

Data analytics: The science of examining raw data with the purpose of drawing conclusions about that information. This information can then be used to make business decisions concerning which services to provide and how to improve patient care

Data capture: The process of recording healthcare-related data in a health record system or clinical database

Data cleansing: The process of checking internal consistency and duplication as well as identifying outliers and missing data. In other words, it means looking for errors or problems with the data, such as duplicate patients

Data comprehensiveness: The patient's health record must be complete and all required data must be included

Data consistency: Ensures that like data are the same on each document or computer screen

Data content standards: Clear guidelines for the acceptable values for specified data fields. These standards make it possible to exchange health information using electronic networks, and they identify the structure and content of data elements to be collected by the EHR

Data currency: Ensures that data are up to date

Data definition language (DDL): A special type of software used to create the tables within a relational database. It translates how data are stored in the computer from the physical view (physical structure of the database) to the logical view (one that is understandable by the user)

Data field: A predefined area within a database in which the same type of information is usually recorded such as the data of birth

Data flow diagrams (DFDs): A diagram that shows how data moves (input, storage, output) within the database. It is a way to show management and other nontechnical users the system design

Data granularity: The level of detail at which the attributes and values of healthcare data are defined

Data integrity: The extent to which healthcare data are complete, accurate, consistent, and timely

Data integrity analyst: Individual who is responsible for ensuring the quality of the data in IIIM information systems. Data integrity analysts must be able to apply data and content standards to data collection and data storage. They must be able to maintain the information systems, ensure compliance with legal and accreditation requirements, and be able to analyze data

Data manipulation language (DML): A special type of software used to retrieve, update, and edit data in a relational database. The DML accesses, makes changes to, and retrieves data from the database

Data manipulation: Allowing the user to add and delete rows in a table and to sort, find, and compare. Another function of the data manipulation component is to update data

Data mapping: Allows for connections between two systems

Data mart: A subset of the data warehouse designed for a single purpose or specialized use

Data mining: The process of extracting and analyzing large volumes of data from a database for the purpose of identifying hidden and sometimes subtle relationships that would be unnoticed without the analysis

Data modelling: The design of the database needed for the organization. The model should be based on the organization's strategic plan and should identify the data elements to be collected and the relationship between them

Data precision: Ensures that there is justification for the need to collect the data

Data quality management: The business processes that ensure the integrity of an organization's data during collection, application (including aggregation), warehousing, and analysis

Data quality measure: Mechanism to assign a quantitative figure to quality of care by comparison to a criterion. Quality measurements typically focus on structures or processes of care that have a demonstrated relationship to positive health outcomes

Data relevancy: Extent to which healthcare-related data are useful for the purposes for which they were collected

Data repository: An open-structure database (not dedicated to the software of any particular vendor or data supplier) in which data from multiple information systems are stored so that an integrated, multidisciplinary (includes a variety of healthcare providers) view of the data can be achieved in a single source

Data standards: Allow data to be shared in a uniform way. It includes data content standards and data exchange standards

Data timeliness: Data should be recorded in an appropriate period of time after the event and should be available to the user when needed

Data warehouse: A database that makes it possible to access data from multiple databases and combine the results into a single query and reporting interface

Database: An organized collection of data, text, references, or pictures in a standardized format, typically stored in a computer system for multiple applications

Database management system (DBMS): Manipulates and controls the data stored within the database to meet the needs of the user; it controls the ability to create, read, write, and delete data stored in the database

Database table: Table that contains all data related to a particular subject or concept such as a patient and is made up of the records and fields

Decision support system (DSS): An information system that gathers data from a variety of sources and assists in providing structure to the data by using various analytical models and visual tools in order to facilitate and improve the ultimate outcome in decision-making tasks associated with the nonroutine and nonrepetitive problems

Degaussing: Application of a magnetic field to the media to render the data on it useless; it renders data impossible to recover and is not reversible

Descriptive statistics: A set of statistical techniques used to describe data such as means, frequency distributions, and standard deviations

Designated standard maintenance organizations (DSMOs): Six organizations to which the Department of Health and Human Services (HHS) has assigned of developing and maintaining standards for the Transaction and Code Sets rule

Diagnostic and Statistical Manual of Mental Disorders (DSM): A classification system of mental disorders used by mental health providers. It is published by the American Psychiatric Association. The current fifth edition is known as *DSM-5*. The purpose of *DSM-5* system is to assist physicians in properly

Dictation system: Used by the physician to verbally record various medical reports such as history and physical examinations, discharge summaries, radiology reports, autopsy reports, catheterization reports, and other designated reports into the dictation system

Digital Imaging and Communications in Medicine (DICOM): Standard retrieves images and other information from imaging equipment of a variety of different vendors. Although DICOM started out in diagnostic medical imaging, it has broadened to include specialties such as cardiology, dentistry, and radiology

Directed exchange: Frequently referred to as a "push exchange" because it pushes authorized and secure information from one HCO to another

Director of clinical informatics: Individual who is the leader in the implementation of the EHR as well as the post-implementation services. The director is the champion for the EHR and works with the implementation team to ensure they have the resources needed

Disclosure management system: A system that tracks the disclosures made throughout the healthcare facility for reporting purposes

Document management system (DMS): An electronic method of capturing and managing documents; used primarily by HIM departments and other departments to handle documents regarding patient care

Dumb terminals: All of the processing is performed at the server or mainframe, used to input patient data, capturing various patient or clinical data for reporting purposes

Edit check: A standard feature in many applications' data entry and data collection software packages. Edit checks are preprogrammed definitions of each data field set up within the application

eHealth Exchange: Originally known as Healtheway, a group of federal agencies and non-federal organizations that came together under a common mission and purpose to improve patient care, streamline disability benefit claims, and improve public health reporting through secure, trusted, and interoperable health information exchange

Electronic data interchange (EDI): The transfer of data from one point to another without human intervention, which can significantly improve the efficiency of healthcare

Electronic health record (EHR): An electronic record of health-related information on an individual that conforms to nationally recognized interoperability standards and that can be created, managed, and consulted by authorized clinicians and staff across more than one healthcare organization

Electronic medical record (EMR): An electronic collection of all of the patient's health information and clinical care that is stored, managed, and referred to by authorized members of one healthcare entity, much like the actual paper health record only in digital or electronic form

Electronic medication administration record (EMAR): A software that automates many of the medication administration processes in a healthcare facility

Electronic protected health information (ePHI): PHI that is created, received, or transmitted electronically by covered entities

Electronic signature: Requires at least a password but can use a two-factor authentication method

Emergency access procedure: There may be times when users need to have access to data they are not normally allowed (also called "break the glass")

Emergency department systems (EDSs): A tool designed to meet the unique needs of the emergency department; they are able to track patients from triage to discharge. The information systems are also able to record test results and other clinical information

Emergency mode operation plan: Encompasses procedures necessary to keep the critical business processes of the covered entity in place during information system downtime

Encoder: A specialty software used by coders to select the appropriate code for the diagnosis(es) and procedure(s) supported by the health record

Encryption: A process that converts data from a readable form to unintelligible text. This is done with the science of cryptography, using mathematics to convert data into unintelligible data and back again

Enterprise master patient index (EMPI): A database that provides access to multiple repositories of information from overlapping patient populations that are maintained in separate information systems and databases

Entity-relationship diagram: A common type of data modeling that focuses on relationships between entities

E-patients: Individuals who are equipped, enabled, empowered, and engaged in their health and health care decisions

Escrow: A situation in which a third party holds a copy of the software in case the vendor goes bankrupt

Evidence-based medicine: Healthcare services based on clinical methods that have been thoroughly tested through controlled, peer-reviewed biomedical studies

Executive information system (EIS): A decision support system that is designed to be used by healthcare administrators

Expander: A tool that allows transcriptionists to type an acronym such as "CHF" and the full phrase "congestive heart failure" will automatically be spelled out, thus saving keystrokes and time

External scanning: Identifying changes outside the healthcare facility that will impact it

Facilities management system: Used by a healthcare facility to manage the physical plant; track routine maintenance such as elevator inspections, fire extinguisher inspections, and equipment preventive maintenance

Facility access controls: Limit physical access to the data center and software to only authorized information system staff

Fact about an entity: An attribute is a fact about an entity

Feasibility study: Study conducted by the healthcare facility to determine if a proposed information system is an appropriate option to meet the objectives of the healthcare facility

Federated (decentralized) model: Occurs where there is not a centralized database of patient information

Financial applications: Software applications that handle patient accounts, budgets, and other financial activities

Financial information system: A critical system to the fiscal health of the healthcare facility; receive accurate financial information in a timely manner to monitor and manage the finances of the healthcare facility

Force majeure: A legal term that refers to an event or effect that cannot be reasonably anticipated or controlled

Foreign key: A primary key from another table

Forward map: A map that translates an ICD-9 code, as source code, to ICD-10 as its target code

Front-end speech recognition (FESR): A speech recognition technology in which the physician or the dictator is the editor of the document that is dictated

Functional requirements: Functionality that an information system should be able to perform

Gantt chart: A project management tool that records specific tasks, their start and end dates, the person responsible for the tasks, and any connections between tasks

General Equivalence Mappings (GEMs): A common mapping system used to convert ICD-9-CM codes to ICD-10-CM and ICD-10-PCS codes or the reverse

Grouper: A computer program that uses specific data elements to assign the diagnostic and procedural codes entered into the encoder into the appropriate Medicare severity diagnosis-related group (MS-DRG) or other diagnosis-related group (DRG)

Health informatics: A scientific discipline that is concerned with the cognitive, information-processing, and communication tasks of healthcare practice, education, and research, including the information science and technology to support these tasks

Health information blocking: Persons or entities knowingly and unreasonably interfere with the exchange or use of electronic health information

Health information exchange (HIE): The exchange of health information electronically between providers and others with the same level of interoperability

Health information organization (HIO): A public-private partnership organization that oversees, governs, and facilitates the transmission of health data between different types of HCOs that have various EHR systems, according to nationally recognized standards. Many HIOs started as local health information

Health information technology (HIT): The hardware, software, integrated technologies or related licenses, intellectual property, upgrades, or packaged solutions sold as services that are designed for or support the use by healthcare entities or patients for the electronic creation, maintenance, access, or exchange of health information

Health Information Technology for Economic and Clinical Health (HITECH) Act: Promotes the adoption and meaningful use of health information technology (Health IT) and provides additional privacy and security requirements that develop and support electronic health information, facilitate information exchange, and strengthen monetary penalties

Health Insurance Portability and Accountability Act of 1996 (HIPAA): A federal law that impacts many areas of healthcare, including insurance portability, code sets, privacy, security, electronic data interchange (EDI), and national identifier standards

Health Level Seven International (HL7): A not-for-profit ANSI-accredited SDO dedicated to providing a comprehensive framework and related standards for the exchange, integration, sharing, and retrieval of electronic health information that supports clinical practice and the management, delivery, and evaluation of health services

Healthcare clearinghouse: Companies that function as intermediaries who collect billing data and process it for the healthcare provider. The healthcare clearinghouse then submits the claim to the health plan for payment

Healthcare quality indicator system: An abstracting system that records information about the patient, the care provided to the patient, and the healthcare practitioner(s) involved in the care delivered

Hierarchical database model: Model that structures the data in a hierarchy very similar to that used for an organizational chart

HIM Reimagined (HIMR): A vision of the future of HIM, created by AHIMA, that has four recommendations: increasing the number of AHIMA members holding graduate degrees, increasing the research related to HIM and health informatics, increasing opportunities for specialization in HIM, and revising the RHIT certification to become RHIT (+Specialty)

Hospital information system: The major information system used by a healthcare facility; is made up of many administrative systems, such as the financial information system and the MPI

Hot spot: Is a type of help message that is triggered when the cursor is placed on top of a data field

Human resources information system (HRIS): A system that tracks employees within the organization. This tracking includes promotions, transfers, terminations, performance appraisal due dates, and absenteeism

Hybrid model: A combination of the advantages of centralized and decentralized models; has an RLS, and some data are stored in a central repository while the remainder stays with the other HCOs within the HIE

Hybrid record: A combination of paper and electronic health records

Identity management: Ensures that the individual who has been identified is who they say they are, that they have the authority to do what they want to do, and that their actions are tracked

Identity matching: Also known as patient matching, the process in which the HIO identifies the right person within the database to exchange information between HCOs

Inferential statistics: A set of statistical techniques that allows researchers to make generalizations about a population's characteristics on the basis of a sample's characteristics, such as HIM professionals' continuing education efforts

Information access management: Involves implementing policies and procedures to determine which employees have access to what information

Information system activity review: Monitors for the inappropriate use or disclosure of ePHI. HIPAA does not mandate the frequency of this review nor the way this review is to be conducted. These reviews should include logs, access, and incident reporting

Information system strategic planning: Plan that identifies information systems needed to meet the healthcare facility's business objectives

Information system trainer: Individual who is responsible for the development and implementation of the training plan

Information systems project steering committee: Group of staff members responsible for every information system acquisition project in the healthcare facility

Interdisciplinary charting systems: A system used by any healthcare professional to collect and store patient assessments, progress notes, and care plans

Internal scanning: Identifying changes within the healthcare facility that will impact the information system

Intrusion detection: Systems that monitor networks and information systems to catch hackers and other intruders

Laboratory information system (LIS): A system that collects, stores, and manages laboratory tests and their respective results; can speed up access to test results through improved efficiency from various locations, including anywhere in the hospital, the physician's office, or even the clinician's home

Logical data model: A complete representation of data requirements and the structural business rules that govern data quality in support of project's requirements. In other words, it ensures that the data are available and in a useful format for the intended purpose

Logical Observation Identifiers Names and Codes (LOINC): The preferred standardized terminology for laboratory data in information systems and provides a standard set of codes and names for the electronic reporting of laboratory results

Longitudinal health record: A permanent record of significant information listed in chronological order and maintained across time, ideally from birth to death

Master patient index (MPI): Part of the hospital information system; it is a patient-identifying directory, referencing all patients related to a healthcare facility; that also serves as a link to the patient health record or information, facilitates patient identification, and assists in maintaining a longitudinal patient record from birth to death

Materials management system: A system that automates the purchasing process, inventory control, menu planning, and food service

Meaningful Use (MU): A regulation that was issued by the Centers for Medicare and Medicaid (CMS) on July 28, 2010, outlining an incentive program for eligible professionals (EPs), eligible hospitals, and critical access hospitals (CAHs) participating in Medicare and Medicaid programs that adopt and successfully demonstrate meaningful use of certified EHR technology(CEHRT)

MEDCIN: A nomenclature and knowledge-based system developed by Peter S. Goltra and is now controlled by Medicomp Systems, Inc. It is the most comprehensive vocabulary for signs and symptoms

Messaging standards: Also called interoperability standards or data exchange standards; its purpose is to support communications between information systems. With messaging standards, proprietary systems are able to talk to one another, allowing the exchange of data

Mitigation: The process of attempting to reduce or eliminate harmful effects of the breach (45 CFR 160, 162, and 164)

Multidimensional database model: Model used in data warehouses in which data are collected from multiple sources, such as other databases, and then summarized

National Council for Prescription Drug Programs (NCPDP): An independent, ANSI-accredited program that is regulated under the Medicare Modernization Act (MMA) of 2003, Medicare Part D e-prescribing SDO and is ANSI-accredited

National drug codes (NDC): Developed by the Food and Drug Administration to act as a universal unique identifier for human drugs; identifies the labeler or vendor, product, and trade package size

National Voluntary Laboratory Accreditation Program (NVLAP): A program that maintains the Healthcare Information Technology Testing Laboratory Accreditation Program and accredits organizations those contract to perform health IT conformance testing in the ONC Health IT Certification Program

Natural language queries: Common words used to tell the database which data are needed

Network database model: Uses pointers to connect data. The nodes are called owners and members rather than parent and child nodes, as in the hierarchical database model

Normalization: Breaking the data elements into the level of detail desired by the healthcare facility

Nursing information system (NIS): A system that assists in the planning and monitoring of overall patient care and documents the nursing care provided to a patient

Object-oriented database model: A database management system that handles text, images, audio, video, and other objects

Office of the National Coordinator for Health Information Technology (ONC): The lead federal agency spearheading this national effort to improve patient safety and health outcomes

ONC–Approved Accreditor (ONC-AA): An entity designated by the ONC to accredit and oversee the certification bodies (ONC-ACBs)

ONC–Authorized Certification Bodies (ONC-ACBs): Under HITECH, an organization or consortium of organizations that has applied to and been authorized by the National Coordinator to perform the certification of complete EHRs, EHR modules, or other types of HIT under the ONC HIT Certification Program

One-factor authentication: Utilizes one level of access control such as a username and password

Online analytical processing (OLAP): A data access architecture that allows the user to retrieve specific information from a large volume of data

Opt-in or opt-out consent: Sets the default for health information of patients to be included in the HIO automatically (opt-in), but the patient can choose not to be included (opt-out) completely. Opt-in consent means that the patient must specifically agree to have the personal health information accessible for the HIE

Order entry and results reporting: A software application in which healthcare professionals can enter patient care orders and then see the test results

Open-structure database: A data repository is created in an open format so it is not tied to any system

Parent and child: The relationships of a hierarchical database model is parent to child

Patient monitoring systems: A system that automatically collects and stores patient data from various information systems used in healthcare. Data collected include fetal monitoring, vital signs, and oxygen saturation rates

Patient portal: An information system established and maintained by the healthcare facility that allows patients to log in to obtain their health information, register for appointments, and perform other functions such as using secure e-mail, downloading forms, updating demographics, scheduling appointments, and requesting a prescription refill

Patient registration systems: Collects information on patients receiving treatment

Patient safety: A discipline that emphasizes safety in health care through the prevention, reduction, reporting, and analysis of medical error that often leads to adverse effects

Patient-provider portal: A secure method of communication between the healthcare provider and the patient, just the providers, or the provider and the payer

Payment milestones: An action that triggers payment to the vendor

Personal health record (PHR): An electronic or paper health record maintained and updated by individuals that can be used to collect, track, and share past and current information about their health or the health of someone in their care

PERT chart: A management tool that evaluates the tasks, the dependencies on other activities, the activity sequence, and the time required to complete the task

Pharmacy information system (PIS): A key tool in providing optimal patient care and assisting providers in ordering, allocating, and administering medication, with a focus on patient safety issues, especially medication errors

Physical data model: Model that shows how the data are physically stored within the database. The users are not involved with this level of the database because of its technical complexity

Physical safeguards: Physical measures, policies, and procedures to protect a CE's electronic information systems, and related buildings and equipment, from natural and environmental hazards and unauthorized intrusion

Physician advisor (PA): A hired staff by the healthcare facility to act as a liaison between the HIM or others and the patient's physician

Picture archival communication system (PACS): An integrated information system that obtains, stores, retrieves, and displays digital images

Point of care (POC): The place or location where the physician administers services to the patient, such as the patient's bedside

Population health reporting: The aggregate data on immunizations, communicable diseases, and other health events and CQMs that healthcare entities, providers, and public health agencies are required to report and is a standard function in EHRs

Population health: The cohesive, integrated, and comprehensive approach to health considering the distribution of health outcomes in a population, the health determinants that influence the distribution of care, and the policies and interventions that impact and are impacted by the determinants

Practice management systems: A software used by physician practices; scheduling, patient accounting, patient collections, claims submission, appointment scheduling, human resources, and other functions all are built into this single information system

Predictive modelling: A process of identifying patterns that can be used to predict the odds of a particular outcome based on the observed data

Primary key: In the electronic health record (EHR) and other clinical information systems, this unique identifier is typically the health record number

Protected health information (PHI): Individually identifiable health information that is transmitted or maintained in any form or format by an organization subject to HIPAA

Query by example (QBE): A query method whereby the user only has to point and click to choose tables and fields contained in the database. The information system then allows the user to choose whether the entries that meet those criteria should be included or excluded from the query

Query-based exchange: A find-and-seek request for information that is sent through the HIO to find any available health information on a specified individual

Radiofrequency identification devices (RFIDs): A microchip implanted in an item to allow tracking of that item

Radiology information system (RIS): A system used to collect, store, and provide information on radiological tests such as x-rays, ultrasound, magnetic resonance imaging (MRI), computed tomography (CT), and positron emission tomography (PET)

Ransomware: A type of malicious software that prohibits access to information systems in an organization

Record locator service (RLS): A master patient index, where the patient's information is detected within the participating HCOs based on patient identity information and record data type

Reengineering: Evaluating the way the healthcare facility does business in order to improve efficiency

Reference Information Model (RIM): A model of information, or data objects, that is shared and reused between domains of care, such as clinical encounters, laboratory testing, prescriptions, billing, public health reporting, and research

Registered Health Information Administrator (RHIA): A type of certification granted after completion of an AHIMA-accredited four-year program in health information management and a credentialing examination

Registered Health Information Technician (RHIT): A type of certification granted after completion of an AHIMA-accredited two-year program in health information management and a credentialing examination

Registration—admission, discharge, transfer (R-ADT): A type of administrative information system that stores demographic information and performs functionality related to registration, admission, discharge, and transfer of patients within the organization

Release of information (ROI) system: A valuable tool designed to manage the processing of requests for protected health information (PHI) received and processed by the HIM department

Remote wipe: Used when data must be deleted from the mobile device remotely because it has been lost or stolen

Request for information (RFI): A formal document requesting information on information system

Request for proposal (RFP): A type of business correspondence asking for very specific product and contract information that is often sent to a narrow list of vendors that have been preselected after a review of requests for information during the design phase of the systems development life cycle

Required standards: Must be implemented by all CEs to protect the ePHI

Revenue cycle: A very complex process involving several departments and many employees who perform tasks of reviewing services provided for claims submitted as well as reviewing outstanding claims, returned claims, denials, missing accounts, bill holds, and other claims involving the revenue of the healthcare facility

Revenue cycle management: The management of the accounts receivable and the accounts payable on a daily basis by the healthcare facility

Role-based authentication: The functions and data available to the user are based on the role of the user

Rules-based encoder: An encoder that requires the user to type in the name or portion of the name of the diagnosis or procedure. This entry into the encoder generates a list of suggestions from which the coder selects

RxNorm: A clinical drug nomenclature developed by the Food and Drug Administration, the Department of Veterans Affairs, and HL7 to provide standard names for clinical drugs and administered dose forms. It also provides normalized names for drugs and links names to commercial drug databases that are frequently used in pharmacy management and information systems in EHRs

Scheduling systems: A method of using scheduling algorithms to control the use of resources throughout the healthcare facility; these resources can include staff, equipment, rooms, and more

Scope creep: Changes that happen when items not included in the original scope are added after the project has begun

Screen design: Developing screens of an IS to meet the needs of the user and to promote job efficiency

Secondary data sources: Data derived from the primary data sources, such as the health record. Secondary data sources include indices, registries, and other databases

Security awareness training: Educates CE employees about the CE's security policies and procedures

Security events: Poor security practices that have not led to harm, whereas security incidents have resulted in harm or a significant risk of harm

Security incident: The attempted or successful unauthorized access, use, disclosure, modification, or destruction of information or interference with system operations in an information system

Security management plan: Includes the policies required to prevent, identify, control, and resolve security incidents (45 CFR 160, 162, and 164 2013); Should be updated periodically to address changes in law, changes in the CE, and other issues

Security Rule: Rules that define the minimum that a CE must do to protect electronic protected health information (ePHI)

Semantics: Branch of linguistics dealing with the study of meaning, including the ways meaning is structured in language and how changes in meanings and form occur over time

Setting configuration: The entry of the desired behaviors of the IS into tables or setting fields

Shared data record: A popular and effective model for a PHR that is maintained by the patient and provider, health plan, or employer

Site preparation: Making any needed changes to the physical location where the computer, workstations, printers, or other hardware will be installed

Site visits: A great way to view the products in a live environment. It consists of a small group of team members visiting a healthcare facility, preferably similar in size and characteristics that has the product implemented to observe the IS in use

SMART methodology: A goal-writing strategy that uses a **S**pecific, **M**easurable, **A**ttainable, **R**elevant, and **T**ime-based methodology

Soundex: A phonetic-based indexing system that is easily incorporated into computer software for searching surnames that sound alike but are spelled differently

Source systems: Information systems that capture and feed data into the electronic health record

Speech recognition: Also known as voice recognition, a technology that translates speech to text. The text must be edited, as speech recognition software may misunderstand words and therefore translate speech into text incorrectly

Spoliation: Intentional destruction, mutilation, alteration, or concealment of evidence or alteration of evidence

Standards development organization (SDO): A private or government agency involved in the development of healthcare informatics standards at a national or international level

Symbiology: The format of a barcode

System development life cycle (SDLC): A model used to represent the ongoing process of developing (or purchasing) information systems

Systematized Nomenclature of Medicine—Clinical Terms (SNOMED-CT): The most comprehensive, multilingual clinical healthcare terminology in the world; contributes to the improvement of patient care by underpinning the development of EHRs that record clinical information in ways that enable meaning-based retrieval

Tangible benefits: Can be quantified monetarily

Target code: The destination map or the data set in which one attempts to find equivalence or establish the code relationship

Target sheets: Pages that contain only a barcode that tell the scanner and, ultimately, the computer the content of the pages that follow

Telehealth: Professional services given to a patient through an interactive telecommunications system by a practitioner at a distant site or a telecommunications system that links healthcare facilities and patients from diverse geographic locations and transmits text and images for (medical) consultation and treatment

Telemedicine: A subset of telehealth that focuses on the provision of care whereas telehealth includes administrative uses and education

Telephone callback: Another form of entity authentication, which is most commonly used when users access the information system remotely, such as from their home

Teleradiology: The ability to view radiology images from any location by the radiologist and other users

Telesurgery: The use of robotics to perform surgery

Template-based data entry: A cross between free text and structured data entry. The user is able to pick and choose data that are entered frequently, thus requiring the entry of data that change from patient to patient. It assists the healthcare provider by providing direction in what is to be documented

Template-based entry: A blending of both free text and structured data entry

Termination process: To eliminate access to the information systems by a member of the workforce when that person's employment with the CE ends—either through resignation or through termination

Token used for security: Usually a physical device that an authorized user of computer services is given to aid in authentication

Train the trainer: A method of training certain individuals who, in turn, will be responsible for training others on a task or skill such as how to use the new IS

Transaction and Code Sets Rule: Designed to standardize transactions performed by CEs; these standards apply to electronic transactions only, such as claim submission, eligibility queries, and many more insurance-related functions; however, paper submissions are similar

Transcription system: Used by the transcriptionist to type the various documents dictated by physicians

Transmission security: Mechanisms designed to protect ePHI while the data are being transmitted between two points

Trauma registry software: An information system that tracks patients with traumatic injuries from initial trauma treatment to death

Triggers: Identify the need for a closer inspection. These trigger events cannot be used as the sole basis of the review, but they can significantly reduce the amount of reviews performed

Trojan: A type of malware that gives the appearance that it is perfectly legitimate software. This tricks the user into accessing it

Trouble ticket: A form that is used to give specific information on problems encountered

Two-factor authentication: Combines two different categories of access control, such as something you know and something you have

Unified Medical Language System (UMLS): A program designed to build an automated system that can understand biomedical concepts, words, and expressions and their interrelationships, and it includes concepts and terms from many different vocabularies

Unstructured data: Also called narrative data, can be entered in a free text format by the user, usually by typing

Unstructured data fields: Data elements that allow for free text entry, which means that the user can type in any data that he or she chooses

Use case: Part of the information system design process; it describes how the user will interact with the system and what the system will do

User preparation: Providing the users with enough information about the IS being implemented so that they are prepared both psychologically and through training to use it

User task force: A group of users, who will ultimately be using the information system (IS), who test the IS and perform other project-related tasks for which the committee receives feedback

User-based authentication: The functions and data available are based on the needs of the individual user, not all users with the same job title

Value-based healthcare: An evolving concept focused on three areas: Better care for the individual, better health for the community, and lower cost of healthcare through improvement of services and delivery methods

Version control: The process whereby a healthcare facility ensures that only the most current version of a patient's health record is available for viewing, updating, and so forth

Vetting: The process of critically appraising the abilities of an organization or person to determine compliance with the stated criteria

Vocabulary standards: A list or collection of clinical words or phrases with their meanings, address the problem of multiple ways to define, classify, and represent language. Language generally refers to a system of communication using an arbitrary set of vocal sounds, written symbols, signs, or gestures in conventional ways with conventional meanings

Weighted decision matrix: A useful method of ascertaining the best electronic health record product and vendor, which can be used to select an information system based on the features that are the most important to the healthcare facility

Wireless on wheels (WOW): See Computer on wheels (COW)

Workforce clearance procedure: Ensures that each member of the workforce's level of access is appropriate

Worm: Standalone software that does not require a host program or human help to propagate. The worm is programmed to install itself onto a computer attached to a computer network and then moves to all computers on the network

Index

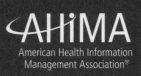